The Unofficial Guide to Radiology

100 Practice Abdominal X-rays

SECOND EDITION

EDITION

2

The Unofficial Guide to Radiology

100 Practice Abdominal X-rays

Edited by

Mary Patrice Eastwood MBChB, PhD, MRCSEd
Paediatric Surgical Registrar
Royal Belfast Hospital for Sick Children
Belfast, United Kingdom

Ali B.A.K. Al-Hadithi MB BChir, MA (Cantab), MRCP (UK), AFHEA, PGCert (Med Ed)
Academic Clinical Fellow (Cardiology and Internal Medicine)
University of Cambridge
Cambridge, United Kingdom
Cambridge University Hospitals NHS Foundation Trust
Cambridge, United Kingdom

Series Editor

Zeshan Qureshi BM, BSc (Hons), MSc, MRCPCH, FAcadMEd, MRCPS (Glasg)
Paediatric Registrar
London Deanery
United Kingdom

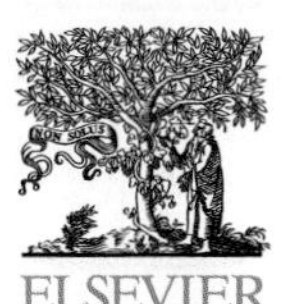

ELSEVIER

First edition 2020. Published by Zeshan Qureshi.

Notices

Practitioners and researchers must always rely on their own experience and knowledge in evaluating and using any information, methods, compounds or experiments described herein. Because of rapid advances in the medical sciences, in particular, independent verification of diagnoses and drug dosages should be made. To the fullest extent of the law, no responsibility is assumed by Elsevier, authors, editors or contributors for any injury and/or damage to persons or property as a matter of products liability, negligence or otherwise, or from any use or operation of any methods, products, instructions, or ideas contained in the material herein.

ISBN: 978-0-443-10918-8

Content Strategist: Trinity Hutton
Content Project Manager: Tapajyoti Chaudhuri
Design: Hitchen Miles
Marketing Manager: Deborah Watkins

Printed in India

Last digit is the print number: 9 8 7 6 5 4 3 2 1

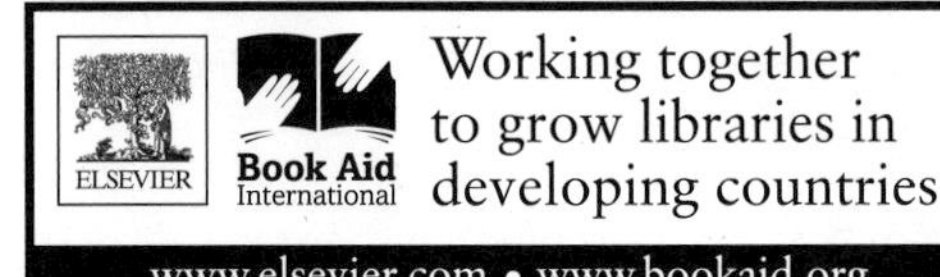

Ali would like to dedicate this book to his family Bara, Suhair, Ahmed and Miriam for their continuous support.

Patrice would like to dedicate this book to her husband and family who always offer her their full support.

Contents

Series Editor Foreword

The Unofficial Guide to Medicine is not just about helping students study, it is also about allowing those that learn to take back control of their own education. Since its inception, it has been driven by the voices of students, and through this, democratized the process of medical education, blurring the line between learners and teachers.

Medical education is an evolving process, and the latest iteration of our titles has been rewritten to bring them up to date with modern curriculums, after extensive deliberation and consultation. We have kept the series up to date, incorporating new guidelines and perspectives from a wide range of students, junior doctors and senior clinicians. There is greater consistency across the titles, more illustrations, and through these and other changes, I hope the books will now be even better study aids.

These books though are a process of continual improvement. By reading this book, I hope that you not only get through your exams but also consider contributing to a future edition. You may be a student now, but you are also the future of medical education.

I wish you all the best with your future career and any upcoming exams.

Zeshan Qureshi
November 2022

Introduction

The Royal College of Radiologists has published iRefer guidelines to assist clinicians in requesting the most appropriate imaging test for patients. These guidelines provide invaluable information, including the clinical indications for which abdominal X-rays should be requested. These include, but are not limited to, preliminary evaluation for bowel obstruction, radiopaque foreign body evaluation, evaluation of radiopaque lines and tubes and assessment for renal calculi.

The key to interpreting X-rays is having a systematic method for assessment, and then getting lots of practice looking at and presenting X-rays.

We have designed this book to allow readers to practice interpreting X-rays in as useful and clinically relevant a way as possible. There are:

- 100 large, high-quality abdominal X-rays to assess.
- Cases presented in the context of a clinical scenario and covering a wide range of common and important findings (in line with the Royal College of Radiologists' Undergraduate Radiology Curriculum).
- Detailed on-image colour annotations to highlight key findings.
- Comprehensive systematic X-ray reports.
- Relevant further investigations and management.
- Our second edition offers an additional 3 questions per case, listed at the end of the book.

The cases in the book are divided by difficulty into standard, intermediate and advanced. Each begins with a clinical scenario and an abdominal X-ray for you to interpret. You can then turn the page and find a fully annotated version of the same X-ray with a comprehensive report. Each systematically structured report is colour coded to match the corresponding labelled image.

Each report is based on a systematic approach to assessing the abdominal X-ray and is as follows:

- Technical information
- Bowel gas pattern
- Bowel wall
- Pneumoperitoneum
- Solid organs
- Vascular
- Bones
- Soft tissues
- Other
- Review areas
- Summary
- Investigations and management

With this textbook, we hope you will become more confident and competent interpreting abdominal X-rays, both in exam situations and in clinical practice.

Case

13

An 11-year-old female attends the gastroenterology outpatient clinic for a routine follow-up appointment. Her past medical history is significant for chronic constipation, for which she takes laxatives. On examination, she has oxygen saturations of 98% in room air and a temperature of 36.7°C. Her HR is 80 bpm, RR is 20 and blood pressure is 110/70mmHg. The abdomen is soft, but slightly distended, with mild tenderness with normal bowel sounds.

An abdominal X-ray is requested to assess for possible bowel obstruction.

Realistic clinical history

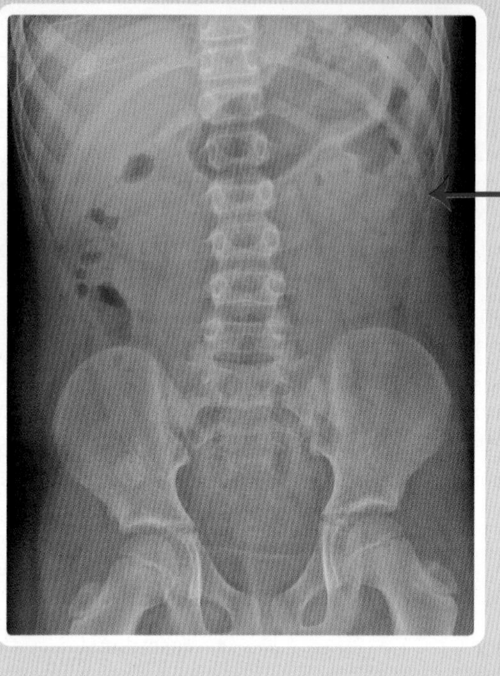

Large, high quality image to assess

REPORT – ANTEGRADE COLONIC STOMA

Detailed report following a standard format

TECHNICAL INFORMATION

Patient ID: Anonymous.
Projection: AP supine.
Rotation: Adequate.
Penetration: Adequate – the spinous processes are visible.
Coverage: Adequate – the anterior ribs are visible superiorly and the pubic rami are visible inferiorly.

BOWEL GAS PATTERN

The bowel gas pattern is normal.

BOWEL WALL

There is no evidence of mural thickening or intramural gas within the large or small bowel.

PNEUMOPERITONEUM

There is no evidence of free intraabdominal gas.

SOLID ORGANS

The solid organ contours are within normal limits with no solid organ calcification.

VASCULAR

No abnormal vascular calcification.

BONES

There are no abnormalities of the imaged thoracic and lumbar spine, or within the pelvis.

There are growth plates at the femoral head, greater trochanter and acetabulum as the ossification centres have not yet fused, which is a normal finding in a child of this age.

SOFT TISSUES

The psoas muscle outline is visible bilaterally.

The extraabdominal soft tissues are unremarkable.

OTHER

There is a rounded radiopaque density projected over the right iliac fossa, which most likely represents the stopper of an Antegrade Colonic Enema (ACE) stoma given the history of chronic constipation.

There are no vascular lines, drains or surgical clips.

REVIEW AREAS

Gallstones/renal calculi: No radiopaque calculi.
Lung bases: Not fully included.
Spine: Normal.
Femoral heads: Normal – growth plates present.

X-ray review areas specifically highlighted

Clear annotations highlighting the major x-ray findings

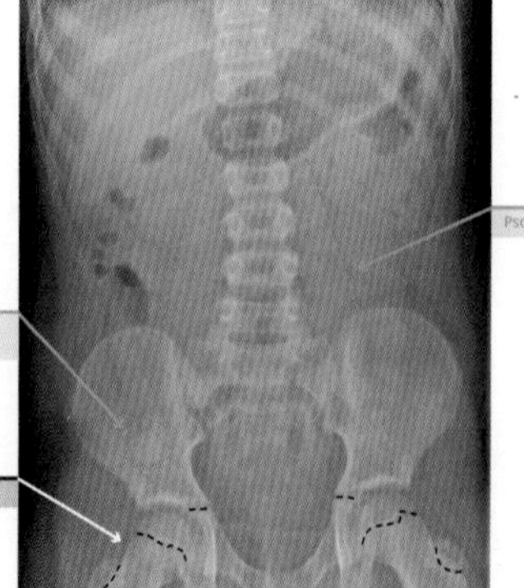

SUMMARY

This X-ray demonstrates no evidence of bowel obstruction. There is a rounded radiopaque density projected over the right iliac fossa, most likely to represent the stopper of an ACE stoma.

INVESTIGATIONS AND MANAGEMENT

Adequate analgesia and hydration should be provided.

If the patient is otherwise well, no further investigation or imaging is required. Referral to the paediatric continence team would be helpful to review her laxative regime.

Investigations and management plan put the x-ray in the context of the overall clinical management

Acknowledgements

Thank you to the following contributors for their contribution to the first edition:

Mark Rodrigues
Daniel Weinberg
Rebecca Best
Lydia Shackshaft

Abbreviations

AAA	abdominal aortic aneurysm
ABCDE	airway, breathing, circulation, disability, and exposure
APD	automated peritoneal dialysis
ACE	antegrade colonic enema
AP supine	anterior–posterior supine
AXR	abdominal X-ray
BMI	body mass index
BPM	beats per minute
CAPD	continuous ambulatory peritoneal dialysis
CKD	chronic kidney disease
CMV	cytomegalovirus
COPD	chronic obstructive pulmonary disease
CRP	c-reactive protein
CSF	cerebrospinal fluid
CT scan	computerized tomography scan
CXR	chest X-ray
DVT	deep vein thrombosis
EBV	Epstein–Barr virus
ECG	electrocardiogram
ED	emergency department
ESR	erythrocyte sedimentation rate
ESWL	extracorporeal shock wave lithotripsy
ET tube	endotracheal tube
EVAR	endovascular aortic aneurysm repair
FBC	full blood count
FIGO	The International Federation of Gynaecology and Obstetrics
FISH	florescence in situ hybridization
GCS	Glasgow coma scale
GP	general practitioner
HD	haemodialysis
HDU	high dependency unit
HR	heart rate
ICU	intensive care unit
IgG	immunoglobulin G
IUCD	intrauterine contraceptive device
IV	intravenous
IVC	inferior vena cava
JJ	ureteric stent
KUB	kidney, ureter and bladder
LDH	lactate dehydrogenase
LFT	liver function tests
MCS	microscopy, culture and sensitivity
MDT	multidisciplinary team
MRI	magnetic resonance imaging
NBM	nil by mouth
NG	nasogastric
NICU	neonatal intensive care unit
NSAIDs	nonsteroidal antiinflammatory drugs
PCR	polymerase chain reaction
PE	pulmonary embolism
PEG	percutaneous endoscopic gastrostomy
PEG-J	percutaneous endoscopic transgastric jejunostomy
PR	rectal examination
RCC	renal cell carcinoma
RCSC	renal cell carcinoma
RIG	radiologically inserted gastrostomy tube
RR	respiratory rate
SCBU	special care baby unit
SSRI	selective serotonin reuptake inhibitor
TFT	thyroid function tests
U&Es	urea and electrolytes
USS	ultrasound scan
UVC	umbilical venous catheter
VP	ventriculoperitoneal
WBC	white blood cell

Contributors

SERIES EDITOR

Zeshan Qureshi
BM, BSc (Hons), MSc, MRCPCH, FAcadMed, MRCPS (Glasg)
Paediatric Registrar, London Deanery, United Kingdom

EDITORS

Mary Patrice Eastwood
MBChB, PhD, MRCSEd
Paediatric Surgical Registrar, Royal Belfast Hospital for Sick Children, Belfast, United Kingdom

Ali B.A.K. Al-Hadithi
MB BChir, MA (Cantab), MRCP (UK), AFHEA, PGCert (Med Ed)
Academic Clinical Fellow (Cardiology and Internal Medicine), University of Cambridge, Cambridge, United Kingdom

Cambridge University Hospitals NHS Foundation Trust, Cambridge, United Kingdom

STANDARD CASES

Case

1

A 36-year-old female presents to ED with a 2-day history of generalized abdominal pain. She has not opened her bowels in that time and feels nauseated but has not vomited. Her past medical history is significant for a recent toothache, for which she has been taking co-codamol and she is a nonsmoker. On examination, she has oxygen saturations of 99% in room air and a temperature of 36.9°C. Her HR is 82 bpm, RR is 15 and blood pressure is 115/66 mmHg. The abdomen is distended with tenderness over the right side. Bowel sounds are normal. Urine dipstick is unremarkable and a pregnancy test is negative.

An abdominal X-ray is requested to assess for possible bowel obstruction.

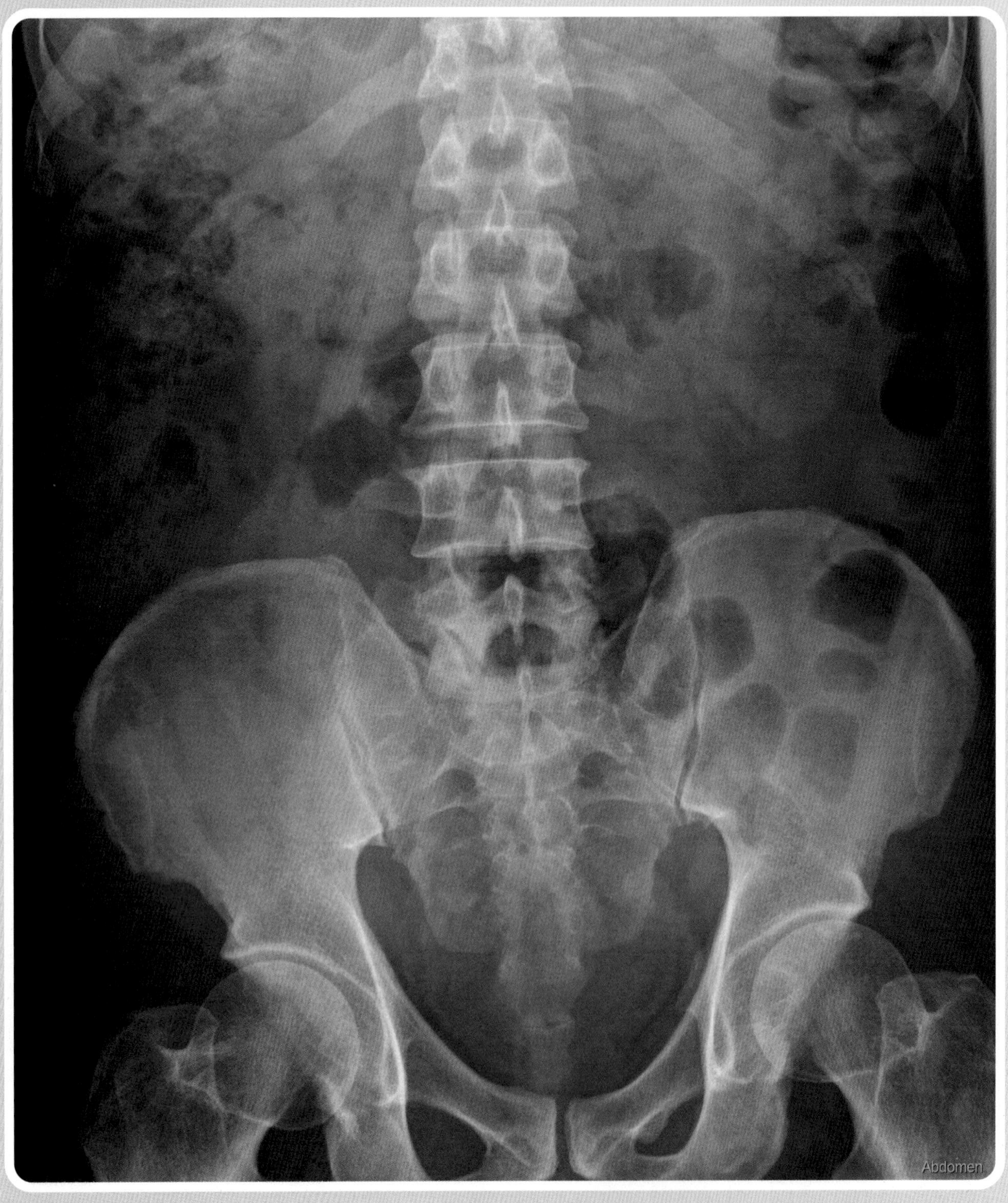

TECHNICAL INFORMATION

Patient ID: Anonymous.
Projection: AP supine.
Rotation: Adequate.
Penetration: Adequate – the spinous processes are visible.
Coverage: Inadequate – the upper abdomen is not fully included.

BOWEL GAS PATTERN

The bowel gas pattern is normal.

There is moderate volume of faecal residue present predominantly from the caecum to the proximal transverse colon.

BOWEL WALL

There is no evidence of mural thickening or intramural gas within the large or small bowel.

PNEUMOPERITONEUM

There is no evidence of free intraabdominal gas.

SOLID ORGANS

The solid organ contours are within normal limits with no solid organ calcification.

VASCULAR

No abnormal vascular calcification.

BONES

There is degenerative change visible in the distal lumbar spine with osteophyte formation.

There is degenerative change in the weight-bearing region of the sacroiliac joints bilaterally.

No fractures or destructive bone lesions are visible in the imaged skeleton.

SOFT TISSUES

The psoas muscle outline is visible bilaterally.

The extraabdominal soft tissues are unremarkable.

OTHER

There are no radiopaque foreign bodies.

There are no vascular lines, drains or surgical clips.

REVIEW AREAS

Gallstones/renal calculi: No radiopaque calculi.
Lung bases: Not fully included.
Spine: Degenerative change in the distal lumbar spine and weight-bearing sacroiliac joints.
Femoral heads: Normal.

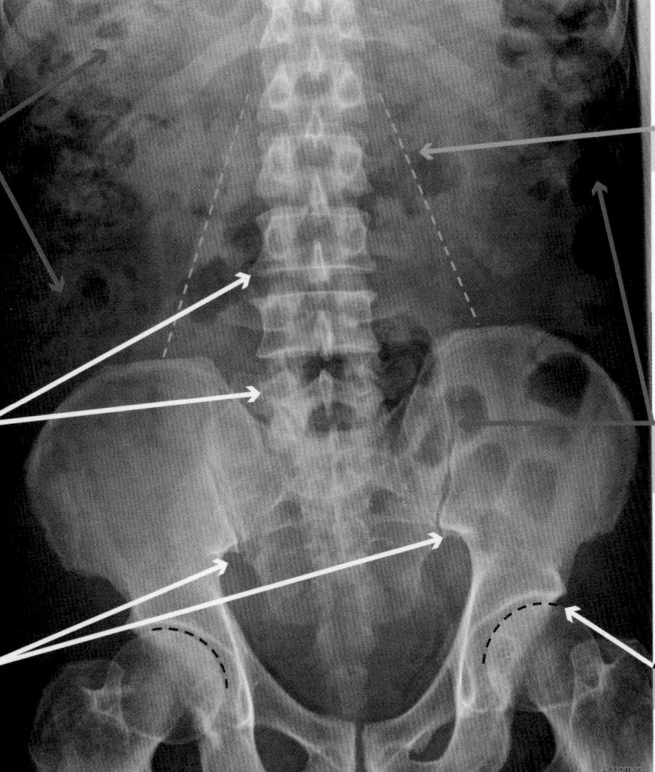

SUMMARY

This X-ray demonstrates a moderate volume of faecal residue predominantly in the ascending and proximal transverse colon. There are mild degenerative changes in the distal lumbar spine and weight-bearing sacroiliac joints bilaterally. There is no evidence of bowel obstruction or pneumoperitoneum.

INVESTIGATIONS AND MANAGEMENT

If the patient is clinically constipated, current medications should be reviewed and laxatives considered. Advice should be given regarding lifestyle adjustments, including adequate fluid intake, sufficient dietary fibre and exercise if clinically appropriate.

If the patient is otherwise well, no further investigation or imaging is required.

Case

2

A 60-year-old male presents to ED with generalized abdominal pain. He has no significant past medical history and is a nonsmoker. On examination, he has oxygen saturations of 97% in room air and a temperature of 36.7°C. His HR is 83 bpm, RR is 17 and blood pressure is 118/80 mmHg. The abdomen is soft and there is tenderness in both flanks with normal bowel sounds. Urine dipstick shows blood +++.

An abdominal X-ray is requested to assess for possible renal calculi.

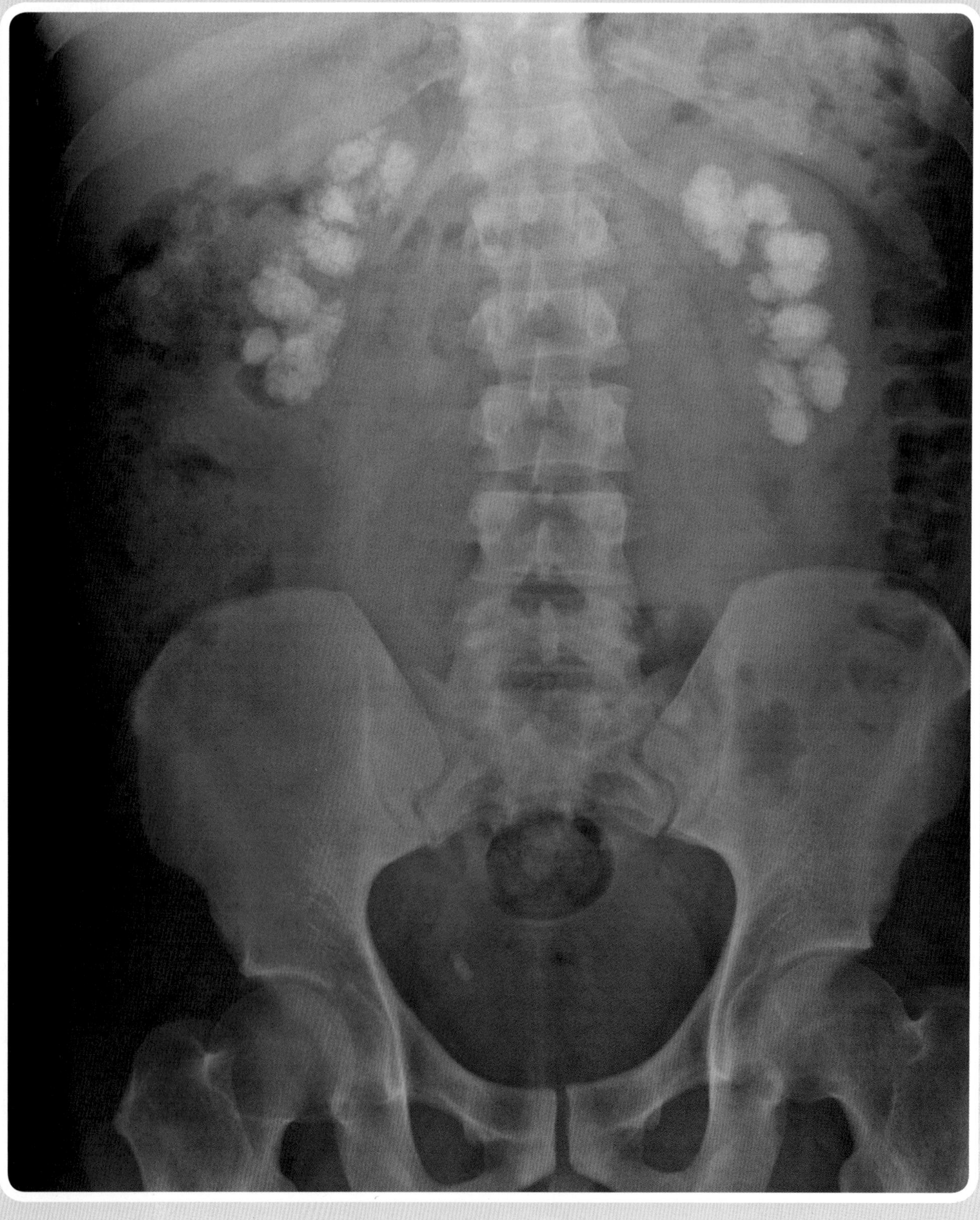

TECHNICAL INFORMATION

Patient ID: Anonymous.
Projection: AP supine.
Penetration: Adequate – the spinous processes are visible.
Coverage: Adequate – the anterior ribs are visible superiorly and the inferior pubic rami are visible.

BOWEL GAS PATTERN

The bowel gas pattern is normal.

There is a moderate volume of faecal residue present in the ascending colon and distal transverse colon.

BOWEL WALL

There is no evidence of mural thickening or intramural gas within the large or small bowel.

PNEUMOPERITONEUM

There is no evidence of free intraabdominal gas.

SOLID ORGANS

There are multiple large well-defined radiopaque densities projected over the renal medullae of both kidneys.

VASCULAR

No abnormal vascular calcification.

BONES

There are no abnormalities of the imaged thoracic and lumbar spine, or within the pelvis.

SOFT TISSUES

The psoas muscle outline is visible bilaterally.

The extraabdominal soft tissues are unremarkable.

OTHER

There is a radiopaque density projected over the region of the right urinary bladder, which most likely represents a bladder calculus.

There are no radiopaque foreign bodies.

There are no vascular lines, drains or surgical clips.

REVIEW AREAS

Gallstones/renal calculi: There are multiple calcific densities projected over the renal medullae.
Lung bases: Not fully included.
Spine: Normal.
Femoral heads: Normal.

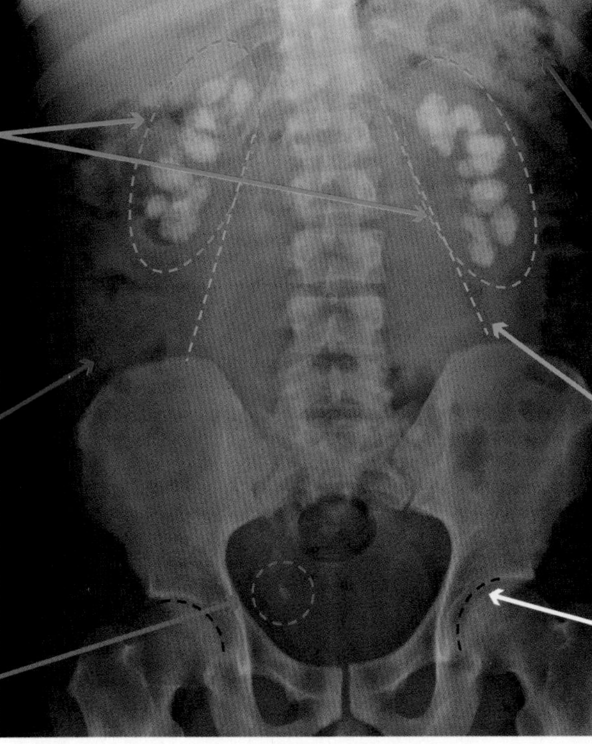

SUMMARY

This X-ray demonstrates multiple radiopaque densities projected over the renal medullae of both kidneys in keeping with medullary nephrocalcinosis. There is a further radiopaque density projected over the urinary bladder, which most likely represents a urinary bladder calculus. There is a moderate volume of faecal loading in the ascending colon and distal transverse colon.

INVESTIGATIONS AND MANAGEMENT

The patient should be resuscitated using an ABCDE approach.

Adequate analgesia and hydration should be provided.

Urgent bloods should be taken, including FBC, U&Es, CRP, LFTs, blood gas and bone profile.

The patient should be assessed for acute kidney injury, and if present, an ultrasound of the urinary tract in the first instance would be beneficial in assessing for hydronephrosis.

A CT scan of the kidneys, ureters and bladder may be useful for better visualization of the anatomy.

The patient should be referred to urology for further assessment of the medullary nephrocalcinosis and presumed urinary bladder calculus.

Case 3

A 45-year-old female presents to ED with acute abdominal pain. She has a history of recurrent pulmonary embolisms and she is a nonsmoker. On examination, she has oxygen saturations of 97% in room air and a temperature of 39°C. Her HR is 92 bpm, RR is 22 and blood pressure is 125/80 mmHg. The abdomen is rigid with voluntary guarding and there is generalized tenderness with normal bowel sounds. Urine dipstick is unremarkable and a pregnancy test is negative. The patient is noted to be obese.

An abdominal X-ray is requested to assess for possible bowel obstruction.

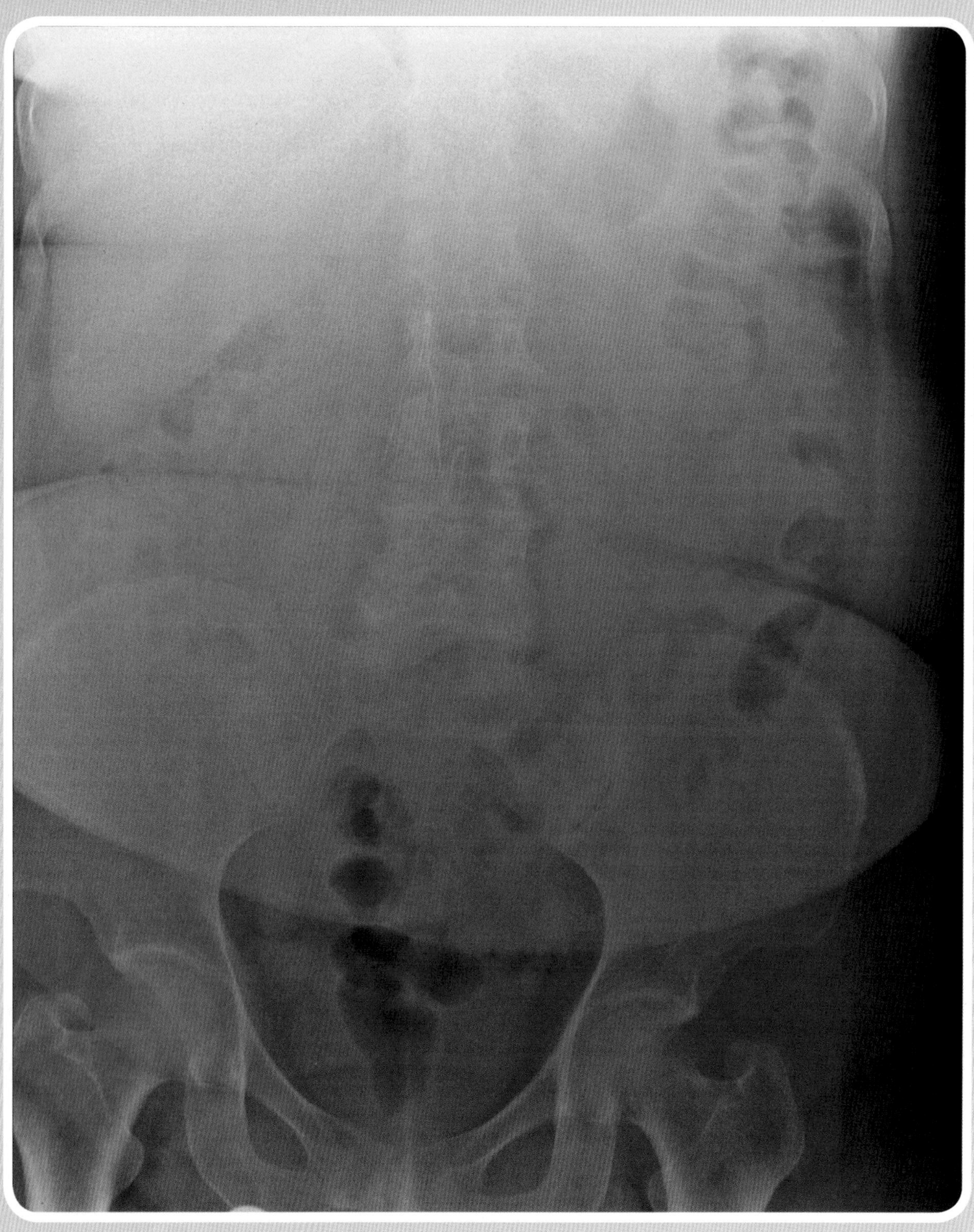

TECHNICAL INFORMATION

Patient ID: Anonymous.
Projection: AP supine.
Rotation: Adequate.
Penetration: Adequate – the spinous processes are visible.
Coverage: Adequate – the anterior ribs are visible superiorly and the inferior pubic rami are visible.

BOWEL GAS PATTERN

The bowel gas pattern is normal.

BOWEL WALL

There is no evidence of mural thickening or intramural gas within the large or small bowel.

PNEUMOPERITONEUM

There is no evidence of free intraabdominal gas.

SOLID ORGANS

The solid organ contours are within normal limits with no solid organ calcification.

VASCULAR

No abnormal vascular calcification.

BONES

There is mild degenerative change seen in the spine.

SOFT TISSUES

The psoas muscle outline is visible bilaterally.

There are cutaneous fat folds projecting over the region of the abdomen.

OTHER

There is a radiopaque foreign object projected over the region of the right pedicles of lumbar vertebrae L2 and L3, within the region of the abdominal inferior vena cava, in keeping with an inferior vena cava filter.

There are no drains or surgical clips.

REVIEW AREAS

Gallstones/renal calculi: No radiopaque calculi.
Lung bases: Not fully included.
Spine: Normal.
Femoral heads: Normal.

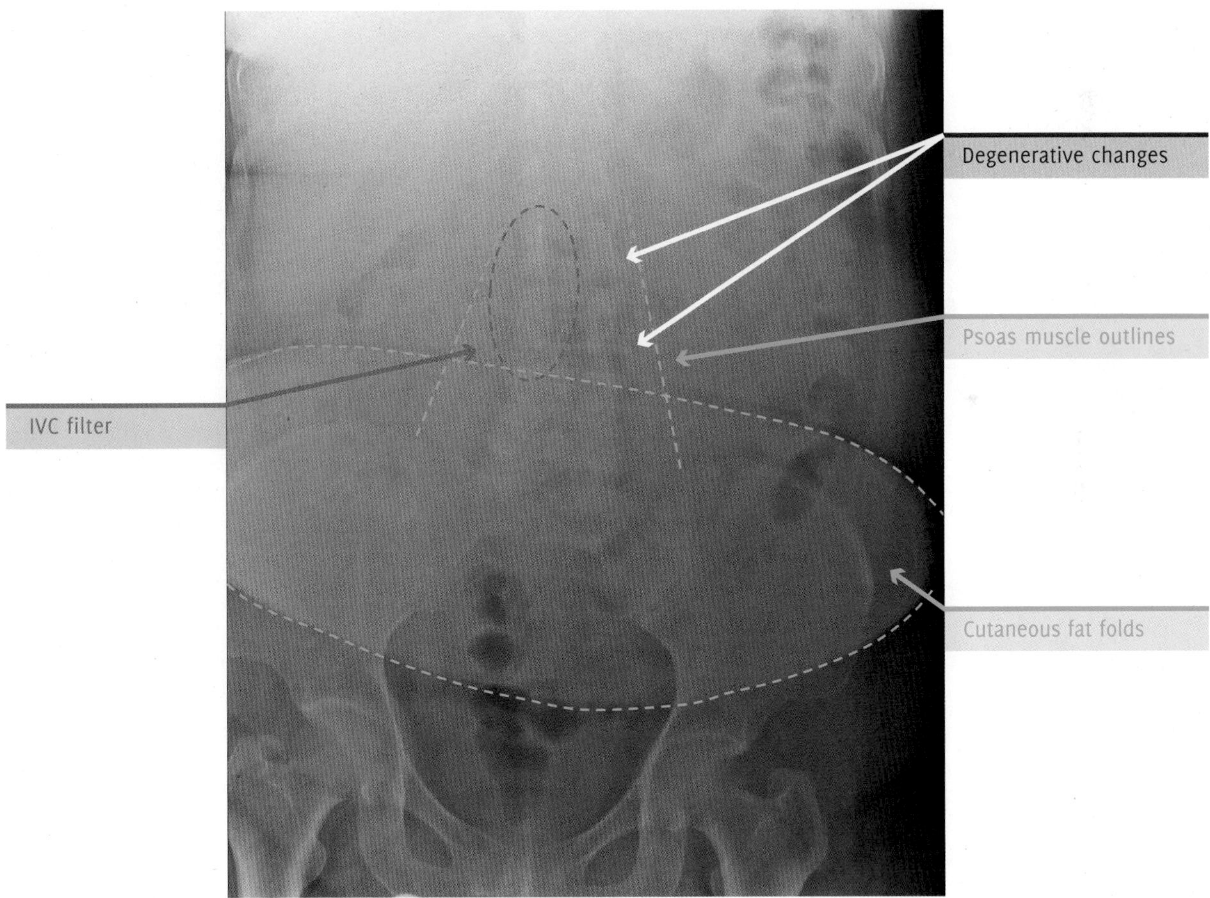

SUMMARY

This X-ray demonstrates no evidence of bowel obstruction. The IVC filter and mild degenerative changes in the spine are incidental findings.

INVESTIGATIONS AND MANAGEMENT

The patient should be resuscitated using an ABCDE approach.

Adequate analgesia and hydration should be provided.

Urgent bloods should be taken including FBC, U&Es, LFTs, amylase, bone profile, coagulation, blood cultures, blood gas and CRP.

Broad-spectrum antibiotics should be prescribed, the patient should be made NBM and started on IV fluids.

There are no clear findings on the abdominal X-ray to explain the patient's clinical presentation. A CT scan of the abdomen/pelvis with IV contrast may be considered for further evaluation of the abdomen and the general surgical team should be involved.

Case

4

A 69-year-old male presents to ED with longstanding abdominal and pelvic pain that has worsened over the last 72 hours. He has been taking co-codamol. He feels nauseated but has not vomited, and his bowels have not opened for 3 days. His past medical history is significant for severe COPD, which has been treated with steroids in the past, and ischaemic heart disease. He is an ex-smoker. On examination, he has oxygen saturations of 94% in room air and a temperature of 37.0°C. His HR is 74 bpm, RR is 16 and blood pressure is 130/75 mmHg. His abdomen is soft and there is no tenderness. Rectal examination reveals hard stools and a urine dipstick is unremarkable.

An abdominal X-ray is requested to assess for possible bowel obstruction.

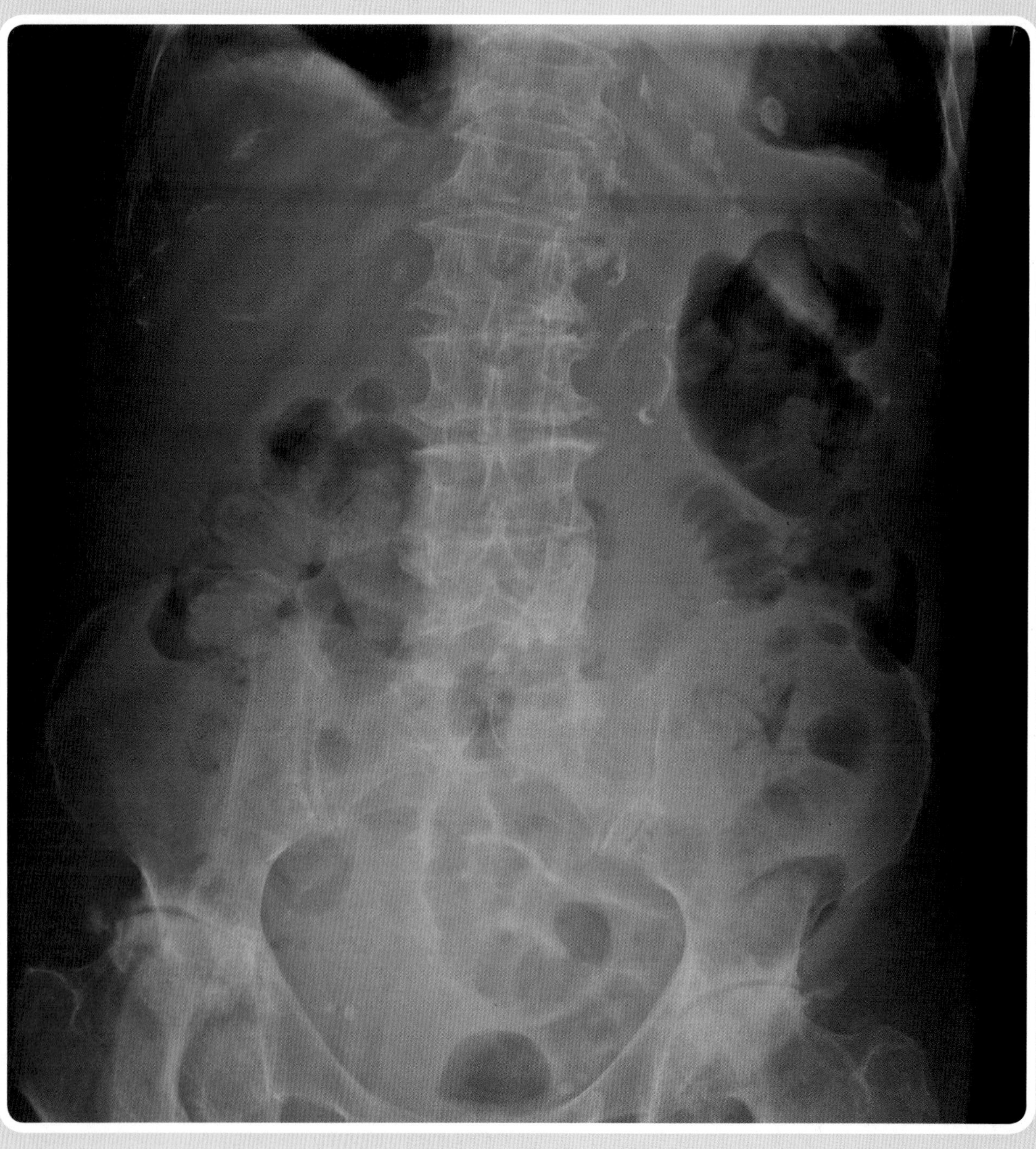

TECHNICAL INFORMATION

Patient ID: Anonymous.
Projection: AP supine.
Rotation: Adequate.
Penetration: Adequate – the spinous processes are visible.
Coverage: Inadequate – the pubic symphysis and inferior pubic rami have not been fully included.

BOWEL GAS PATTERN

Bowel gas pattern is normal.

There is a moderate volume of faecal residue throughout the colon. The rectum contains gas.

BOWEL WALL

There is no evidence of mural thickening or intramural gas within the large or small bowel.

PNEUMOPERITONEUM

There is no evidence of free intraabdominal gas.

SOLID ORGANS

The solid organ contours are within normal limits with no solid organ calcification.

VASCULAR

There is atherosclerotic calcification of the abdominal aorta and iliac arteries.

BONES

There is moderate to severe degenerative change in the imaged lumbar spine, with lateral osteophytes visible.

There is severe bilateral degenerative change in the hip joints, including complete loss of joint space, subchondral sclerosis and subchondral lucencies in keeping with subchondral cyst formation.

Both femoral heads are deformed, with flattened, abnormal contours.

There is widespread age-related costochondral calcification.

SOFT TISSUES

The psoas muscle outline is not visible on the left side, which is nonspecific.

The extraabdominal soft tissues are unremarkable.

OTHER

There are several rounded calcific radiopaque densities projected over the region of the pelvis, which most likely represent phleboliths.

There are no vascular lines, drains or surgical clips.

REVIEW AREAS

Gallstones/renal calculi: No radiopaque calculi.
Lung bases: Normal left lung base. Right lung base is not visible.
Spine: Degenerative change in lumbar spine.
Femoral heads: Bilateral degenerative and dysplastic changes.

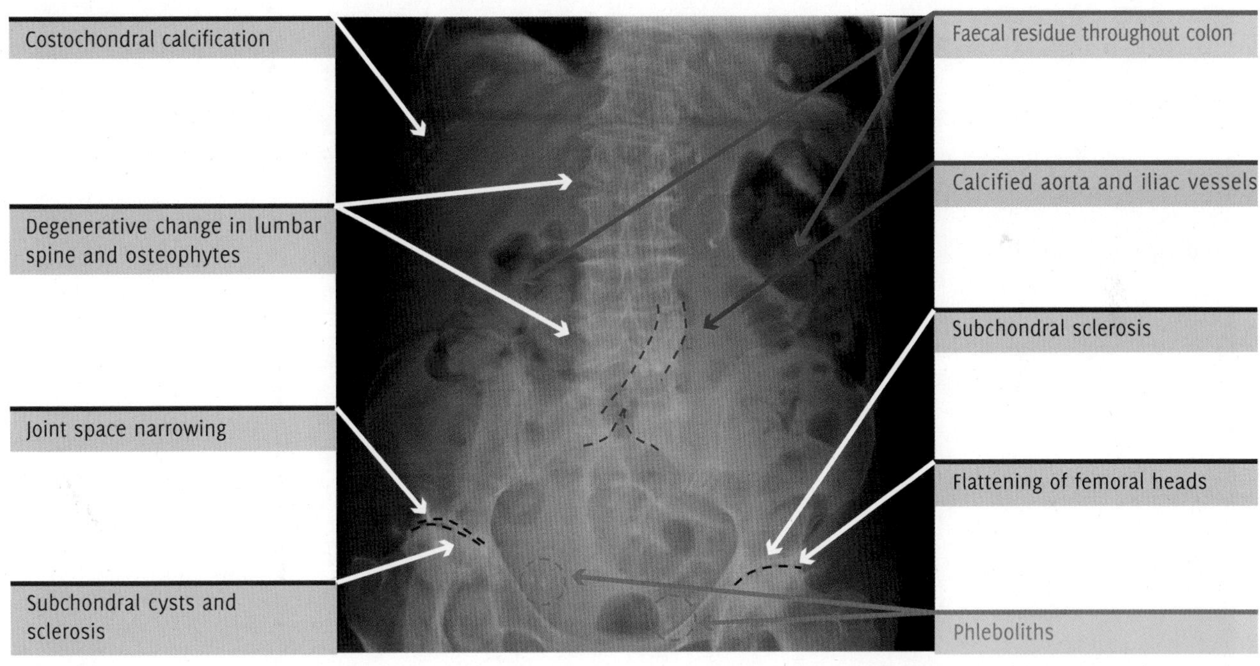

SUMMARY

This X-ray demonstrates a normal bowel gas pattern with a moderate volume of faecal residue throughout the colon, however no evidence of obstruction. There are severe bilateral degenerative changes in the hip joints involving the femoral heads and acetabula in keeping with stage IV avascular necrosis. The degenerative changes in the lumbar spine, costochondral calcification and phleboliths are also incidental findings.

INVESTIGATIONS AND MANAGEMENT

The patient should be resuscitated using an ABCDE approach.

Adequate analgesia and hydration should be provided. Co-codamol may be contributing to the constipation.

Urgent bloods should be taken, including FBC, U&Es, CRP, LFTs, coagulation, amylase, blood gas, and group and save.

If the patient is clinically constipated, current medications should be reviewed and laxatives considered. Advice should be given regarding lifestyle adjustments, including adequate fluid intake, sufficient dietary fibre and exercise if clinically appropriate.

Additionally, the patient should be referred to the orthopaedic outpatient clinic for assessment of the avascular necrosis and degenerative changes, and for consideration of treatment, such as total hip replacement. An AP pelvis should be performed to assess the hip properly.

Case

5

A 32-year-old female presents to ED with a 2-day history of lower abdominal pain. She has not opened her bowels in that time, feels nauseated and reports vomiting numerous times. Her past medical history is significant for generalized anxiety disorder, for which she takes fluoxetine (an SSRI). She is a nonsmoker. On examination, she has oxygen saturations of 99% in room air and a temperature of 36.8°C. Her HR is 74 bpm, RR is 19 and blood pressure is 120/72 mmHg. The abdomen is distended and there is tenderness in the lower abdomen with voluntary guarding. Bowel sounds are sluggish. Urine dipstick is unremarkable and a pregnancy test is negative.

An abdominal X-ray is requested to assess for possible bowel obstruction.

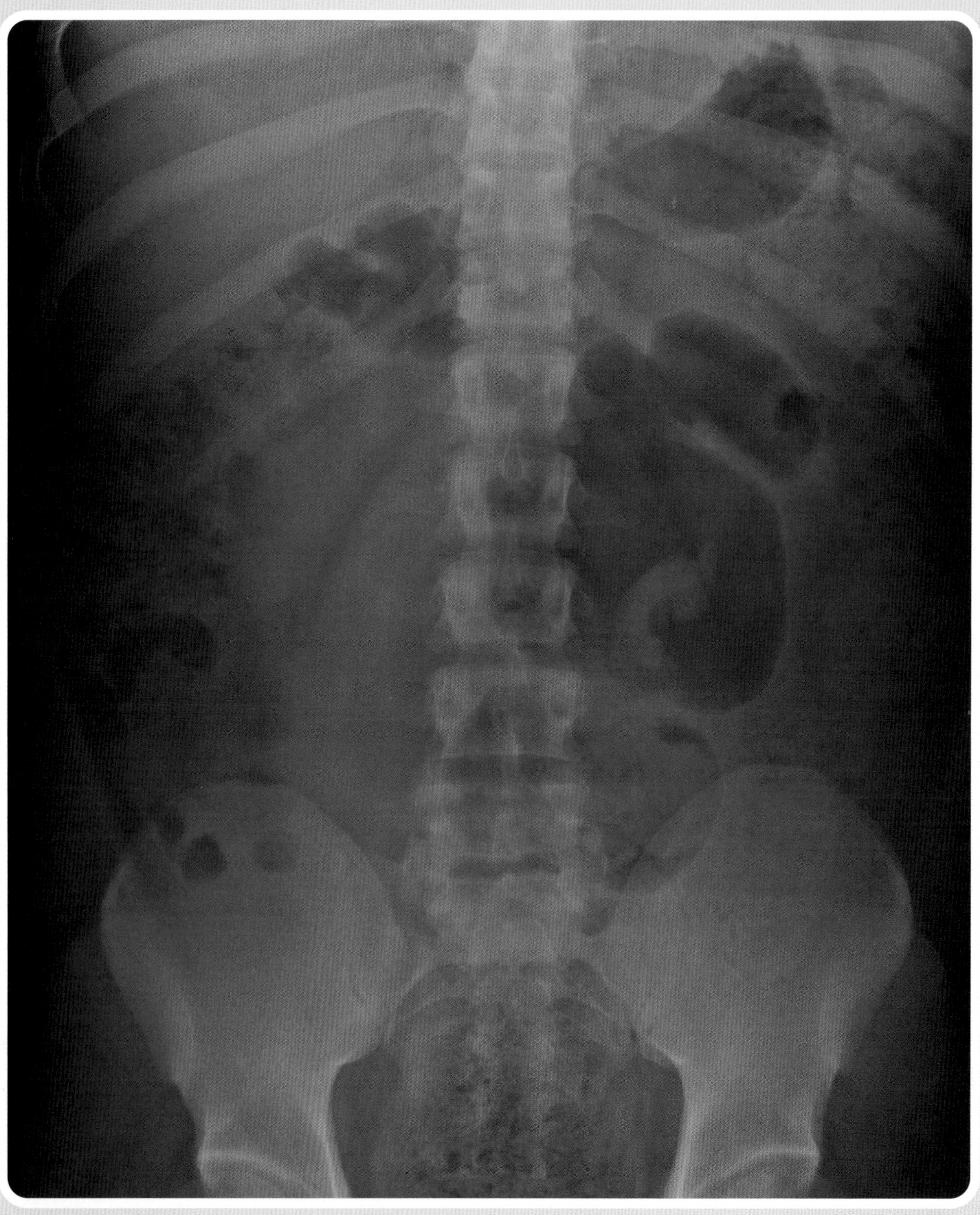

TECHNICAL INFORMATION

Patient ID: Anonymous.
Projection: AP supine.
Rotation: Adequate.
Penetration: Adequate – the spinous processes are visible.
Coverage: Inadequate – the pubic symphysis and inferior pubic rami have not been fully included.

BOWEL GAS PATTERN

The sigmoid colon is mildly distended with gas but no bowel obstruction is evident.

There is a significant volume of faecal residue present throughout the large bowel. The rectum is prominent and contains faeces.

BOWEL WALL

There is no evidence of mural thickening or intramural gas within the large or small bowel.

PNEUMOPERITONEUM

There is no evidence of free intraabdominal gas.

SOLID ORGANS

The solid organ contours are within normal limits with no solid organ calcification.

VASCULAR

No abnormal vascular calcification.

BONES

There are no abnormalities of the imaged thoracic and lumbar spine, or within the pelvis.

SOFT TISSUES

The psoas muscle outline is preserved.

The extraabdominal soft tissues are unremarkable.

OTHER

There are no radiopaque foreign bodies.

There are no vascular lines, drains or surgical clips.

REVIEW AREAS

Gallstones/renal calculi: No radiopaque calculi.
Lung bases: Not fully included.
Spine: Normal.
Femoral heads: Normal.

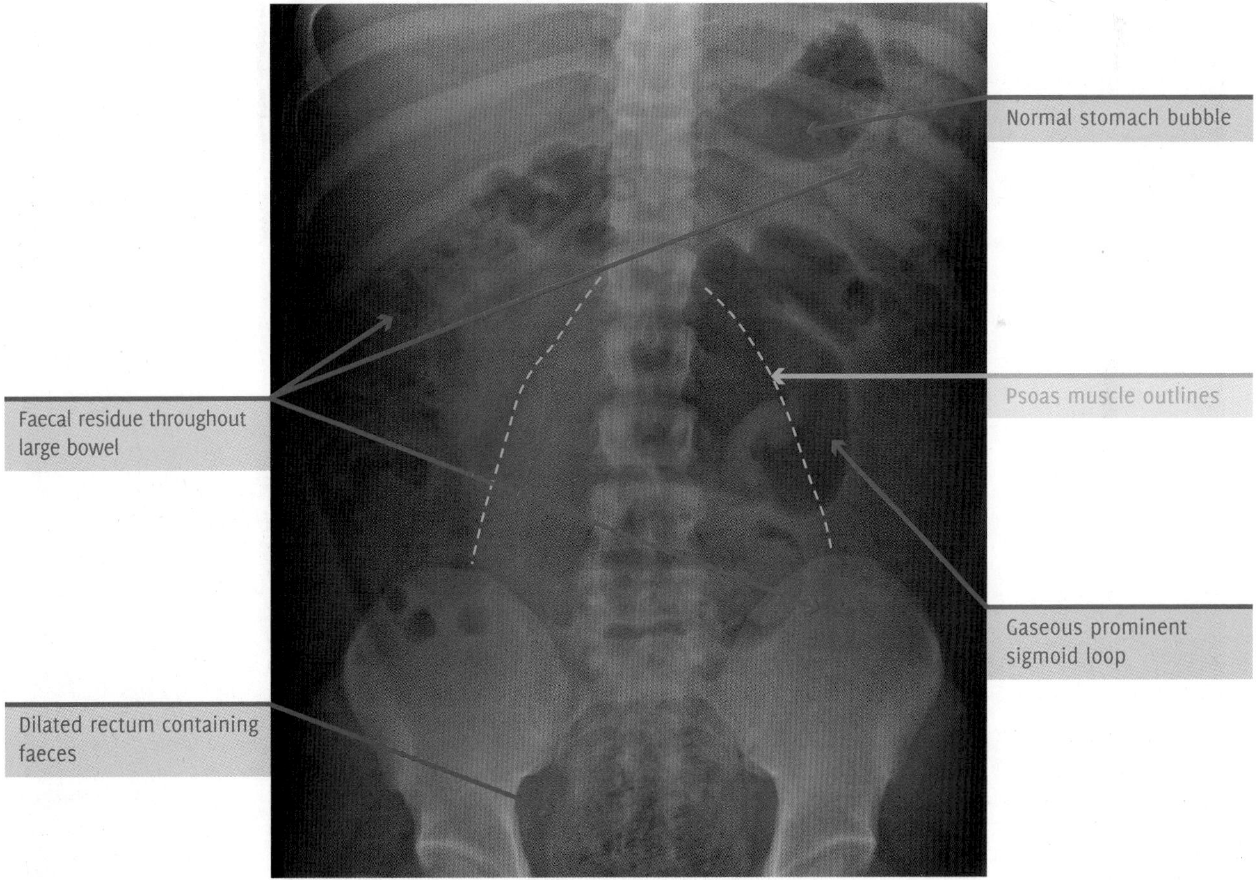

SUMMARY

This X-ray demonstrates a significant volume of faecal residue throughout the large bowel, with prominence of the rectum containing faeces. There is a mildly prominent gaseous sigmoid loop, however no evidence of bowel obstruction or pneumoperitoneum.

INVESTIGATIONS AND MANAGEMENT

If the patient is clinically constipated, current medications should be reviewed and laxatives considered. An enema may be required acutely. Advice should be given regarding lifestyle adjustments, including adequate fluid intake, sufficient dietary fibre and exercise if clinically appropriate.

If the patient is otherwise well, no further investigation or imaging is required.

Case

6

A 69-year-old female presents to ED with worsening abdominal distension. She has not opened her bowels for the past 48 hours. Her past medical history is significant for a previous hysterectomy 10 years ago for endometrial cancer and she is a nonsmoker. On examination, she has oxygen saturations of 96% in room air and a temperature of 37.6°C. Her HR is 102 bpm, RR is 30 and blood pressure is 110/65 mmHg. The abdomen is rigid and there is generalized tenderness with tinkling bowel sounds. Urine dipstick is unremarkable.

An abdominal X-ray is requested to assess for possible bowel obstruction.

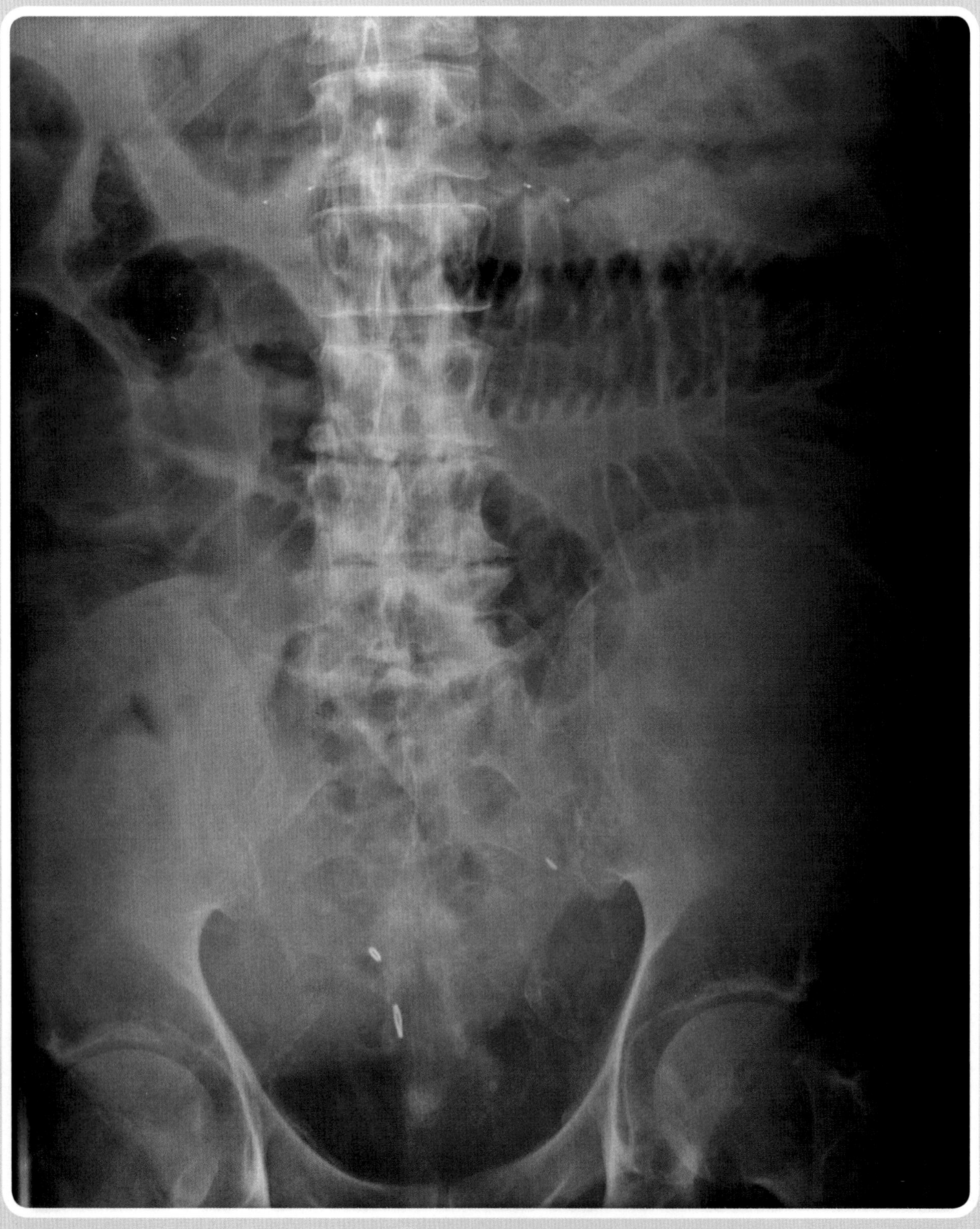

TECHNICAL INFORMATION

Patient ID: Anonymous.
Projection: AP supine.
Rotation: Adequate.
Penetration: Adequate – the spinous processes are visible.
Coverage: Inadequate – the pubic symphysis, right flank and upper abdomen have not been fully included.

BOWEL GAS PATTERN

There are multiple loops of dilated bowel seen centrally in the abdomen, which demonstrate valvulae conniventes in keeping with small bowel obstruction.

BOWEL WALL

There is no evidence of mural thickening or intramural gas within the large or small bowel.

PNEUMOPERITONEUM

There is no evidence of free intraabdominal gas.

SOLID ORGANS

The solid organ contours are within normal limits with no solid organ calcification.

VASCULAR

There is calcification of the iliac arteries bilaterally.

BONES

There is moderate degenerative change in the lower lumbar spine with osteophyte formation and intervertebral disc space narrowing.

SOFT TISSUES

The psoas muscle outline is not visible bilaterally, which is nonspecific.

The extraabdominal soft tissues are unremarkable.

OTHER

There are three radiopaque densities projected over the pelvis that appear to be surgical clips, in keeping with previous gynaecological surgery.

There are no vascular lines or drains.

REVIEW AREAS

Gallstones/renal calculi: No radiopaque calculi.
Lung bases: Not fully included.
Spine: Moderate degenerative change in lower lumbar spine.
Femoral heads: Normal.

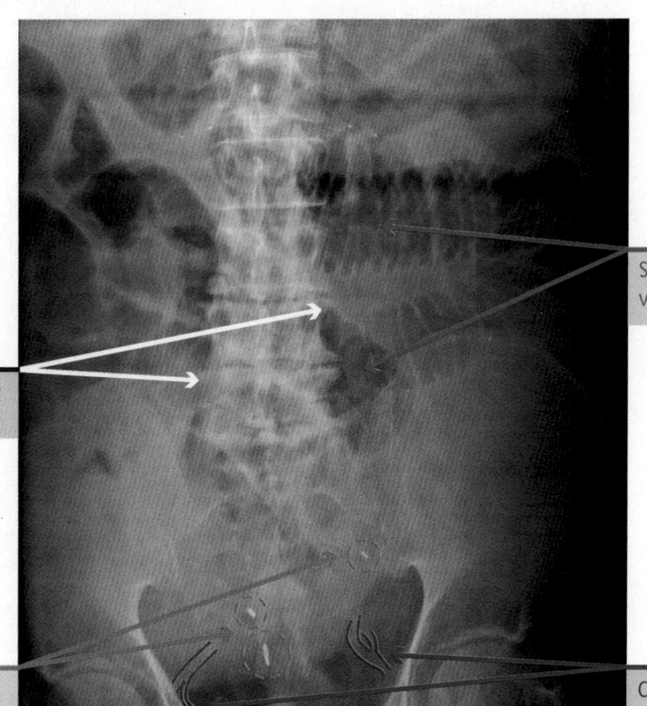

SUMMARY

This X-ray demonstrates multiple loops of dilated bowel seen centrally within the abdomen demonstrating valvulae conniventes, in keeping with small bowel obstruction. No cause for this is visible; however, given the clinical history, this is likely secondary to adhesions from previous surgery. The bilateral iliac artery calcifications, moderate degenerative changes in the lower lumbar spine and pelvic surgical clips are incidental findings.

INVESTIGATIONS AND MANAGEMENT

The patient should be resuscitated using an ABCDE approach.

Adequate analgesia and hydration should be provided.

The patient should be kept NBM and an NG tube inserted on free drainage to decompress the small bowel. IV fluids should be commenced.

Urgent bloods should be taken, including FBC, U&Es, CRP, LFTs, coagulation, blood gas, and group and save.

The general surgical team should be contacted urgently and a CT scan of the abdomen/pelvis with IV contrast should be considered for better visualization of the anatomy and further assessment.

Case

7

A 25-year-old female presents to ED with worsening abdominal pain. Her past medical history is significant for severe constipation (on multiple laxatives) and she is a nonsmoker. A spinal cord stimulator has been inserted previously for severe neuropathic pain. On examination, she has oxygen saturations of 97% in room air and a temperature of 37.2°C. Her HR is 97 bpm, RR is 24 and blood pressure is 132/74 mmHg. The abdomen is soft with generalized tenderness and normal bowel sounds. Urine dipstick is unremarkable and a pregnancy test is negative.

An abdominal X-ray is requested to assess for possible bowel obstruction.

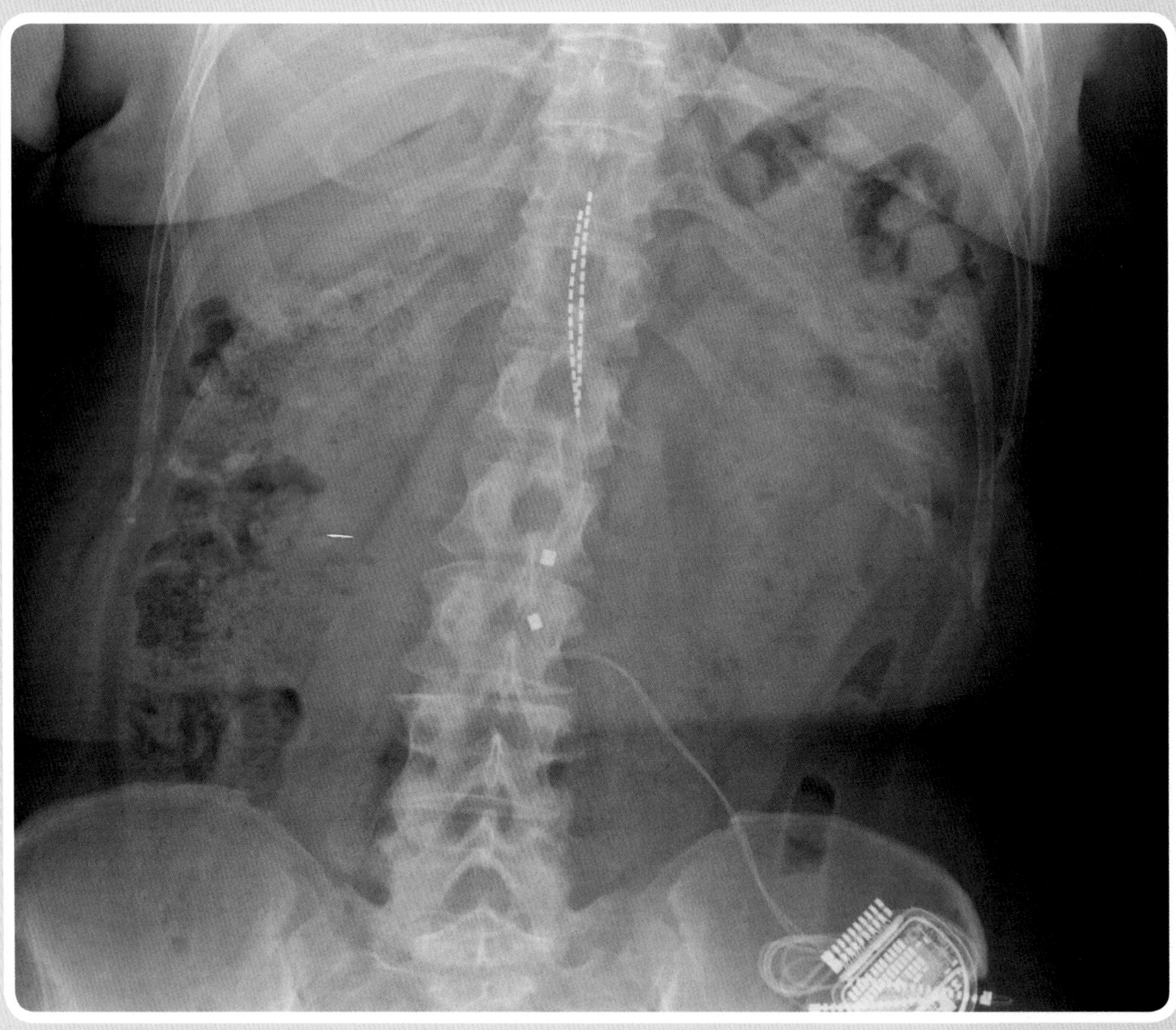

TECHNICAL INFORMATION

Patient ID: Anonymous.
Projection: AP supine.
Rotation: Adequate.
Penetration: Adequate – the spinous processes are visible.
Coverage: Inadequate – the pubic symphysis, inferior pubic rami and hip joints have not been included.

BOWEL GAS PATTERN

The bowel gas pattern is normal.

There is extensive faecal residue present throughout the ascending colon.

BOWEL WALL

The descending colon is featureless.

There is no evidence of mural thickening or intramural gas within the large or small bowel.

PNEUMOPERITONEUM

There is no evidence of free intraabdominal gas.

SOLID ORGANS

The solid organ contours are within normal limits with no solid organ calcification.

VASCULAR

No abnormal vascular calcification.

BONES

There is very mild lumbar scoliosis seen convex to the right, centred at the L2/3 level. No fractures or destructive bone lesions are visible in the imaged skeleton.

SOFT TISSUES

The psoas muscle outline is visible bilaterally.

The extraabdominal soft tissues are unremarkable.

OTHER

There is a radiopaque foreign object projected over the region of the left iliac fossa, with wires extending up towards the midline of the spine, in keeping with a spinal cord stimulator.

The preperitoneal fat is clearly visible, which should not be mistaken for free gas.

There are no vascular lines, drains or surgical clips.

REVIEW AREAS

Gallstones/renal calculi: No radiopaque calculi.
Lung bases: The right lung base is not fully included.
Spine: Very mild lumbar scoliosis seen convex to the right, centred at L2/L3.
Femoral heads: Not visible.

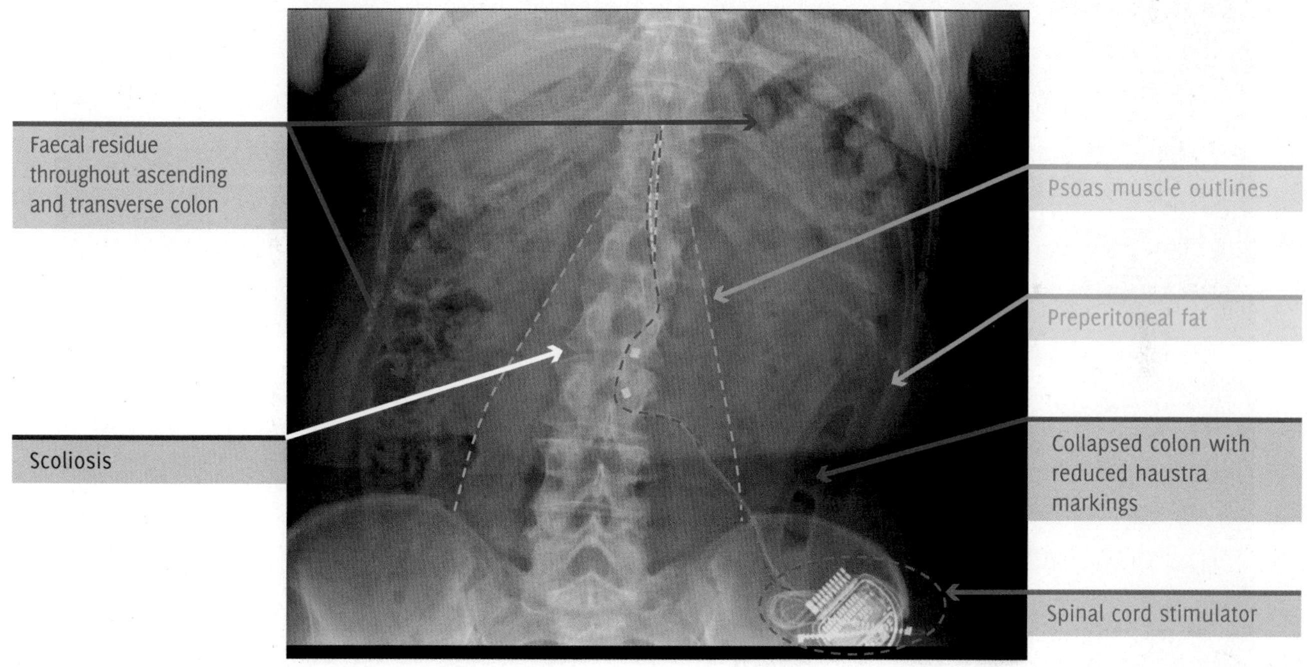

SUMMARY

This X-ray demonstrates extensive faecal residue within the ascending and transverse colon, which given the clinical history is suggestive of constipation. It also demonstrates a spinal cord stimulator in situ. The very mild lumbar scoliosis seen convex to the right, centred at the L2/L3 level, is an incidental finding.

INVESTIGATIONS AND MANAGEMENT

Adequate analgesia and hydration should be provided.

If the patient is otherwise well, no further investigations or imaging is required.

If the patient is clinically constipated, current medications should be reviewed and additional laxatives considered. Advice should be given regarding lifestyle adjustments, including adequate fluid intake, sufficient dietary fibre and exercise if clinically appropriate.

Case

8

A 50-year-old female is currently admitted on the urology ward with ureteric colic. Her past medical history is significant for renal calculi and she previously had a right-sided ureteric stent inserted. She is a nonsmoker. On examination, she has oxygen saturations of 96% in room air and a temperature of 36.5°C. Her HR is 82 bpm, RR is 13 and blood pressure is 118/80 mmHg. The abdomen is soft and there is mild tenderness in the right iliac fossa with normal bowel sounds. Urine dipstick is unremarkable.

An abdominal X-ray is requested to assess the position of the ureteric stent and to assess for possible renal calculi.

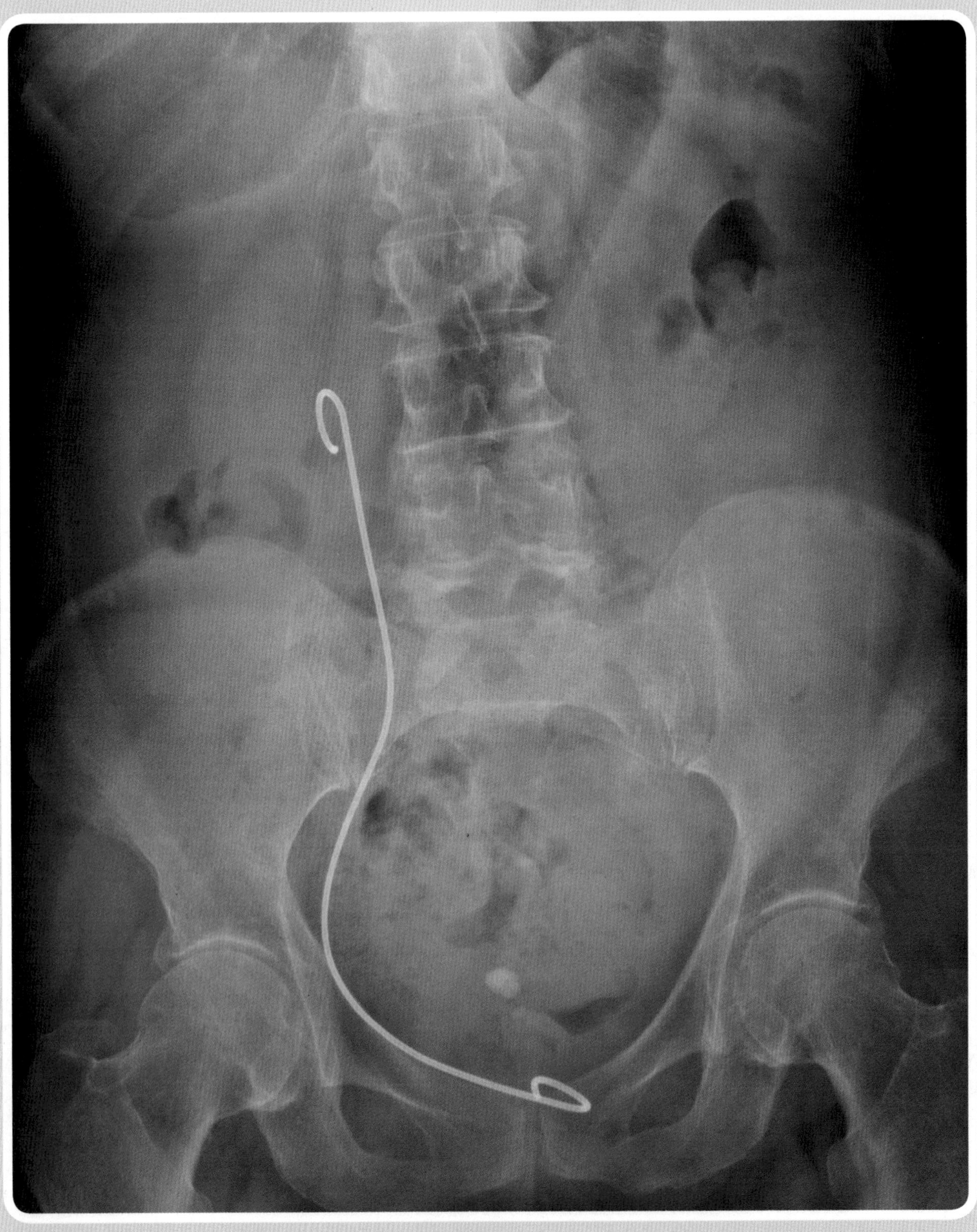

TECHNICAL INFORMATION

Patient ID: Anonymous.
Projection: AP supine.
Rotation: Adequate.
Penetration: Adequate – the spinous processes are visible.
Coverage: Adequate – the anterior ribs are visible superiorly and the inferior pubic rami are visible.

BOWEL GAS PATTERN

The bowel gas pattern is normal.

BOWEL WALL

There is no evidence of mural thickening or intramural gas within the large or small bowel.

PNEUMOPERITONEUM

There is no evidence of free intraabdominal gas.

SOLID ORGANS

The solid organ contours are within normal limits with no solid organ calcification.

VASCULAR

No abnormal vascular calcification.

BONES

There is mild degenerative change seen in the spine.

SOFT TISSUES

The psoas muscle outline is visible bilaterally.

The extraabdominal soft tissues are unremarkable.

OTHER

There is a radiopaque line projected over the region of the right ureter in keeping with a correctly sited JJ ureteric stent. The proximal end is projected over the right renal pelvis and the distal end over the bladder.

There is a well-defined radiopaque density projected over the region of the bladder, which most likely represents a bladder calculus. Other differentials include calcified pelvic lymph node, ovarian teratoma calcification or fibroid calcification.

There are no other radiopaque foreign bodies.

There are no vascular lines or surgical clips.

REVIEW AREAS

Gallstones/renal calculi: Likely bladder calculus.
Lung bases: Normal.
Spine: Mild degenerative changes.
Femoral heads: Normal.

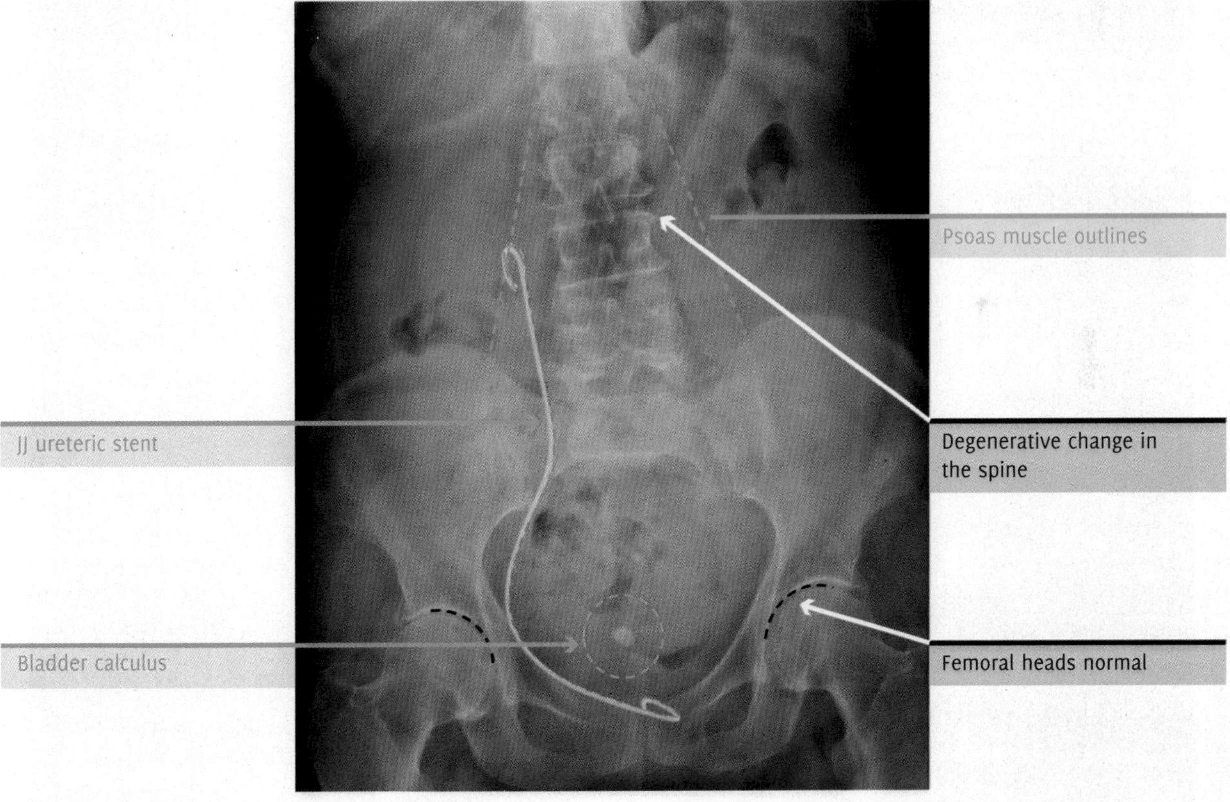

SUMMARY

This X-ray demonstrates a right-sided appropriately sited JJ ureteric stent and a well-defined radiopaque density projected over the region of the bladder most likely in keeping with a calculus.

INVESTIGATIONS AND MANAGEMENT

Adequate analgesia and hydration should be provided.

Urgent bloods should be taken, including FBC, U&Es, CRP, LFTs, blood gas and bone profile.

The patient should be assessed for acute kidney injury, and if present, an ultrasound of the urinary tract in the first instance would be beneficial in assessing for hydronephrosis.

Smaller stones may pass spontaneously, but referral to urology may be required for further assessment.

A CT scan of the kidneys, ureters and bladder may be useful for better visualization of the anatomy. The appearances should be compared with previous imaging to assess for interval change.

Case

9

An 84-year-old male presents to ED with generalized abdominal pain on a background of a 2-month history of hip pain and reduced mobility. His past medical history is significant for prostate cancer and he is a nonsmoker. A nephrostomy tube has previously been inserted on the left for hydronephrosis. On examination, he has oxygen saturations of 99% in room air and a temperature of 36.7°C. His HR is 92 bpm, RR is 20 and blood pressure is 115/65 mmHg. The abdomen is soft and there is mild generalized tenderness with normal bowel sounds. Urine dipstick is unremarkable. There is tenderness over the right hip and pain on hip flexion.

An abdominal X-ray is requested to assess for possible bowel obstruction.

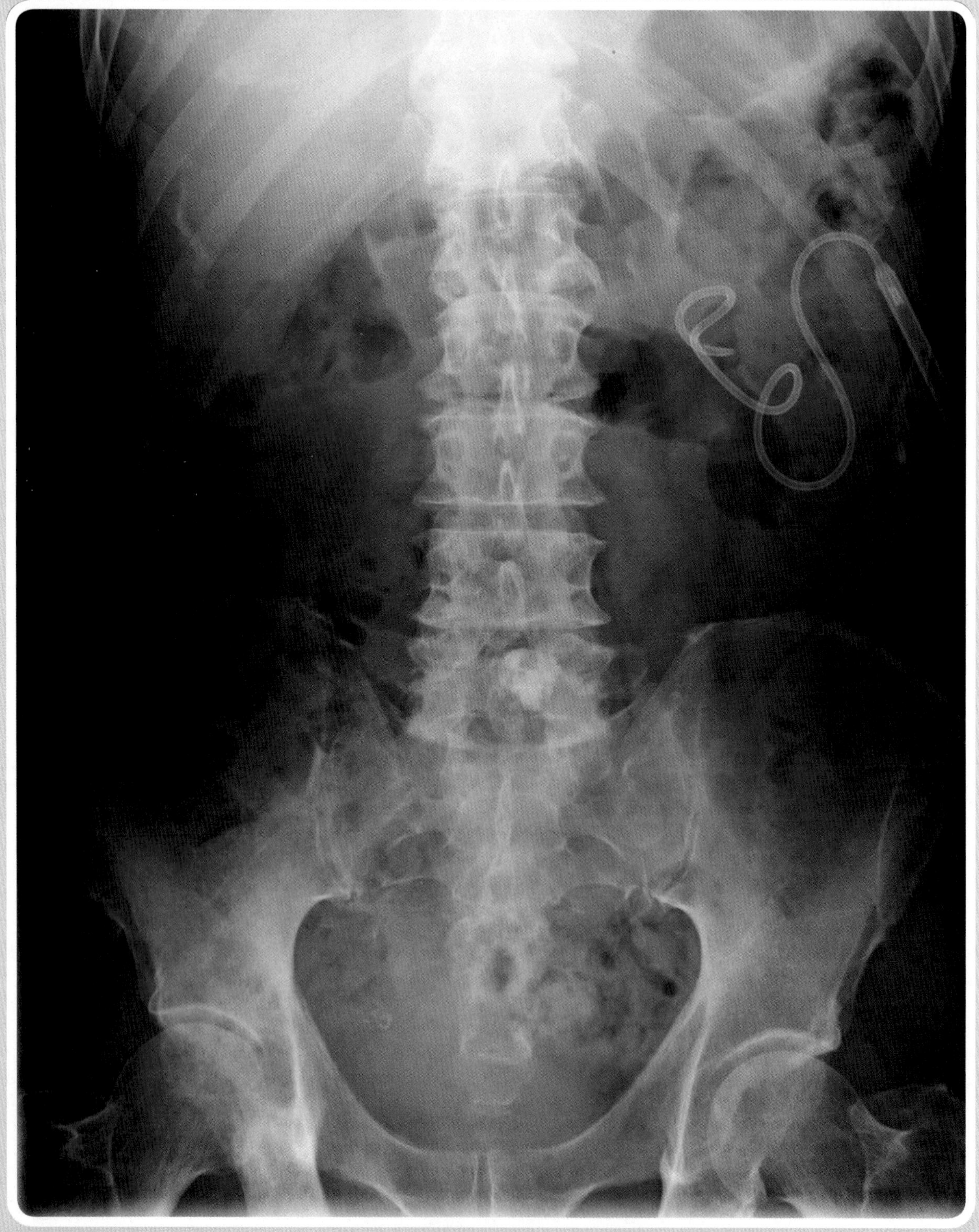

TECHNICAL INFORMATION

Patient ID: Anonymous.
Projection: AP supine.
Rotation: Adequate.
Penetration: Adequate – the spinous processes are visible.
Coverage: Inadequate – the pubic symphysis and inferior pubic rami have not been fully included.

BOWEL GAS PATTERN

The bowel gas pattern is normal.

BOWEL WALL

There is no evidence of mural thickening or intramural gas within the large or small bowel.

PNEUMOPERITONEUM

There is no evidence of free intraabdominal gas.

SOLID ORGANS

There is a left-sided catheter projected over the region of the left kidney, in keeping with a nephrostomy tube.

VASCULAR

There is calcification of the right-sided iliac arteries.

BONES

There is a well-circumscribed sclerotic lesion projected over the L5 vertebral body with loss of the L5 spinous process, which most likely represents a vertebral metastasis given the clinical history. There is a sclerotic ill-defined lesion projected over the region of the inferior aspect of the right acetabulum with sclerosis of the ilioischial line. The location is not typical for degenerative change and most likely represents a further metastasis given the clinical history.

No fractures are visible in the imaged skeleton.

SOFT TISSUES

The psoas muscle outline is visible bilaterally.

The extraabdominal soft tissues are unremarkable.

OTHER

There is a left-sided catheter projected over the region of the left kidney, in keeping with a nephrostomy tube.

There are no other vascular lines, drains or surgical clips.

REVIEW AREAS

Gallstones/renal calculi: No radiopaque calculi.
Lung bases: Not fully included.
Spine: Lesion at L5 vertebral body as previously described.
Femoral heads: Sclerotic lesion at inferior aspect of right acetabulum as previously described.

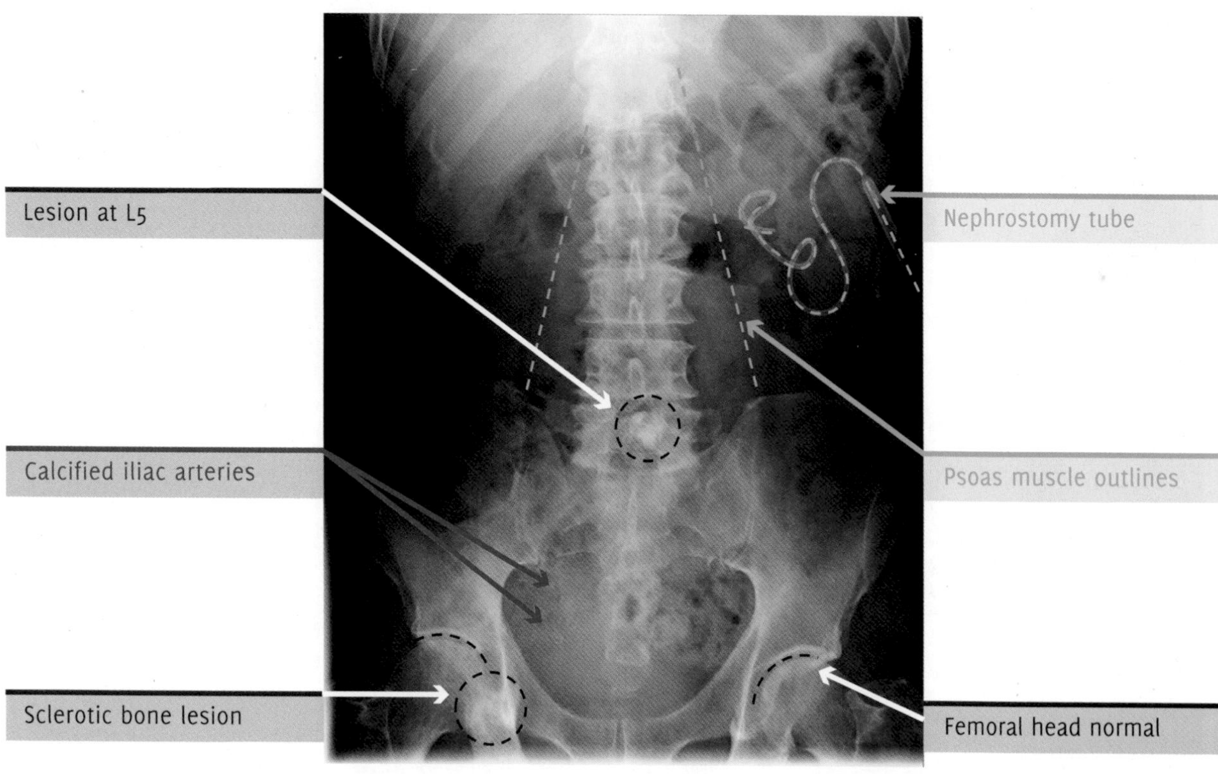

SUMMARY

This X-ray demonstrates two sclerotic bone lesions: one in the L5 vertebra and one at the right-sided acetabulum. These are suspicious for metastases given the clinical history of prostate cancer. There is a left-sided nephrostomy catheter in situ. There is no evidence of bowel obstruction.

INVESTIGATIONS AND MANAGEMENT

The patient should be resuscitated using an ABCDE approach.

Adequate analgesia and hydration should be provided.

Bloods should be taken, including FBC, U&Es, CRP, LFTs, bone profile, blood gas and tumour markers.

If no recent scan has been performed, an up-to-date staging CT scan of the chest, abdomen and pelvis with IV contrast should be considered to evaluate for disease progression.

The patient should be referred to urology and oncology services for further management, which may include biopsy and MDT discussion.

Treatment, which may include surgery, radiotherapy, chemotherapy or palliative treatment, will depend on the outcome of the MDT investigations and the patient's wishes.

Case

10

A 30-year-old male presents to ED with left-sided loin pain radiating to the left groin. His past medical history is significant for previous renal calculi and he is a nonsmoker. He has previously had a left-sided ureteric stent inserted. On examination, he has oxygen saturations of 96% in room air and a temperature of 36.8°C. His HR is 102 bpm, RR is 24 and blood pressure is 130/80 mmHg. The abdomen is soft with tenderness in the left loin radiating to the left groin. Bowel sounds are normal. Urine dipstick shows blood +++.

An abdominal X-ray is requested to assess for possible renal calculi.

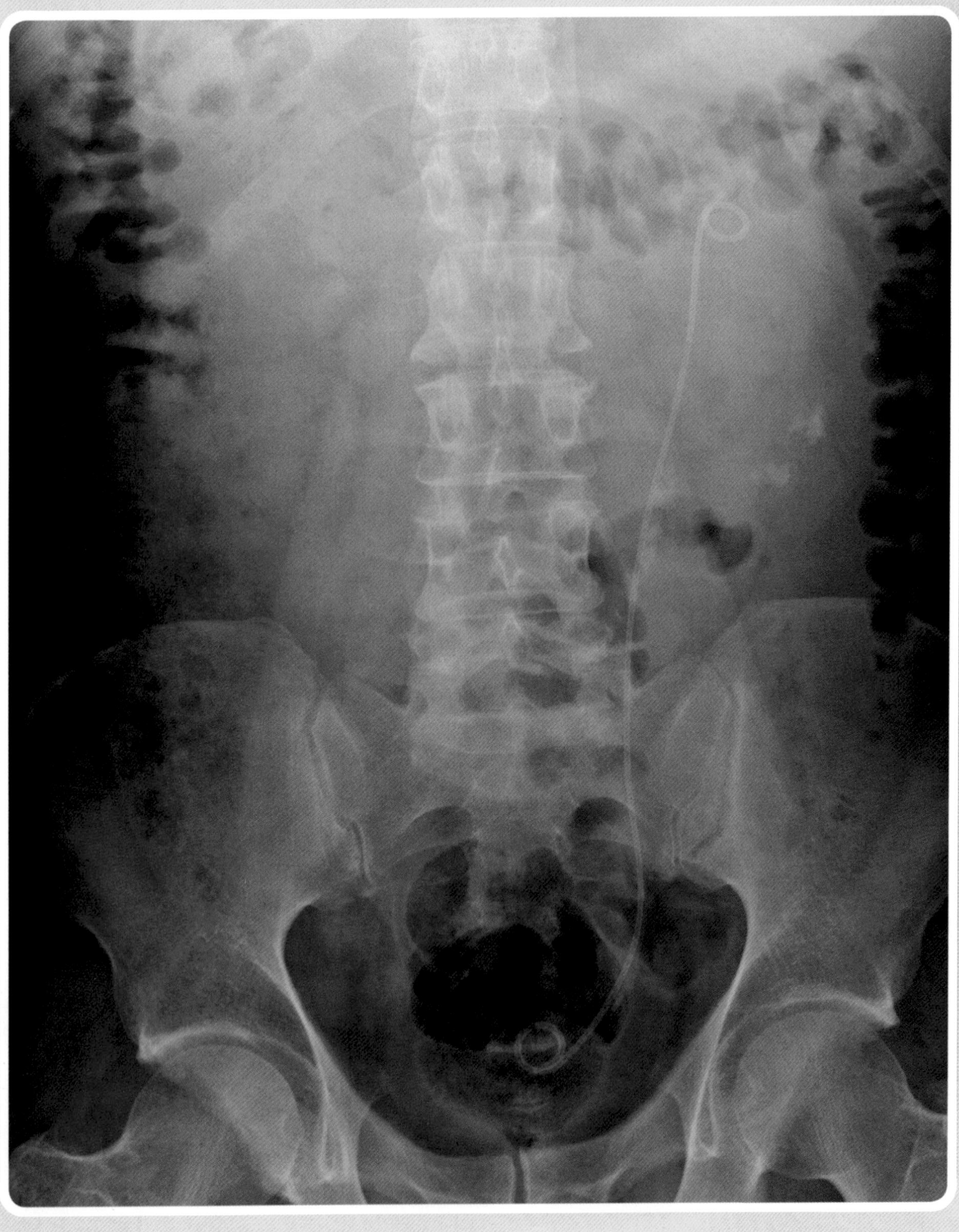

TECHNICAL INFORMATION

Patient ID: Anonymous.
Projection: AP supine.
Rotation: Adequate.
Penetration: Adequate – the spinous processes are visible.
Coverage: Inadequate – the inferior pubic rami have not been fully included.

BOWEL GAS PATTERN

The bowel gas pattern is normal.

There is a mild volume of faecal residue present throughout the ascending colon.

BOWEL WALL

There is no evidence of mural thickening or intramural gas within the large or small bowel.

PNEUMOPERITONEUM

There is no evidence of free intraabdominal gas.

SOLID ORGANS

There are two small radiopaque densities projected over the region of the inferior pole of the left kidney, in keeping with renal calculi.

VASCULAR

No abnormal vascular calcification.

BONES

There are no abnormalities of the imaged thoracic and lumbar spine, or within the pelvis.

SOFT TISSUES

The psoas muscle outline is visible bilaterally.

The extraabdominal soft tissues are unremarkable.

OTHER

There is a radiopaque line projected over the region of the left ureter, which represents a correctly sited JJ ureteric stent.

There are several radiopaque densities projected to the left side of the ureteric stent at the level of L3/4, in keeping with ureteric calculi.

There are no vascular lines, drains or surgical clips.

REVIEW AREAS

Gallstones/renal calculi: Renal calculi in inferior pole of left kidney and left ureter.
Lung bases: Not fully included.
Spine: Normal.
Femoral heads: Normal.

Psoas muscle outlines

Faecal residue in ascending colon

Femoral heads normal

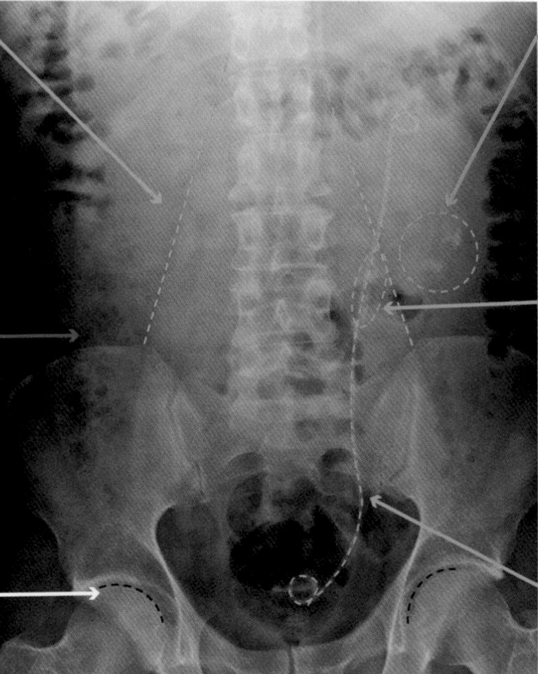

Renal calculi

Calcification within left ureter

JJ ureteric stent

SUMMARY

This X-ray demonstrates two small radiopaque densities projected over the region of the inferior pole of the left kidney, in keeping with renal calculi. It also demonstrates a left-sided JJ ureteric stent in situ with associated ureteric calculi. There is a mild volume of faecal residue within the ascending colon.

INVESTIGATIONS AND MANAGEMENT

The patient should be resuscitated using an ABCDE approach.

Adequate analgesia and hydration should be provided.

Urgent bloods should be taken, including FBC, U&Es, CRP, LFTs, blood gas and bone profile.

The patient should be assessed for acute kidney injury, and if present, an ultrasound of the urinary tract in the first instance would be beneficial in assessing for hydronephrosis.

Smaller stones may pass spontaneously, but referral to urology is required for possible further intervention. A CT scan of the kidneys, ureters and bladder might be useful for better visualization of the anatomy.

Case

11

A 45-year-old female presents to ED with pain on urination. Her past medical history is significant for previous bowel surgery and she is a nonsmoker. On examination, she has oxygen saturations of 98% in room air and a temperature of 36.8°C. Her HR is 85 bpm, RR is 16 and blood pressure is 120/80 mmHg. The abdomen is soft and there is tenderness in the right flank with normal bowel sounds. Urine dipstick shows blood ++ and a pregnancy test is negative.

An abdominal X-ray is requested to assess for possible renal calculi.

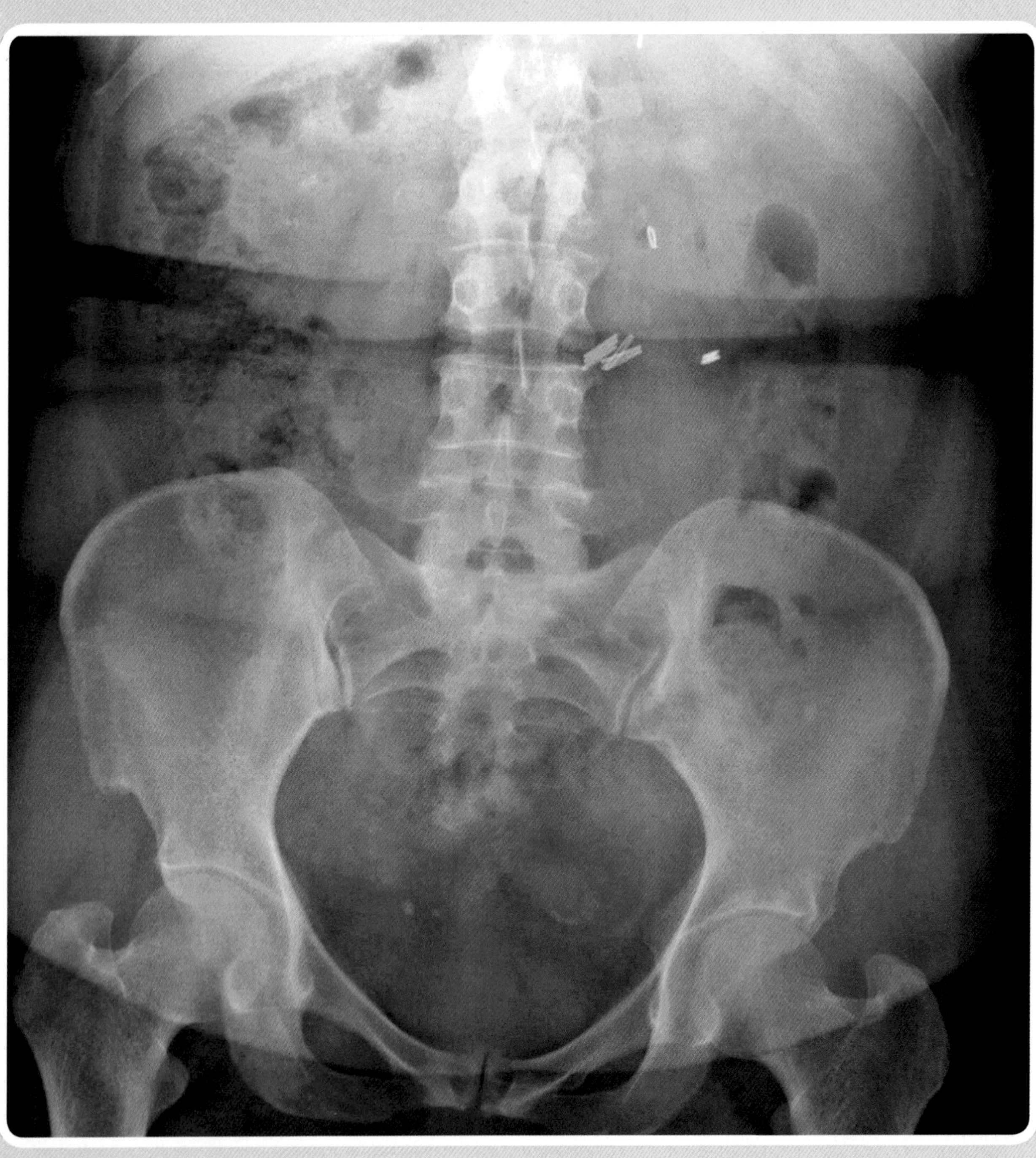

TECHNICAL INFORMATION

Patient ID: Anonymous.
Projection: AP supine.
Rotation: Adequate.
Penetration: Adequate – the spinous processes are visible.
Coverage: Adequate – the anterior ribs are visible superiorly and the inferior pubic rami are visible.

BOWEL GAS PATTERN

There is a paucity of bowel gas but no bowel dilatation is visible.

There is a moderate volume of faecal residue present throughout the large bowel, extending from caecum to rectum.

BOWEL WALL

There is no evidence of mural thickening or intramural gas within the large or small bowel.

PNEUMOPERITONEUM

There is no evidence of free intraabdominal gas.

SOLID ORGANS

There are several small radiopaque densities projected over the region of the right kidney, in keeping with renal calculi.

VASCULAR

No abnormal vascular calcification.

BONES

There are no abnormalities of the imaged thoracic and lumbar spine, or within the pelvis.

SOFT TISSUES

The psoas muscle outline is visible bilaterally.

The extraabdominal soft tissues are unremarkable.

OTHER

There are no vascular lines or drains.
There are several rounded radiopaque densities projected over the region of the pelvis, which most likely represent phleboliths.

There are several surgical clips, including in the epigastric region and to the left of L2/3 to L3/4.

REVIEW AREAS

Gallstones/renal calculi: Several likely renal calculi in the region of the right kidney.
Lung bases: Not fully included.
Spine: Normal.
Femoral heads: Normal.

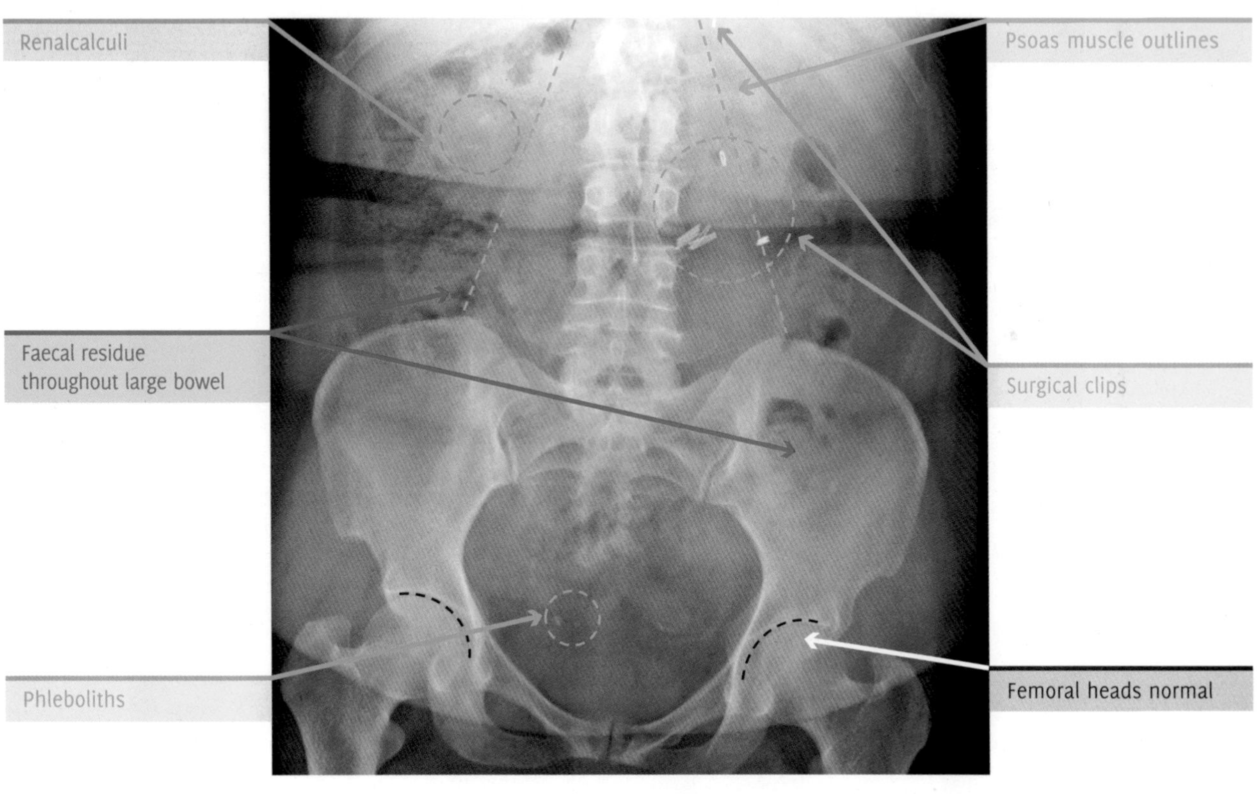

SUMMARY

This X-ray demonstrates several small radiopaque densities projected over the region of the right kidney, in keeping with renal calculi. The moderate volume of faecal residue throughout the large bowel, pelvic phleboliths and surgical clips projecting over the epigastrium and to the left of L2/3 and L3/4 are incidental findings.

INVESTIGATIONS AND MANAGEMENT

The patient should be resuscitated using an ABCDE approach.

Adequate analgesia and hydration should be provided.

Urgent bloods should be taken, including FBC, U&Es, CRP, LFTs, blood gas and bone profile.

The patient should be assessed for acute kidney injury, and if present, an ultrasound of the urinary tract in the first instance would be beneficial in assessing for hydronephrosis.

Smaller stones may pass spontaneously, but referral to urology may be required for possible further intervention. A CT scan of the kidneys, ureters and bladder would be useful for better visualization of the anatomy, depending on the clinical picture and blood test results.

Case

12

A 15-year-old female presents to ED with severe constipation, having not opened her bowels for 6 days or passed flatus for 24 hours. She feels nauseated and reports vomiting that morning. She has no significant past medical history and is a nonsmoker. On examination, she has oxygen saturations of 99% in room air and a temperature of 37.1°C. Her HR is 82 bpm, RR is 16 and blood pressure is 110/65 mmHg. The abdomen is mildly distended and there is tenderness and voluntary guarding in the lower abdomen with normal bowel sounds. Urine dipstick is unremarkable and a pregnancy test is negative.

An abdominal X-ray is requested to assess for possible bowel obstruction.

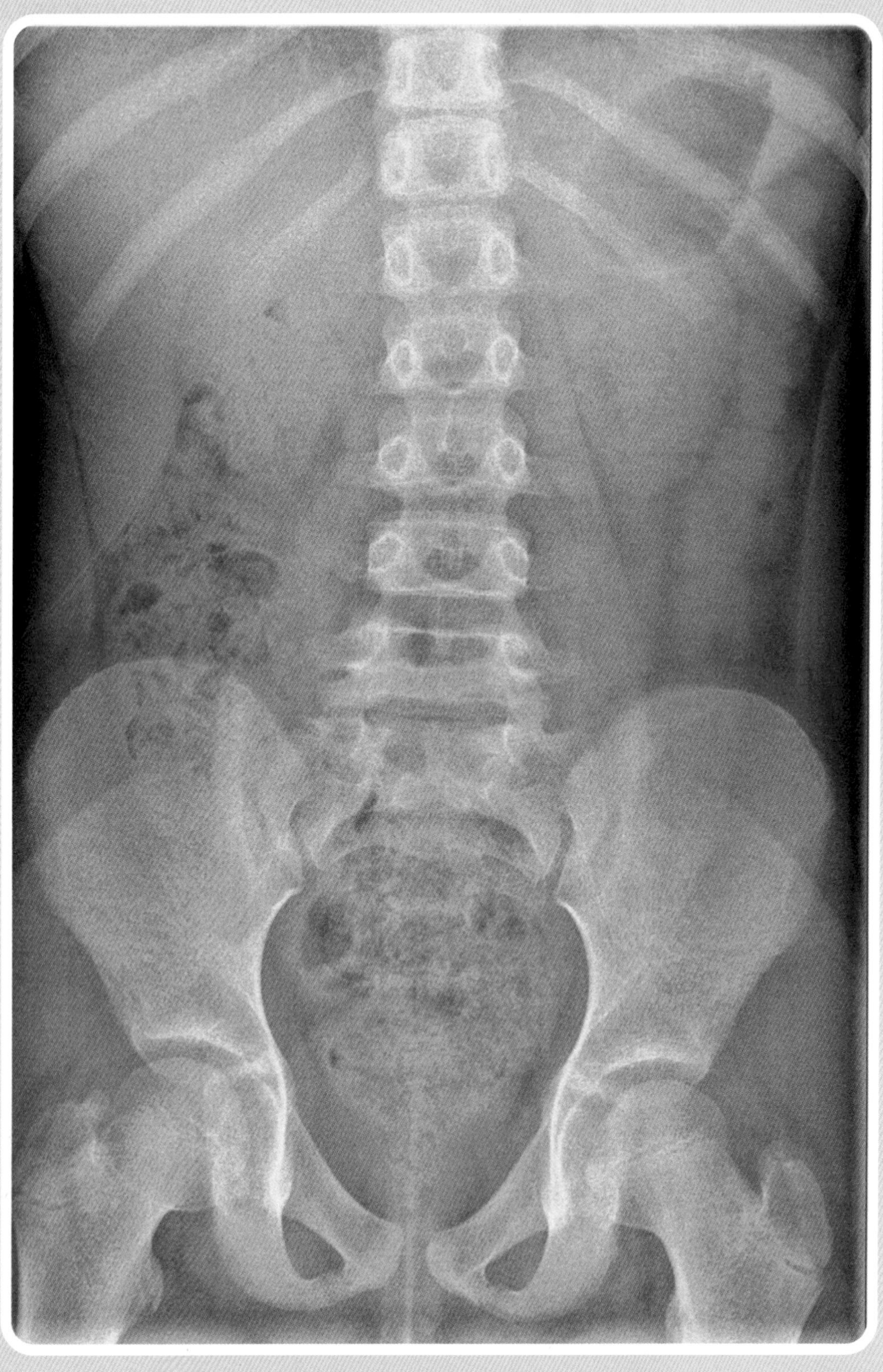

TECHNICAL INFORMATION

Patient ID: Anonymous.
Projection: AP supine.
Rotation: Adequate.
Penetration: Adequate – the spinous processes are visible.
Coverage: Adequate – the anterior ribs are visible superiorly and the inferior pubic rami are visible.

BOWEL GAS PATTERN

There is a paucity of bowel gas but no bowel dilatation is visible.

There is a moderate volume of faecal residue present predominantly in the ascending and distal sigmoid colon and rectum.

BOWEL WALL

There is no evidence of mural thickening or intramural gas within the large or small bowel.

PNEUMOPERITONEUM

There is no evidence of free intraabdominal gas.

SOLID ORGANS

The right lobe of the liver extends inferiorly beyond the lower margin of the right kidney, with a tongue-like appearance, in keeping with a Riedel's lobe.

VASCULAR

No abnormal vascular calcification.

BONES

There are no abnormalities of the imaged thoracic and lumbar spine, or within the pelvis. There are growth plates at the femoral head, trochanters and acetabulum as the ossification centres have not yet fused, which is a normal finding in a child of this age.

SOFT TISSUES

The psoas muscle outline is visible bilaterally.

The extraabdominal soft tissues are unremarkable.

OTHER

There is a urethral urinary catheter in situ.

There are no radiopaque foreign bodies.

There are no vascular lines, drains or surgical clips.

REVIEW AREAS

Gallstones/renal calculi: No radiopaque calculi.
Lung bases: Not fully included.
Spine: Normal.
Femoral heads: Normal.

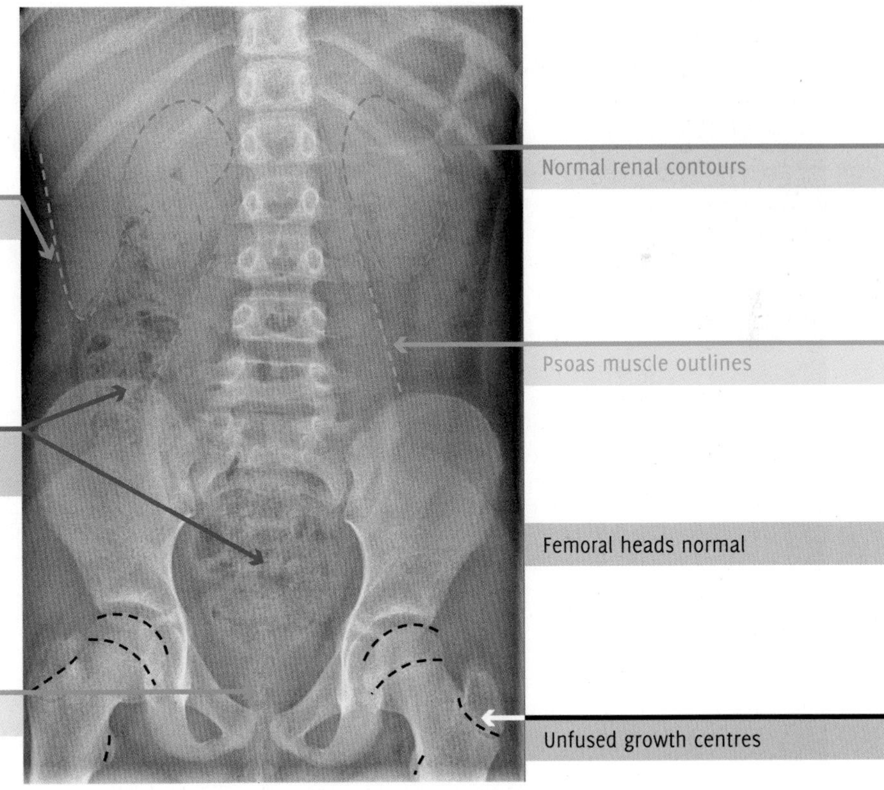

SUMMARY

This X-ray demonstrates a moderate volume of faecal residue predominantly in the ascending and distal sigmoid colon and rectum. There is a normal variant Riedel's lobe of the liver. There is no evidence of bowel obstruction or pneumoperitoneum.

INVESTIGATIONS AND MANAGEMENT

If the patient is clinically constipated, current medications should be reviewed and laxatives considered. Advice should be given regarding lifestyle adjustments, including adequate fluid intake, sufficient dietary fibre and exercise if clinically appropriate.

If the patient is otherwise well, no further investigation or imaging is required.

Case

13

An 11-year-old female attends the gastroenterology outpatient clinic for a routine follow-up appointment. Her past medical history is significant for chronic constipation, for which she takes laxatives. On examination, she has oxygen saturations of 98% in room air and a temperature of 36.7°C. Her HR is 80 bpm, RR is 20 and blood pressure is 110/70 mmHg. The abdomen is soft, but slightly distended, with mild tenderness with normal bowel sounds.

An abdominal X-ray is requested to assess for possible bowel obstruction.

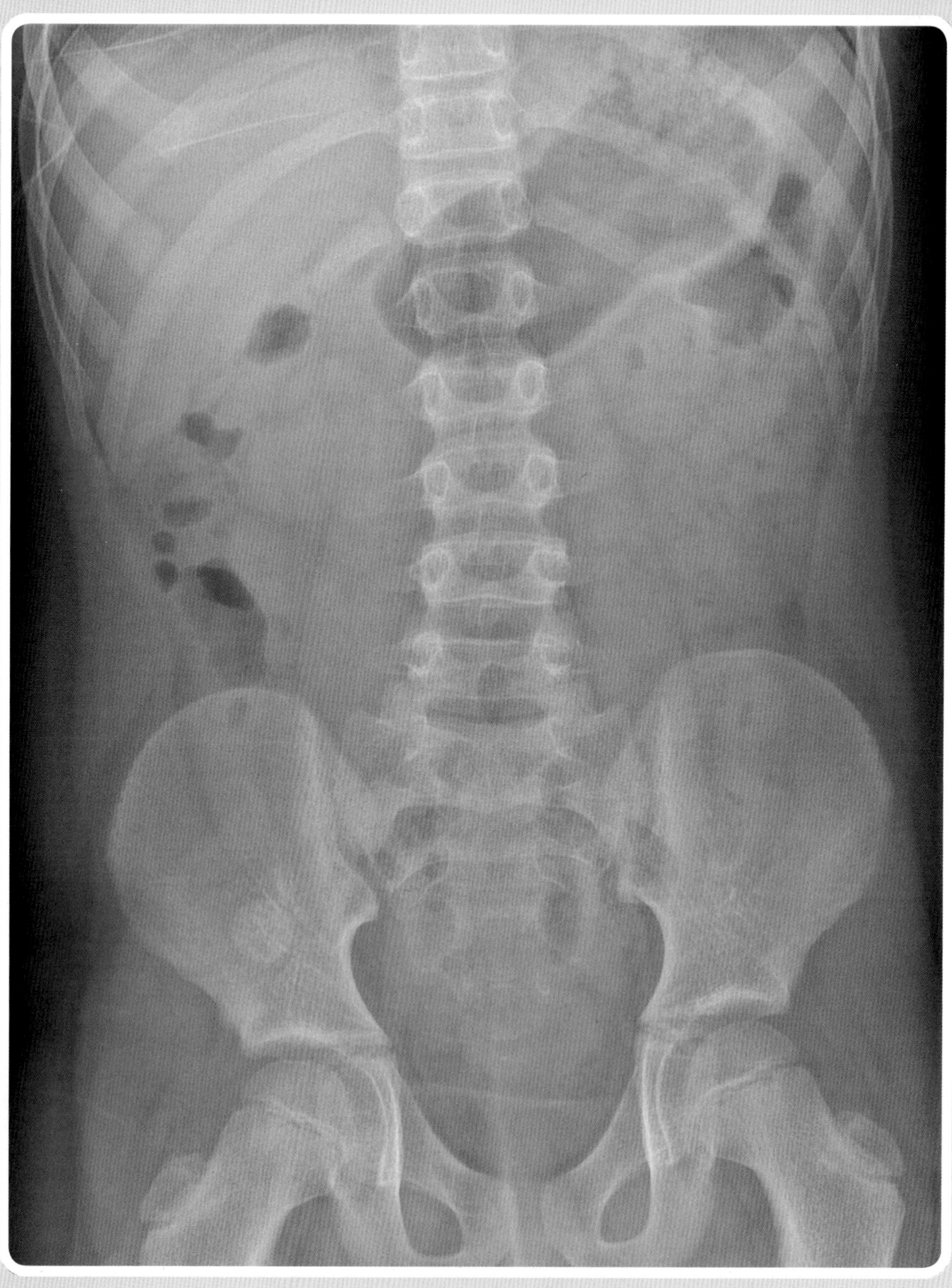

TECHNICAL INFORMATION

Patient ID: Anonymous.
Projection: AP supine.
Rotation: Adequate.
Penetration: Adequate – the spinous processes are visible.
Coverage: Adequate – the anterior ribs are visible superiorly and the pubic rami are visible inferiorly.

BOWEL GAS PATTERN

The bowel gas pattern is normal.

BOWEL WALL

There is no evidence of mural thickening or intramural gas within the large or small bowel.

PNEUMOPERITONEUM

There is no evidence of free intraabdominal gas.

SOLID ORGANS

The solid organ contours are within normal limits with no solid organ calcification.

VASCULAR

No abnormal vascular calcification.

BONES

There are no abnormalities of the imaged thoracic and lumbar spine, or within the pelvis.

There are growth plates at the femoral head, greater trochanter and acetabulum as the ossification centres have not yet fused, which is a normal finding in a child of this age.

SOFT TISSUES

The psoas muscle outline is visible bilaterally.

The extraabdominal soft tissues are unremarkable.

OTHER

There is a rounded radiopaque density projected over the right iliac fossa, which most likely represents the stopper of an Antegràde Colonic Enema (ACE) stoma given the history of chronic constipation.

There are no vascular lines, drains or surgical clips.

REVIEW AREAS

Gallstones/renal calculi: No radiopaque calculi.
Lung bases: Not fully included.
Spine: Normal.
Femoral heads: Normal – growth plates present.

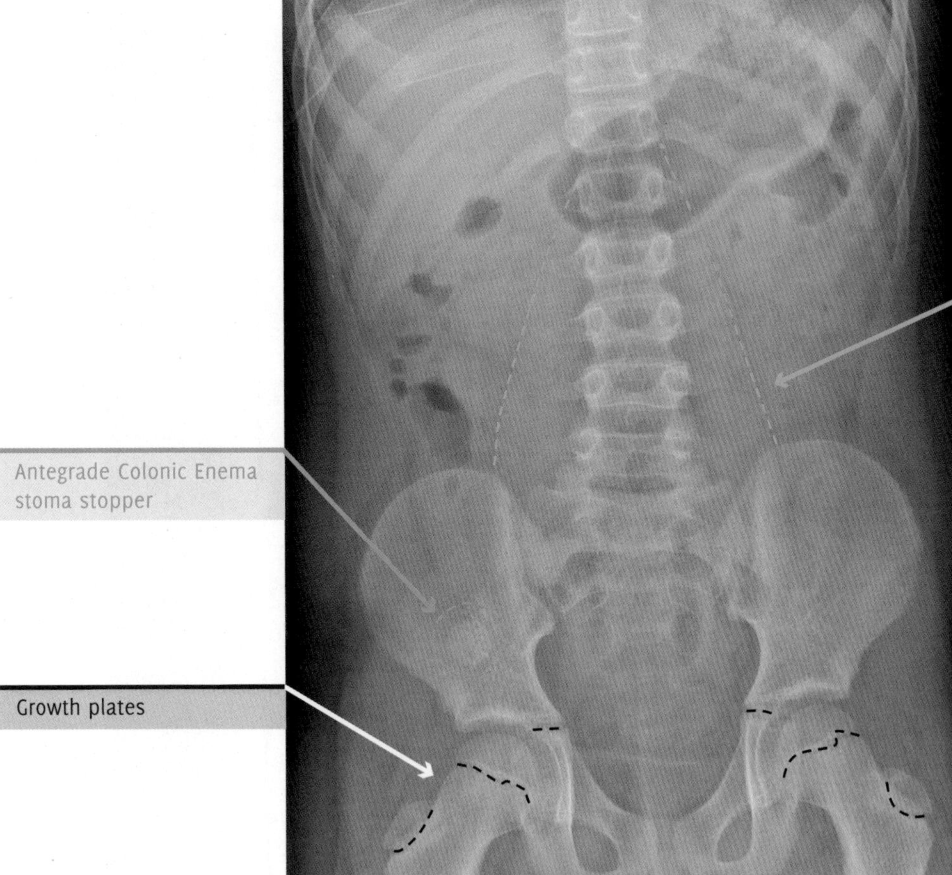

SUMMARY

This X-ray demonstrates no evidence of bowel obstruction. There is a rounded radiopaque density projected over the right iliac fossa, most likely to represent the stopper of an ACE stoma.

INVESTIGATIONS AND MANAGEMENT

Adequate analgesia and hydration should be provided.

If the patient is otherwise well, no further investigation or imaging is required. Referral to the paediatric continence team would be helpful to review her laxative regime.

Case 14

A 12-year-old female presents to ED with abdominal distension and vomiting. She has a PEG-J tube in situ to manage severe gastrooesophageal reflux. On examination, she has oxygen saturations of 99% in room air and a temperature of 37.1°C. Her HR is 90 bpm, RR is 18 and blood pressure is 120/80 mmHg. The abdomen is soft, bowel sounds are normal, the jejunostomy site is clean and there is some mild diffuse tenderness with no evidence of peritonism. Urine dipstick and pregnancy test are both negative.

An abdominal X-ray is requested to assess for the position of the jejunostomy tube, and for possible bowel obstruction.

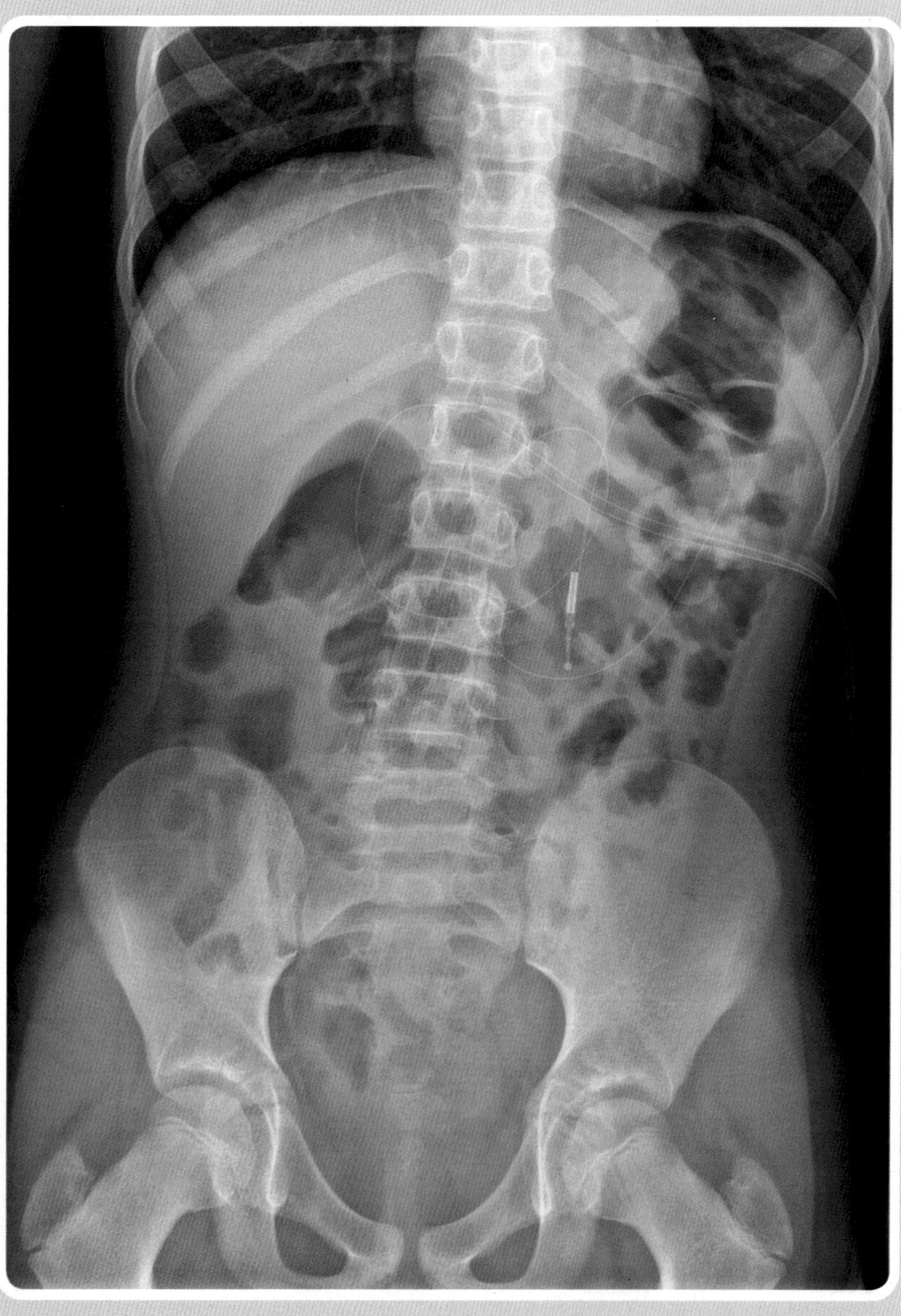

TECHNICAL INFORMATION

Patient ID: Anonymous.
Projection: AP supine.
Rotation: Adequate.
Penetration: Adequate – the spine is visible.
Coverage: Adequate – the anterior ribs are visible superiorly and the inferior pubic rami are visible.

BOWEL GAS PATTERN

Bowel gas pattern is normal.

BOWEL WALL

There is no evidence of mural thickening or intramural gas within the large or small bowel.

PNEUMOPERITONEUM

There is no evidence of free intraabdominal gas.

SOLID ORGANS

The solid organ contours are within normal limits with no solid organ calcification.

VASCULAR

No abnormal vascular calcification.

BONES

There are no abnormalities of the imaged thoracic and lumbar spine, or within the pelvis.

There are growth plates at the femoral head, greater trochanter and acetabulum (triradiate cartilage) as the ossification centres have not yet fused which is a normal finding in a child of this age.

SOFT TISSUES

The psoas muscle outline is visible bilaterally.

Extraabdominal soft tissues are unremarkable.

OTHER

There is a radiopaque port and two internal–external lines projecting in the left upper quadrant. The tip of the shorter line is projected over the stomach in keeping with a PEG and the longer line follows the same course through the expected course of the duodenum with its tip projecting over the proximal jejunum in keeping with a PEG-J.

There are no vascular lines, drains or surgical clips.

REVIEW AREAS

Gallstones/renal calculi: No radiopaque calculi.
Lung bases: Normal.
Spine: Normal. The sacrum is not yet fused which is a normal finding in a child of this age.
Femoral heads: Normal – growth plates present.

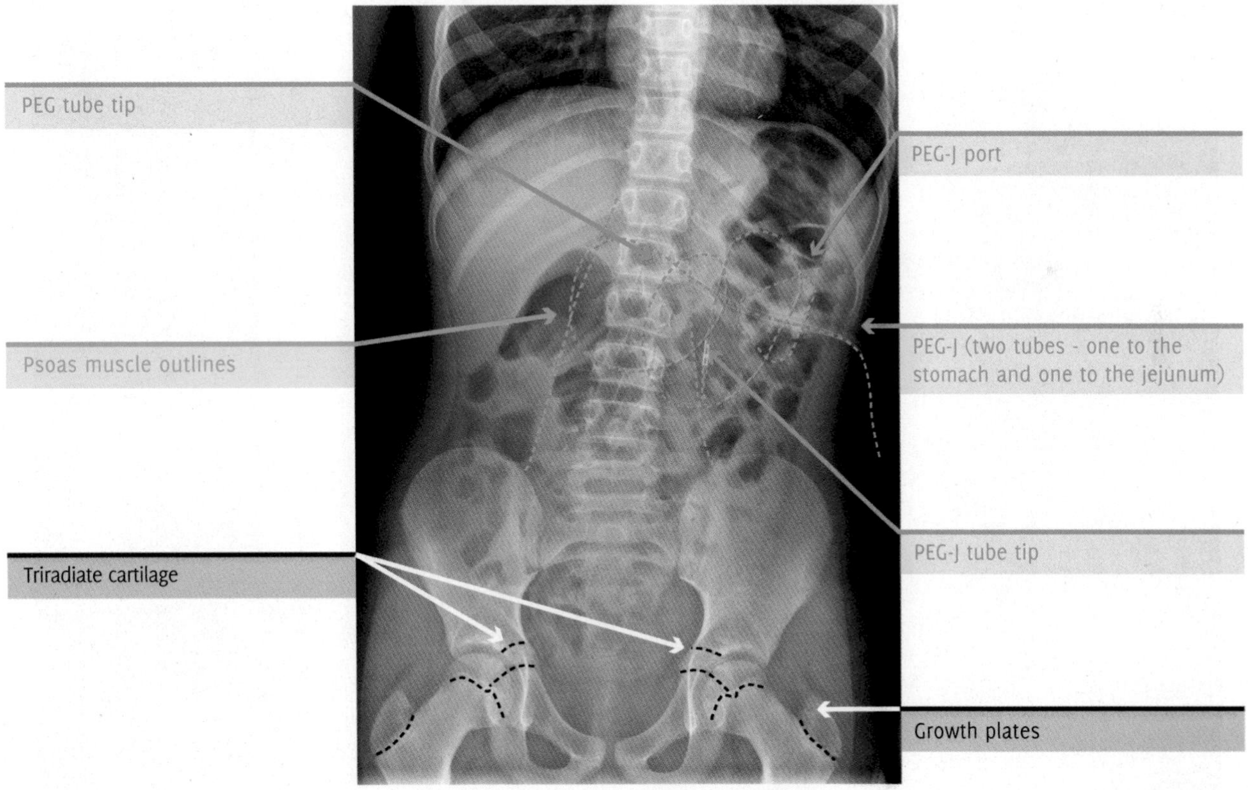

SUMMARY

This abdominal X-ray demonstrates appropriately sited PEG and PEG-J lines, although this cannot be certain from a single view. The bowel gas pattern is normal and there is no evidence of bowel obstruction.

INVESTIGATIONS AND MANAGEMENT

The patient should be resuscitated using an ABCDE approach.

Adequate analgesia and antiemetics should be provided.

The patient should be made NBM, the gastrostomy limb of the PEG-J put on free drainage and the patient should be started on IV fluids.

Urgent bloods should be taken for FBC, U&Es, CRP, bone profile, LFTs, coagulation, blood gas, blood cultures and cross match.

The paediatric general surgical team should be involved, and if there is no improvement, a contrast study could be considered.

Case

15

A 45-year-old male presents to ED with worsening abdominal distension. He has not passed flatus or opened his bowels for over 48 hours. He has no significant past medical history. On examination, he has oxygen saturations of 97% in room air and a temperature of 37.6°C. His HR is 94 bpm, RR is 20 and blood pressure is 134/92 mmHg. The abdomen is rigid and there is generalized tenderness with tinkling bowel sounds. Urine dipstick is unremarkable.

An abdominal X-ray is requested to assess for possible bowel obstruction.

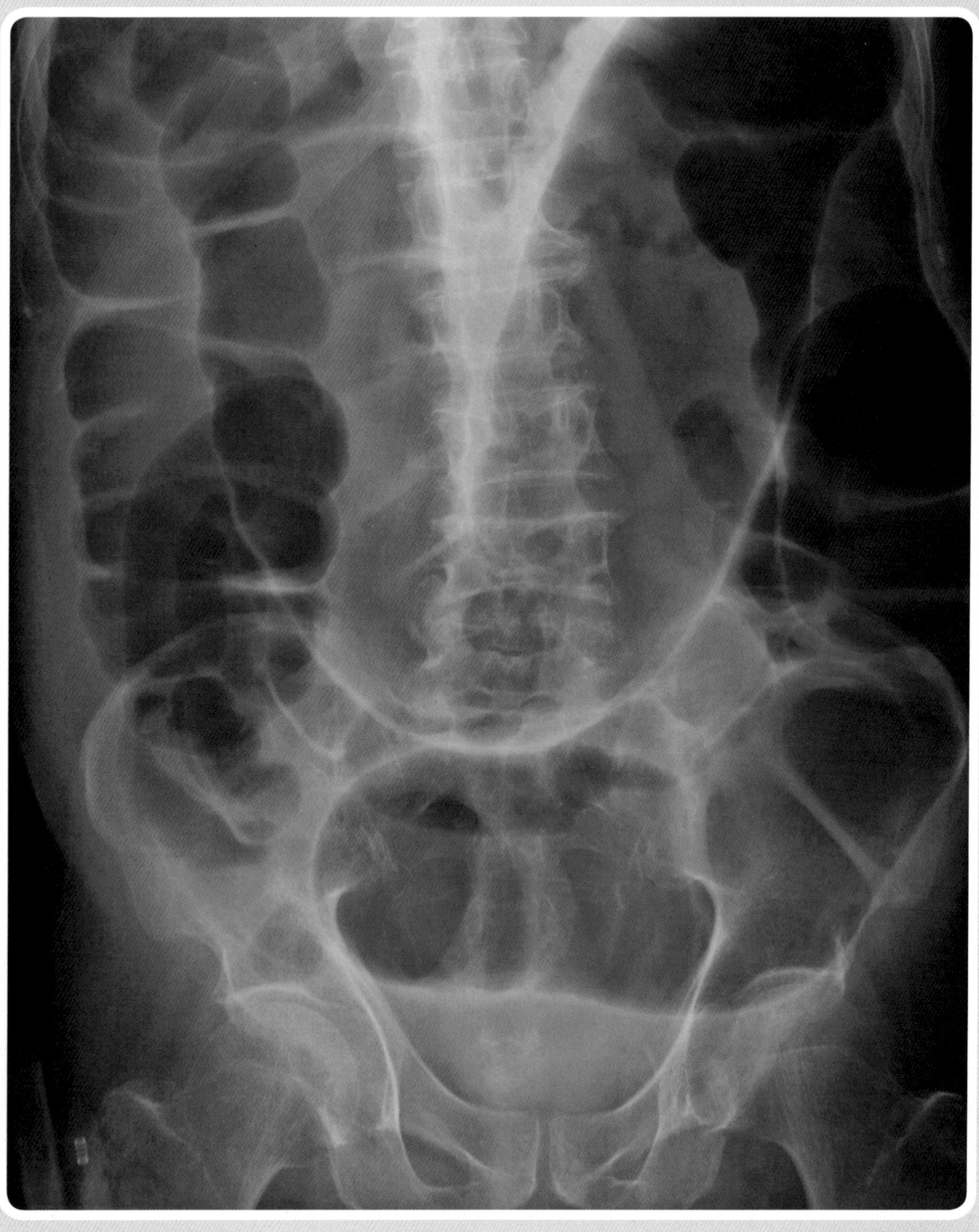

TECHNICAL INFORMATION

Patient ID: Anonymous.
Projection: AP supine.
Rotation: Adequate.
Penetration: Adequate – the spinous processes are visible.
Coverage: Inadequate – the anterior ribs have not been included.

BOWEL GAS PATTERN

There are multiple loops of dilated bowel seen in the abdomen demonstrating haustra, in keeping with large bowel obstruction. A dilated small bowel loop is visible in the right lower quadrant.

Bowel gas is not seen in the rectum.

BOWEL WALL

There is no evidence of mural thickening or intramural gas within the large or small bowel.

PNEUMOPERITONEUM

There is no evidence of free intraabdominal gas.

SOLID ORGANS

The solid organ contours are within normal limits with no solid organ calcification.

VASCULAR

No abnormal vascular calcification.

BONES

There are degenerative changes in the lumbar spine with lateral osteophytes at L1/L2 and a mild scoliosis convex to the left at L4/L5. The L3 and L4 vertebral bodies have reduced height with concave endplates, in keeping with endplate fractures of indeterminate age.

SOFT TISSUES

The psoas muscle outline is visible bilaterally.

The extraabdominal soft tissues are unremarkable.

OTHER

There are no radiopaque foreign bodies.

There are no vascular lines, drains or surgical clips.

REVIEW AREAS

Gallstones/renal calculi: No radiopaque calculi.
Lung bases: Not fully included.
Spine: Degenerative changes and endplate fractures as described.
Femoral heads: Normal.

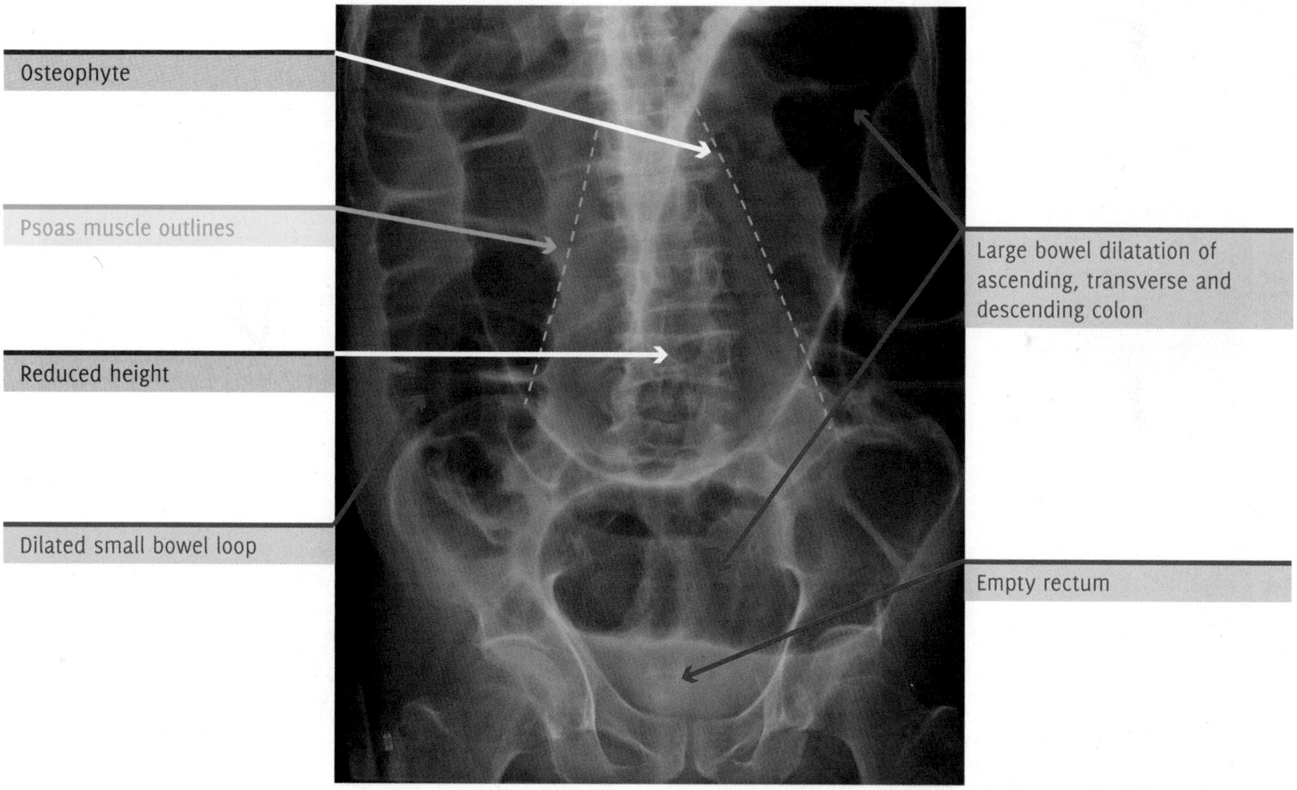

SUMMARY

This X-ray demonstrates multiple loops of dilated bowel seen within the abdomen demonstrating haustra, in keeping with large bowel obstruction, as well as a loop of dilated small bowel. The absence of gas in the small intestine indicates a competent ileo-caecal valve creating a closed-loop obstruction. The absence of bowel gas in the rectum suggests a distal obstructing point. Given the absence of previous abdominal or pelvic surgery, findings may be secondary to a benign or malignant stricture. Vertebral endplate fractures of indeterminate age are also noted, which may be related to malignancy.

INVESTIGATIONS AND MANAGEMENT

The patient should be resuscitated using an ABCDE approach.

Adequate analgesia and hydration should be provided.

The patient should be kept NBM and an NG tube inserted on free drainage. IV fluids should be commenced.

Urgent bloods should be taken, including FBC, U&Es, CRP, LFTs, coagulation, blood gas, and group and save.

The general surgical team should be contacted urgently and a CT scan of the abdomen/pelvis with IV contrast should be considered for better visualization of the anatomy and further assessment. With regard to the bony changes, further history should be taken, and previous images reviewed.

Case 16

A 36-year-old female presents to her doctor with a 6-week history of mild generalized abdominal pain. Her past medical history is significant for type I diabetes mellitus and a previous cholecystectomy. She is a nonsmoker. On examination, she has oxygen saturations of 98% in room air and a temperature of 36.6°C. Her HR is 65 bpm, RR is 15 and blood pressure is 120/68 mmHg. The abdomen is soft with mild generalized tenderness with normal bowel sounds. Urine dipstick is unremarkable and a pregnancy test is negative.

An abdominal X-ray is requested to assess for possible bowel obstruction.

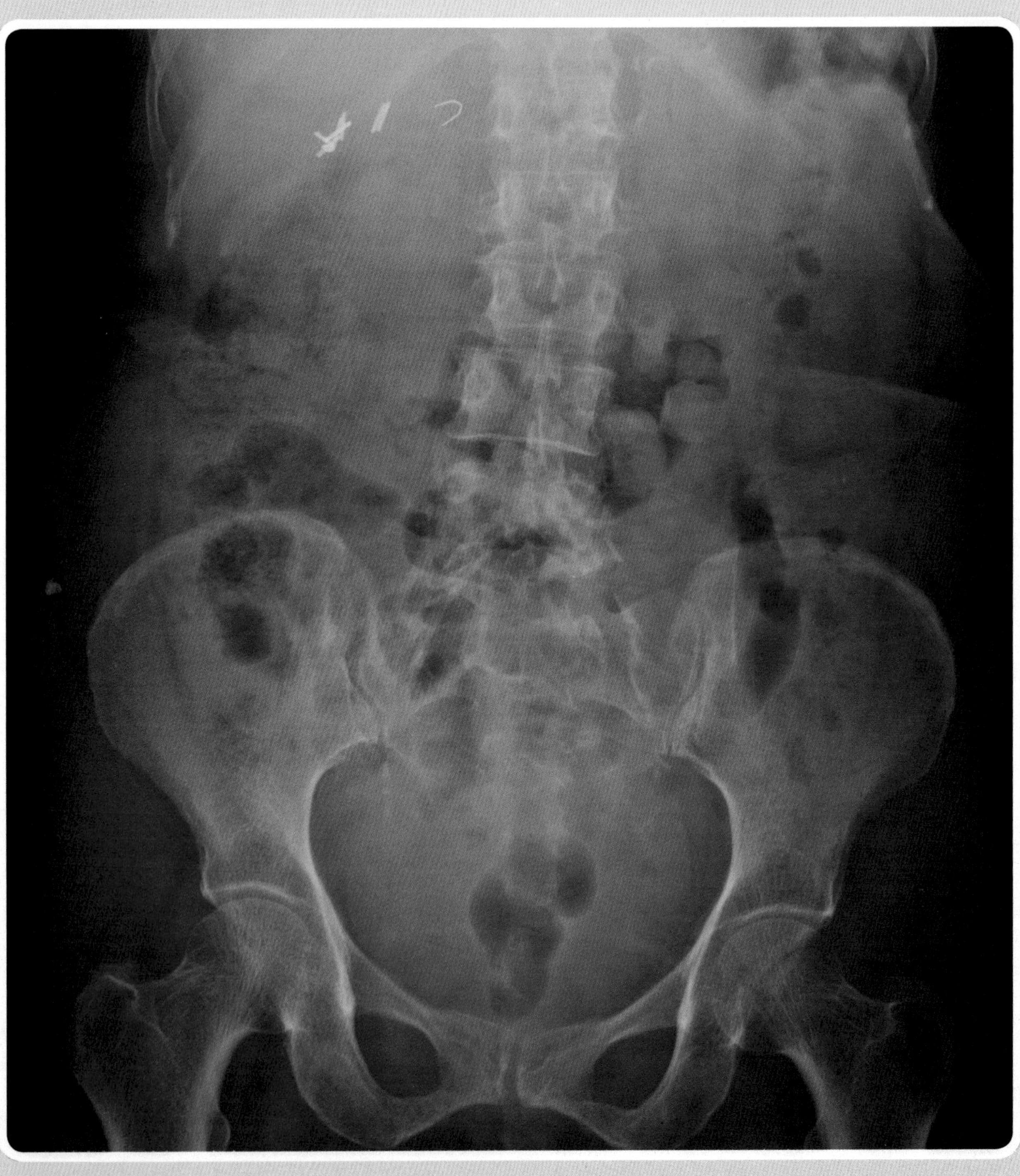

TECHNICAL INFORMATION

Patient ID: Anonymous.
Projection: AP supine.
Rotation: Adequate.
Penetration: Adequate – the spinous processes are visible.
Coverage: Adequate – the anterior ribs are visible superiorly and the pubic rami are visible inferiorly.

BOWEL GAS PATTERN

The bowel gas pattern is normal.

There is a moderate volume of faecal residue present throughout the ascending colon with hard faeces within the transverse colon.

BOWEL WALL

There is no evidence of mural thickening or intramural gas within the large or small bowel.

PNEUMOPERITONEUM

There is no evidence of free intraabdominal gas.

SOLID ORGANS

The solid organ contours are within normal limits with no solid organ calcification.

VASCULAR

There is mild calcification of the right common iliac artery.

BONES

There are moderate degenerative changes seen within the imaged lumbar spine, particularly at the L5/S1 level. There is mild scoliosis convex to the left in the lumbar spine. No fractures or destructive bone lesions are visible in the imaged skeleton.

SOFT TISSUES

The psoas muscle outline is visible bilaterally.

The extraabdominal soft tissues are unremarkable.

OTHER

There are radiopaque surgical clips seen projected over the region of the inferior aspect of the liver, in keeping with cholecystectomy clips.

There are no vascular lines or drains.

REVIEW AREAS

Gallstones/renal calculi: No radiopaque calculi.
Lung bases: Not fully included.
Spine: Moderate degenerative changes particularly at L5/S1 level.
Femoral heads: Normal.

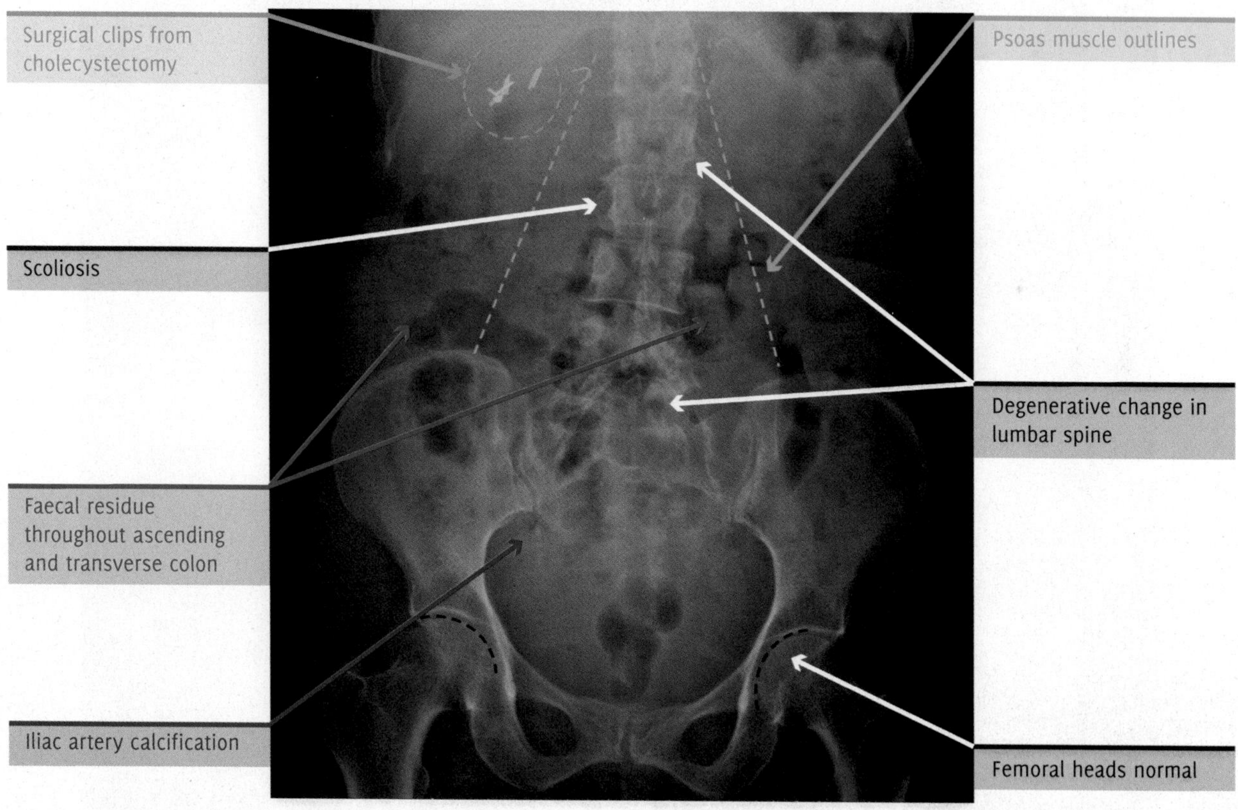

SUMMARY

This X-ray demonstrates no evidence of bowel obstruction. There is moderate faecal loading throughout the ascending and transverse colon with hard faeces present. The cholecystectomy surgical clips, spinal degenerative changes and mild lumbar scoliosis convex to the left are incidental findings.

INVESTIGATIONS AND MANAGEMENT

Adequate analgesia and hydration should be provided.

If the patient is clinically constipated, current medications should be reviewed and laxatives considered. Advice should be given regarding lifestyle adjustments, including adequate fluid intake, sufficient dietary fibre and exercise if clinically appropriate.

Case

17

A 5-year-old male presents to ED with worsening abdominal distension, nausea and vomiting. He has not opened his bowels for the past 24 hours. He has no significant past medical history. On examination, he has oxygen saturations of 99% in room air and a temperature of 36.8°C. His HR is 150 bpm, RR is 32 and blood pressure is 95/50 mmHg. The abdomen is rigid and there is generalized tenderness with tinkling bowel sounds. Urine dipstick is unremarkable.

An abdominal X-ray is requested to assess for possible obstruction.

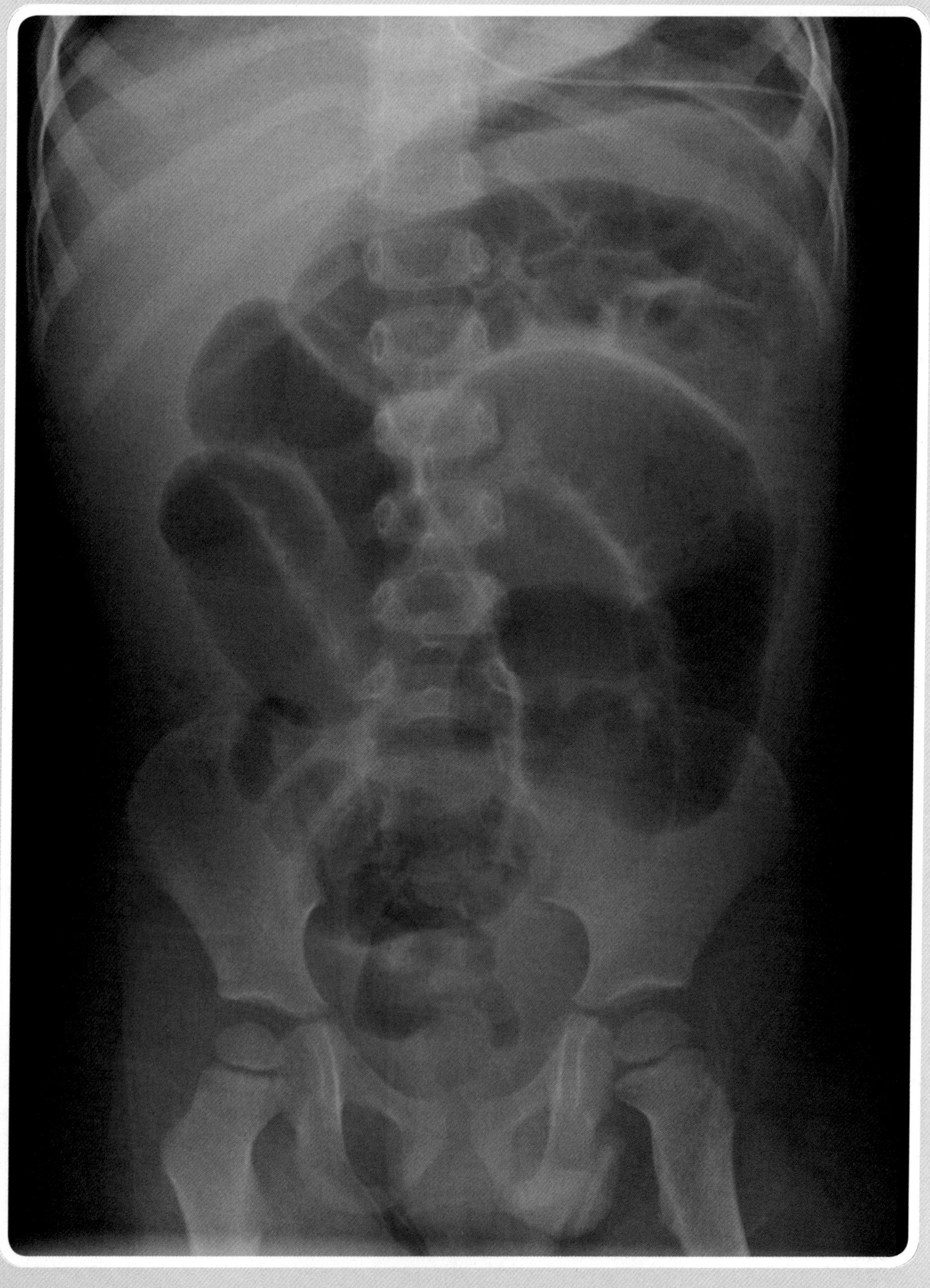

TECHNICAL INFORMATION

Patient ID: Anonymous.
Projection: AP supine.
Rotation: Adequate.
Penetration: Adequate – the spinous processes are visible.
Coverage: Adequate – the anterior ribs are visible superiorly and the inferior pubic rami are visible.

BOWEL GAS PATTERN

There are multiple loops of dilated bowel seen centrally in the abdomen, in keeping with small bowel obstruction. The normal pattern of valvulae conniventes has been lost in several (but not all) dilated small bowel loops.

BOWEL WALL

There is no evidence of mural thickening or intramural gas within the large or small bowel.

PNEUMOPERITONEUM

There is no evidence of free intraabdominal gas.

SOLID ORGANS

The solid organ contours are within normal limits with no solid organ calcification.

VASCULAR

No abnormal vascular calcification.

BONES

There are no abnormalities of the imaged thoracic and lumbar spine, or within the pelvis.

There are growth plates at the femoral head and acetabulum as the ossification centres have not yet fused, which is a normal finding in a child of this age.

SOFT TISSUES

The psoas muscle outline is not visible bilaterally, which is nonspecific, particularly in a child of this age.

The extraabdominal soft tissues are unremarkable.

OTHER

There is an NG tube in situ, with its tip projecting in the left upper quadrant, in the stomach.

There are no vascular lines, drains or surgical clips.

REVIEW AREAS

Gallstones/renal calculi: No radiopaque calculi.
Lung bases: Not fully included.
Spine: Normal.
Femoral heads: Normal – growth plates present.

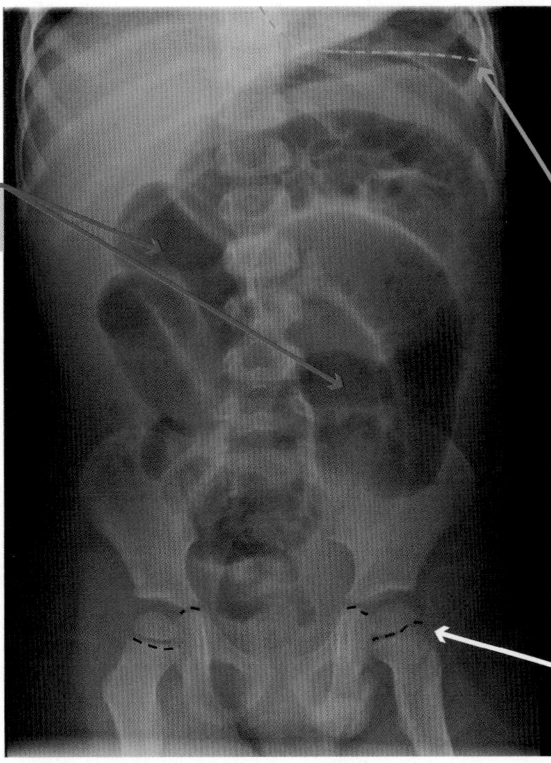

SUMMARY

This X-ray demonstrates multiple loops of dilated bowel seen centrally in the abdomen, with loss of some of the normal valvulae conniventes, in keeping with small bowel obstruction, although no cause is obvious on the radiograph. There is an NG tube in situ with its tip in the stomach.

INVESTIGATIONS AND MANAGEMENT

The patient should be resuscitated using an ABCDE approach.

Adequate analgesia and hydration should be provided.

The patient should be kept NBM, have the NG tube put on free drainage and be started on IV fluids.

Urgent bloods should be taken, including FBC, U&Es, CRP, LFTs, coagulation, blood gas, and group and save.

The paediatric surgical team should be contacted urgently and further radiological imaging of the abdomen and pelvis should be considered for better visualization of the anatomy and further assessment.

Case

18

A 4-year-old male presents to ED with worsening abdominal pain and distension. He has no significant past medical history. On examination, he has oxygen saturations of 97% in room air and a temperature of 37.3°C. His HR is 152 bpm, RR is 36 and blood pressure is 120/75 mmHg. The abdomen is rigid and there is generalized tenderness with tinkling bowel sounds. Urine dipstick is unremarkable.

An abdominal X-ray is requested to assess for possible obstruction.

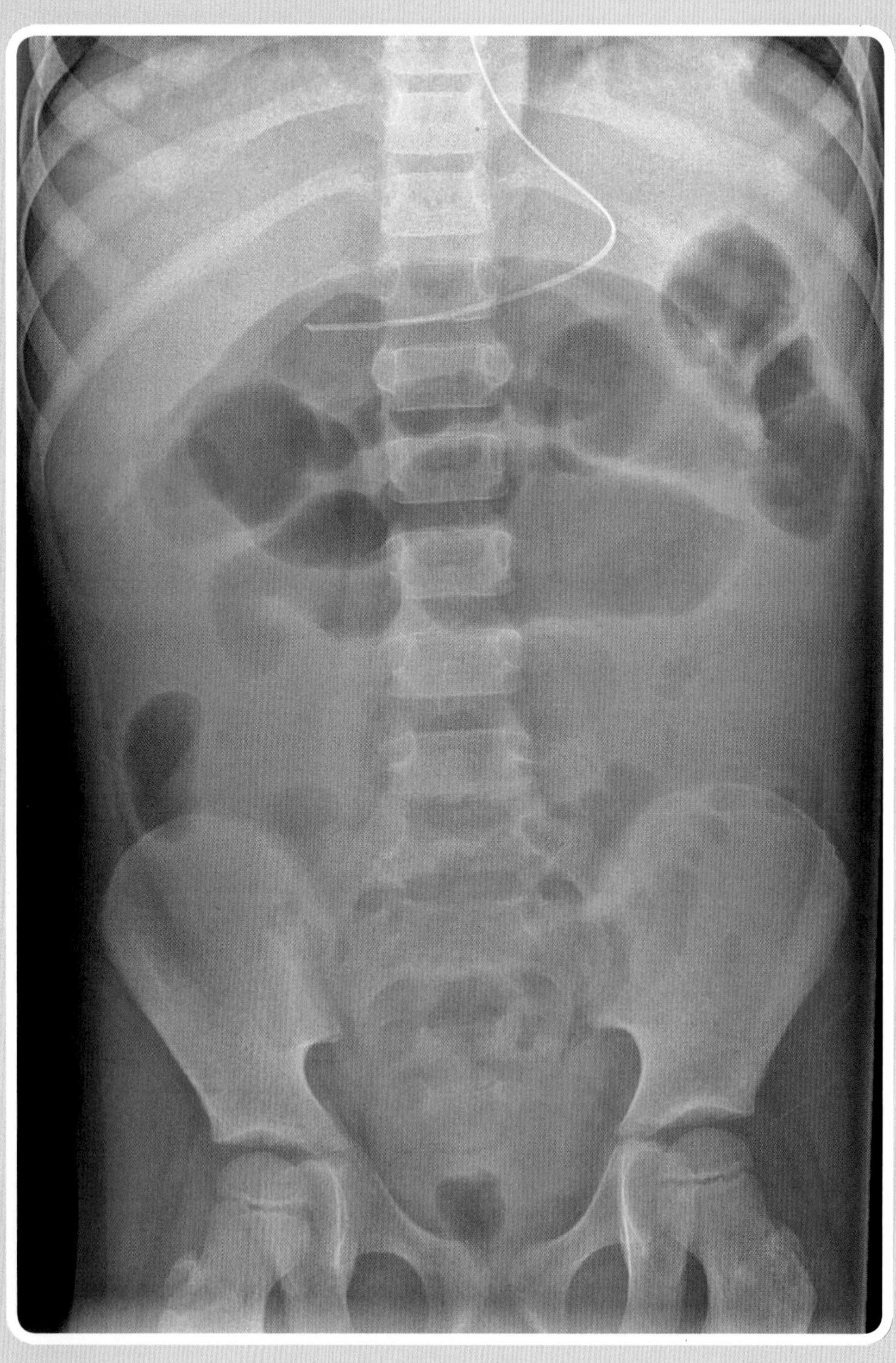

TECHNICAL INFORMATION

Patient ID: Anonymous.
Projection: AP supine.
Rotation: Adequate.
Penetration: Adequate – the spinous processes are visible.
Coverage: Adequate – the anterior ribs are visible superiorly and the pubic rami are visible inferiorly.

BOWEL GAS PATTERN

There are multiple loops of dilated bowel seen centrally in the abdomen, suggestive of bowel obstruction.

BOWEL WALL

There is no evidence of mural thickening or intramural gas within the large or small bowel.

PNEUMOPERITONEUM

There is no evidence of free intraabdominal gas.

SOLID ORGANS

The solid organ contours are within normal limits with no solid organ calcification.

VASCULAR

No abnormal vascular calcification.

BONES

There are no abnormalities of the imaged thoracic and lumbar spine, or within the pelvis.

There are growth plates at the femoral head and acetabulum as the ossification centres have not yet fused, which is a normal finding in a child of this age.

SOFT TISSUES

The psoas muscle outline is visible bilaterally.

The extraabdominal soft tissues are unremarkable.

OTHER

There is an NG tube in situ, with its tip projected over the right upper quadrant of the abdomen, within the antrum of the stomach.

There are no vascular lines, drains or surgical clips.

REVIEW AREAS

Gallstones/renal calculi: No radiopaque calculi.
Lung bases: There is a radiopacity projecting within the right lung base of indeterminate significance.
Spine: Normal.
Femoral heads: Normal – growth plates present.

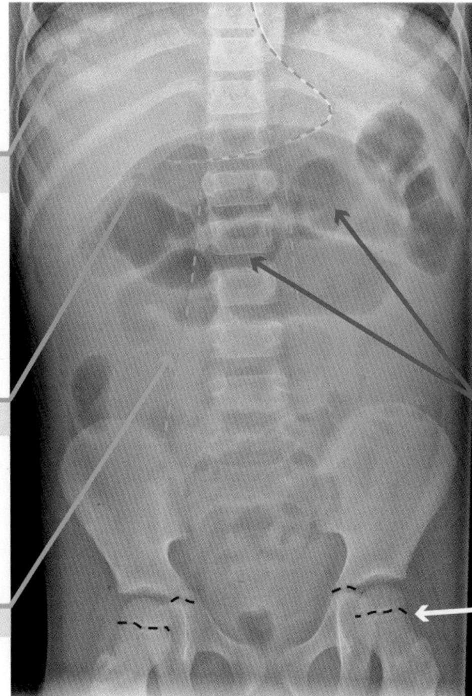

SUMMARY

This X-ray demonstrates multiple loops of dilated bowel seen centrally within the abdomen, in keeping with likely small bowel obstruction, although no cause is visible on X-ray. There is an NG tube in situ which could be pulled back slightly. The right lung base radiopacity is of indeterminate significance and is an incidental finding.

INVESTIGATIONS AND MANAGEMENT

The patient should be resuscitated using an ABCDE approach.

Adequate analgesia and hydration should be provided.

The patient should be kept NBM, have their NG tube put on free drainage and started on IV fluids.

Urgent bloods should be taken, including FBC, U&Es, CRP, LFTs, coagulation, blood gas, and group and save. Assuming this is a new finding, a chest X-ray should be performed to further assess the radiopacity projecting over the right lung base.

The paediatric surgical team should be contacted urgently and further radiological imaging of the abdomen and pelvis should be considered for better visualization of the anatomy and further assessment.

Case

19

A 21-year-old female presents to ED with a 2-day history of generalized, worsening abdominal pain. She has not opened her bowels in that time and feels nauseated but has not vomited. Her past medical history is significant for cystic fibrosis, which is well controlled and she is not on laxatives. She is a nonsmoker. On examination, she has oxygen saturations of 97% in room air and a temperature of 37.2°C. Her HR is 75 bpm, RR is 12 and blood pressure is 115/65 mmHg. The chest is resonant throughout and breath sounds are clear. The abdomen is mildly distended with generalized abdominal tenderness and voluntary guarding. Bowel sounds are normal. Urine dipstick is unremarkable and a pregnancy test is negative.

An abdominal X-ray is requested to assess for possible bowel obstruction.

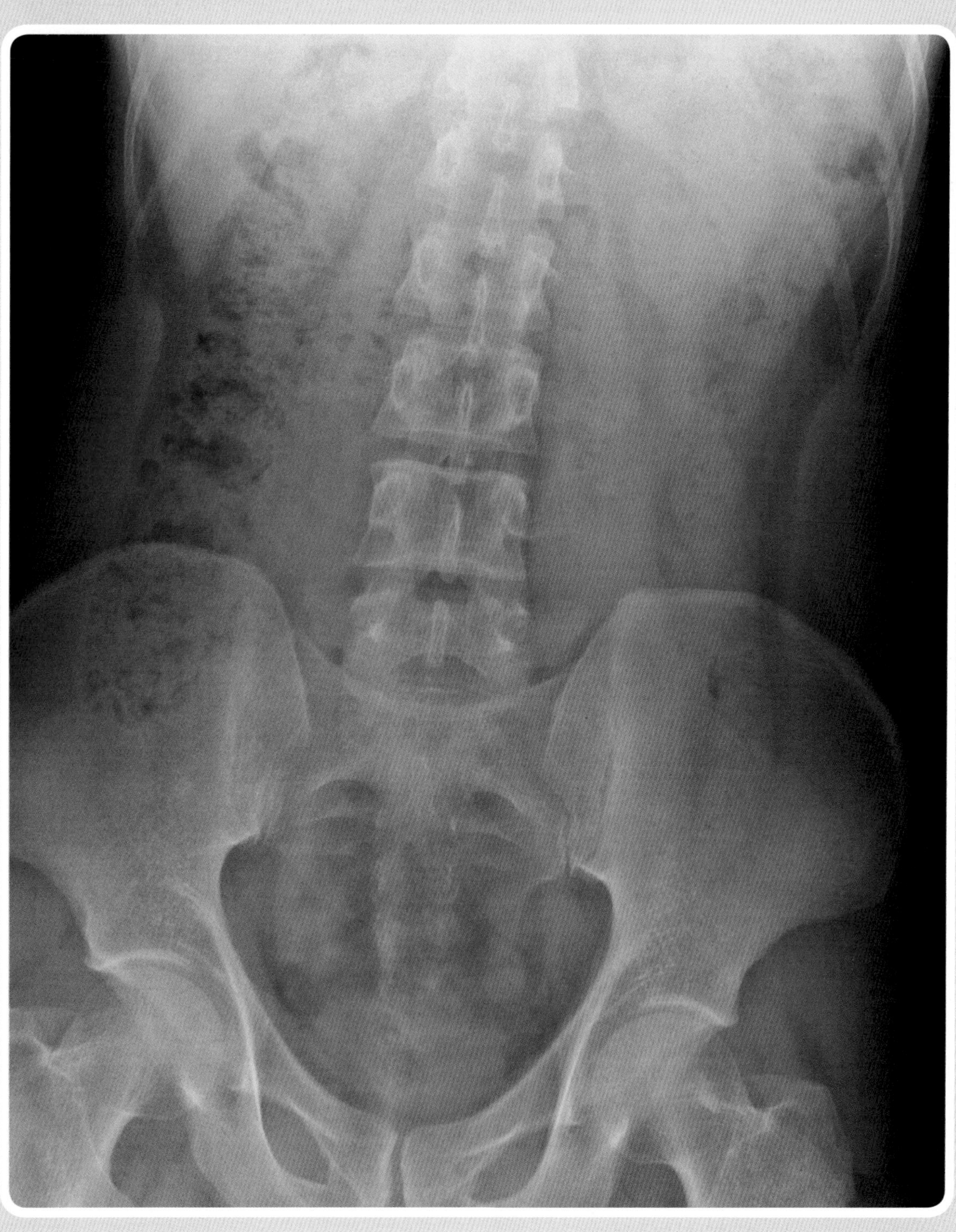

TECHNICAL INFORMATION

Patient ID: Anonymous.
Projection: AP supine.
Rotation: Adequate.
Penetration: Adequate – the spinous processes are visible.
Coverage: Adequate – the anterior ribs are visible superiorly and the inferior pubic rami are visible.

BOWEL GAS PATTERN

There is a paucity of bowel gas but no bowel dilatation is visible.

There is a moderate amount of faecal residue present predominantly in the ascending colon and also throughout the visualized transverse and descending colon. The rectum is relatively empty.

BOWEL WALL

There is no evidence of mural thickening or intramural gas within the large or small bowel.

PNEUMOPERITONEUM

There is no evidence of free intraabdominal gas.

SOLID ORGANS

The solid organ contours are within normal limits with no solid organ calcification.

VASCULAR

No abnormal vascular calcification.

BONES

There are no abnormalities of the imaged thoracic and lumbar spine, or within the pelvis.

SOFT TISSUES

The psoas muscle outline is visible bilaterally.

The extraabdominal soft tissues are unremarkable.

OTHER

There are no radiopaque foreign bodies.

There are no vascular lines, drains or surgical clips.

REVIEW AREAS

Gallstones/renal calculi: No radiopaque calculi.
Lung bases: Normal.
Spine: Normal.
Femoral heads: Normal.

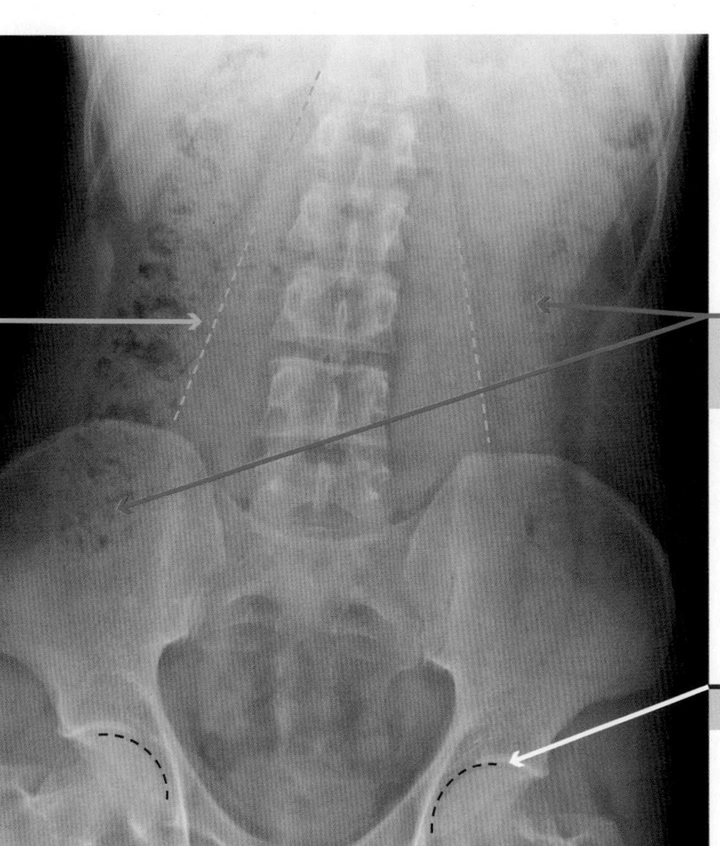

SUMMARY

This X-ray demonstrates a moderate volume of faecal residue predominantly in the ascending colon, and also in the visualized transverse and descending colon. There is no evidence of bowel obstruction or pneumoperitoneum.

INVESTIGATIONS AND MANAGEMENT

If the patient is clinically constipated, current medications should be reviewed and laxatives considered. Advice should be given regarding lifestyle adjustments, including adequate fluid intake, sufficient dietary fibre and exercise if clinically appropriate.

If the patient is otherwise well, no further investigation or imaging is required.

Case

20

A 30-year-old female presents to ED with right-sided pain radiating from her loin to her groin. She has no significant past medical history and is a nonsmoker. On examination, she has oxygen saturations of 99% in room air and a temperature of 37.1°C. Her HR is 90 bpm, RR is 18 and blood pressure is 120/80 mmHg. The abdomen is soft and there is tenderness in the right flank with normal bowel sounds. Urine dipstick shows blood +++ and a pregnancy test is negative.

An abdominal X-ray is requested to assess for possible renal calculi.

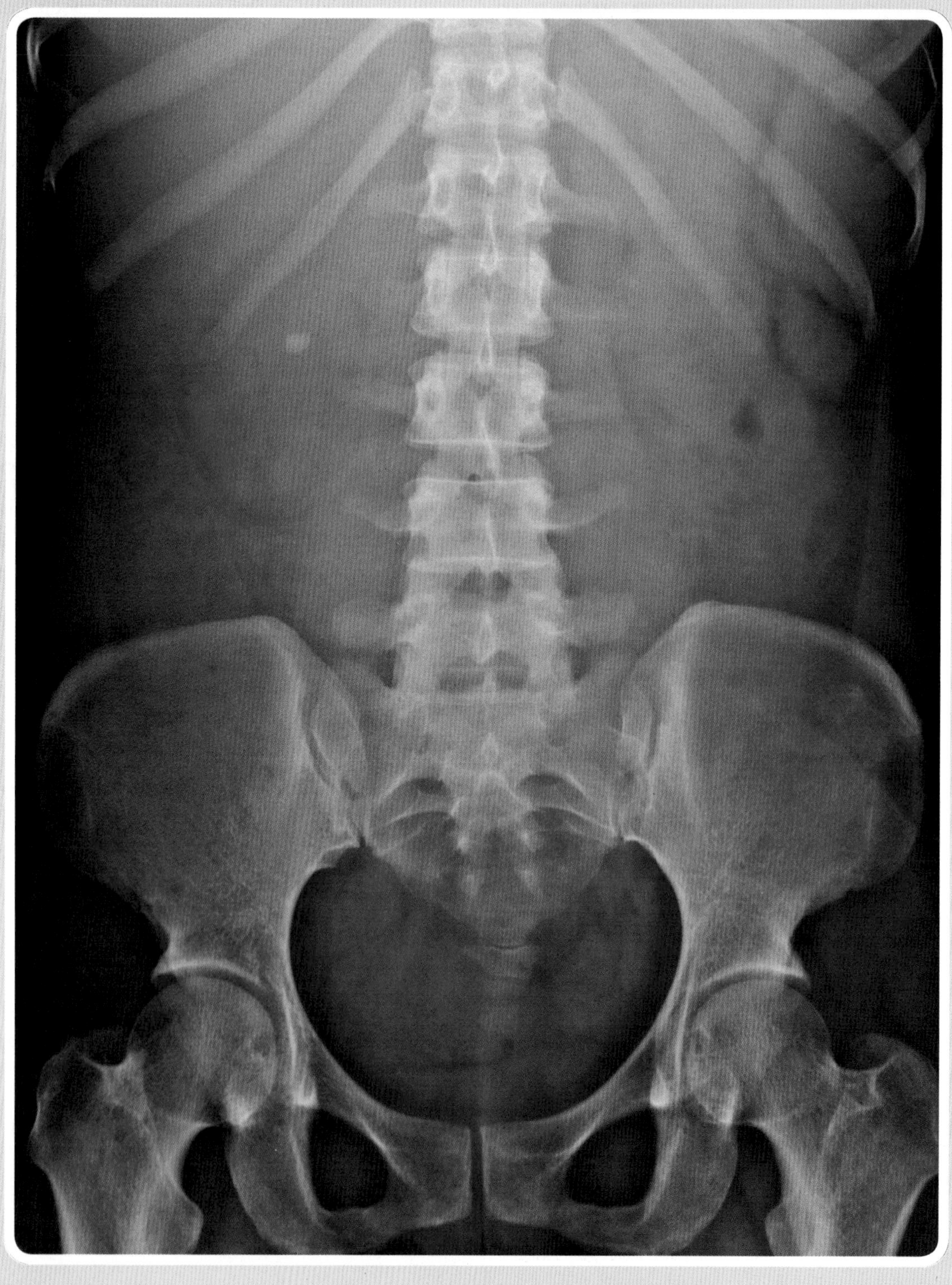

TECHNICAL INFORMATION

Patient ID: Anonymous.
Projection: AP supine.
Rotation: Adequate.
Penetration: Adequate – the spinous processes are visible.
Coverage: Adequate – the anterior ribs are visible superiorly and the inferior pubic rami are visible.

BOWEL GAS PATTERN

There is a paucity of bowel gas, which is nonspecific.

BOWEL WALL

There is no evidence of mural thickening or intramural gas within the large or small bowel.

PNEUMOPERITONEUM

There is no evidence of free intraabdominal gas.

SOLID ORGANS

There is a well-defined radiopaque density projected over the upper pole of the right kidney, in keeping with a renal calculus.

VASCULAR

No abnormal vascular calcification.

BONES

There are no abnormalities of the imaged thoracic and lumbar spine, or within the pelvis.

SOFT TISSUES

The psoas muscle outline is visible bilaterally.

The extraabdominal soft tissues are unremarkable.

OTHER

There are no radiopaque foreign bodies.

There are no vascular lines, drains or surgical clips.

REVIEW AREAS

Gallstones/renal calculi: Likely renal calculus in the upper pole of the right kidney.
Lung bases: Not fully included.
Spine: Normal.
Femoral heads: Normal.

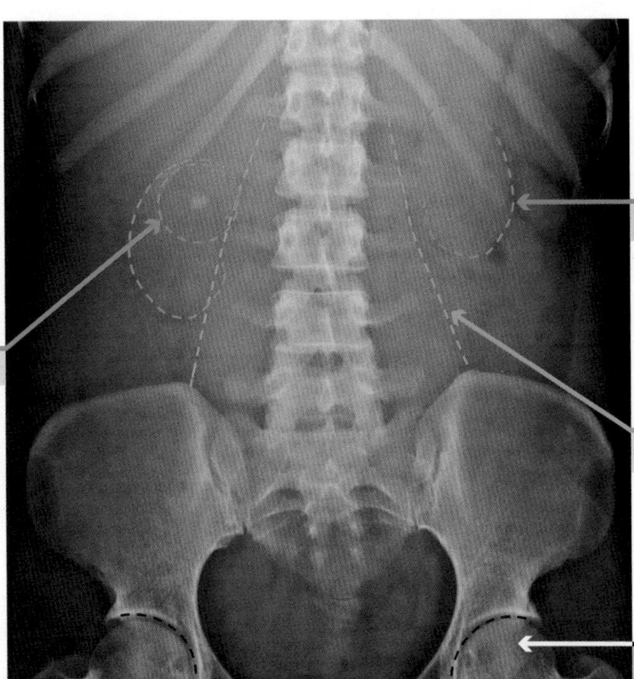

SUMMARY

This X-ray demonstrates a well-defined radiopaque density projecting over the upper pole of the right kidney. Given the clinical history, the most likely diagnosis is a renal calculus. Other differentials include calcification of an artery, lymph node or a radiopaque gallstone within a distended gallbladder. There is a paucity of bowel gas, which is nonspecific.

INVESTIGATIONS AND MANAGEMENT

The patient should be resuscitated using an ABCDE approach.

Adequate analgesia and hydration should be provided.

Urgent bloods should be taken, including FBC, U&Es, CRP, LFTs, blood gas and bone profile.

The patient should be assessed for acute kidney injury, and if present, an ultrasound of the urinary tract in the first instance would be beneficial in assessing for hydronephrosis.

Smaller stones may pass spontaneously, but the patient should be referred to urology for possible further intervention and follow-up. A CT scan of the kidneys, ureters and bladder may be useful for better visualization of the anatomy.

Case 21

A 35-year-old female presents to ED with colicky abdominal pain. Her past medical history is significant for Crohn's disease and she is a nonsmoker. On examination, she has oxygen saturations of 99% in room air and a temperature of 36.6°C. Her HR is 85 bpm, RR is 18 and blood pressure is 118/66 mmHg. The abdomen is soft and there is generalized mild tenderness with normal bowel sounds. An ileostomy is present which appears healthy on examination with normal bag contents. Urine dipstick is unremarkable and a pregnancy test is negative.

An abdominal X-ray is requested to assess for possible bowel obstruction.

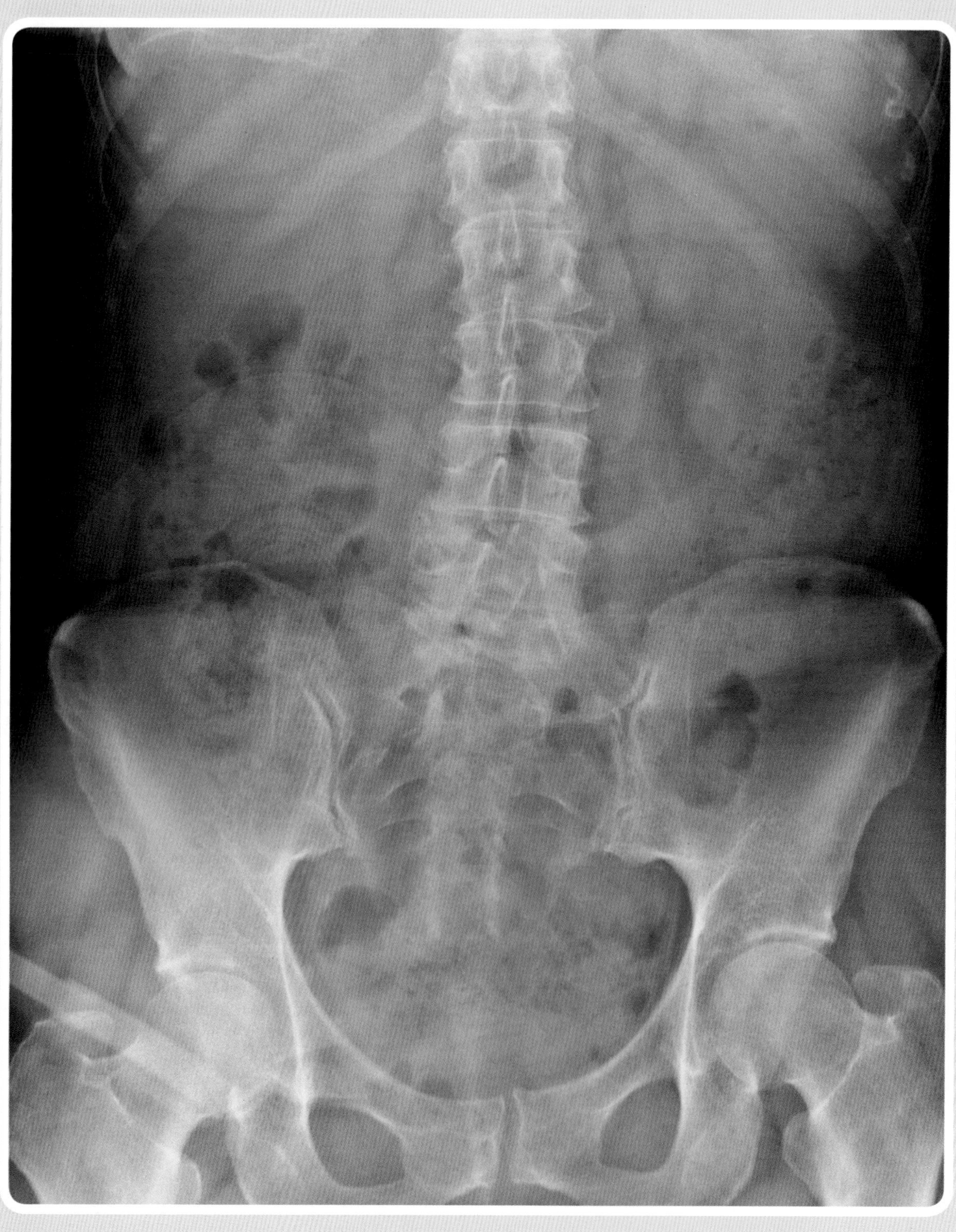

TECHNICAL INFORMATION

Patient ID: Anonymous.
Projection: AP supine.
Rotation: Adequate.
Penetration: Adequate – the spinous processes are visible.
Coverage: Adequate – the anterior ribs are visible superiorly and the inferior pubic rami are visible.

BOWEL GAS PATTERN

The bowel gas pattern is normal.

There is a mild to moderate volume of faecal residue present throughout the large bowel.

BOWEL WALL

There is no evidence of mural thickening or intramural gas within the large or small bowel.

PNEUMOPERITONEUM

There is no evidence of free intraabdominal gas.

SOLID ORGANS

The solid organ contours are within normal limits with no solid organ calcification.

VASCULAR

No abnormal vascular calcification.

BONES

There is mild lumbar scoliosis seen convex to the left, centred at the L2/L3 level.

No fractures or destructive bone lesions are visible in the imaged skeleton.

SOFT TISSUES

The psoas muscle outline is visible bilaterally.

The extraabdominal soft tissues are unremarkable.

OTHER

There is a rounded radiopaque density projected over the right iliac fossa, in keeping with an ileostomy. Superior to this, there is a curvilinear radiopaque density in keeping with an ileostomy bag external to the patient.

There is a radiopaque density in the lower right region of the X-ray, representing an external artefact.

REVIEW AREAS

Gallstones/renal calculi: No radiopaque calculi.
Lung bases: Not fully included.
Spine: Lumbar scoliosis seen convex to the left, centred at the L2/3 level.
Femoral heads: Normal.

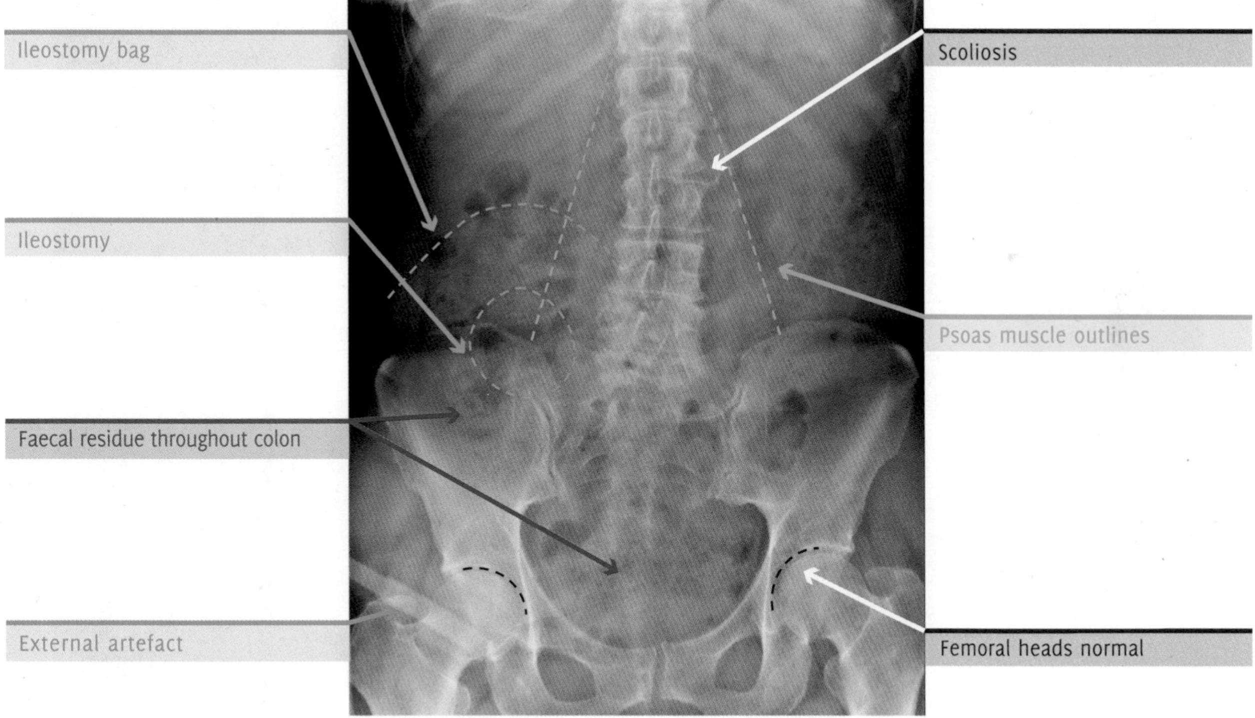

SUMMARY

This X-ray demonstrates an ileostomy. It also demonstrates a mild to moderate volume of faecal residue throughout the large bowel. There is no evidence of bowel obstruction. The scoliosis seen at the L3 vertebral body is an incidental finding.

INVESTIGATIONS AND MANAGEMENT

Adequate analgesia and hydration should be provided.

Urgent bloods should be taken, including FBC, U&Es, CRP, LFTs, amylase, blood gas and bone profile.

This may represent a flare-up of her Crohn's disease, warranting further investigation. A CT scan of the abdomen/pelvis with IV contrast may be considered for further evaluation of the abdomen and surgical/gastroenterology input should be considered.

Case

22

A 55-year-old male presents to ED with a 4-day history of left iliac fossa pain that is worse on straining. He has no significant past medical history and is a nonsmoker. On examination, he has oxygen saturations of 99% in room air and a temperature of 37.1°C. His HR is 80 bpm, RR is 15 and blood pressure is 120/65 mmHg. The abdomen is soft and there is tenderness in the left iliac fossa with normal bowel sounds. Urine dipstick is unremarkable.

An abdominal X-ray is requested to look for possible bowel obstruction.

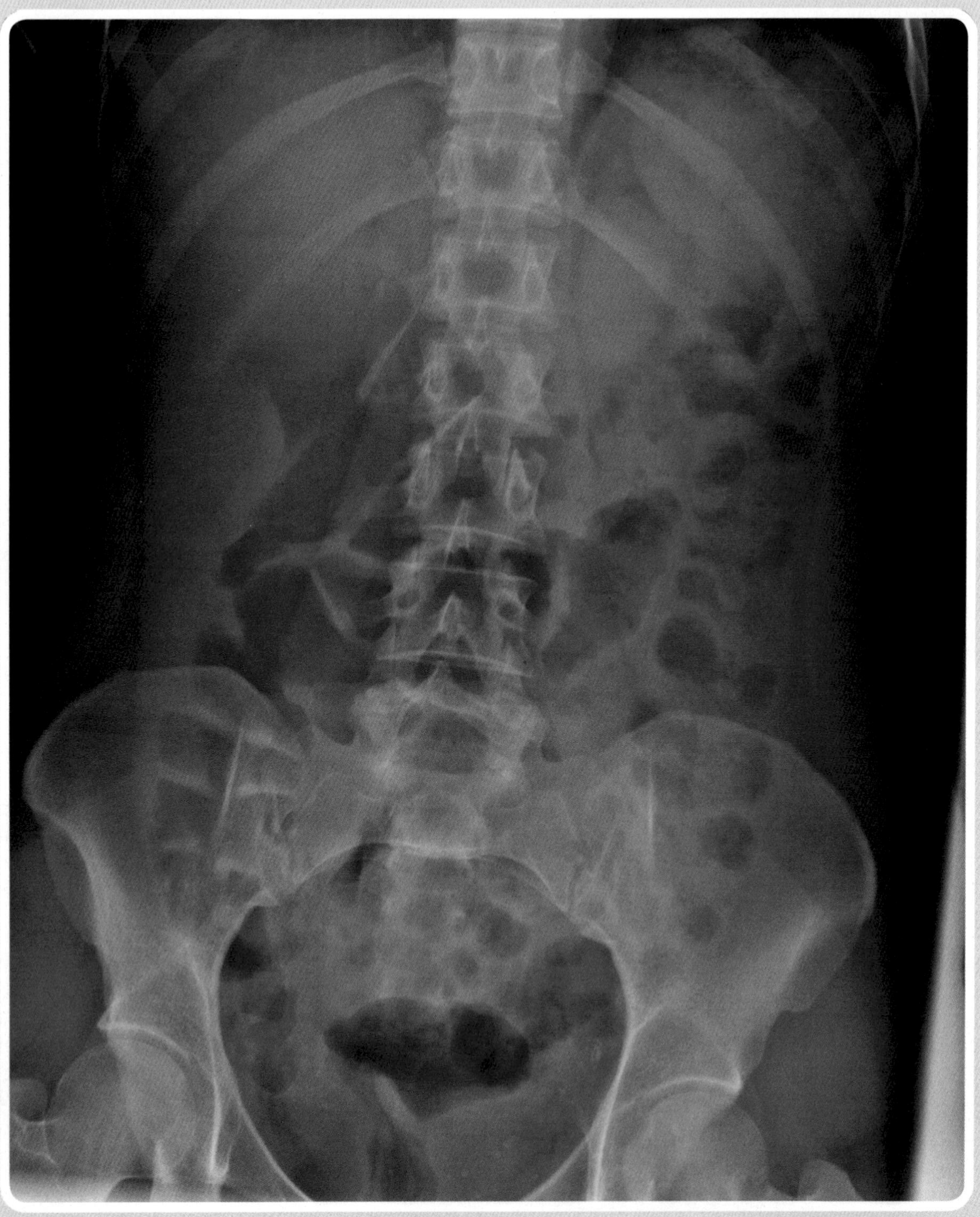

TECHNICAL INFORMATION

Patient ID: Anonymous.
Projection: AP supine.
Rotation: Adequate
Penetration: Adequate – the spinous processes are visible.
Coverage: Inadequate – the inferior pubic rami have not been included.

BOWEL GAS PATTERN

The bowel gas pattern is normal.

BOWEL WALL

There is no evidence of mural thickening or intramural gas within the large or small bowel.

PNEUMOPERITONEUM

There is no evidence of free intraabdominal gas.

SOLID ORGANS

The solid organ contours are within normal limits with no solid organ calcification.

VASCULAR

No abnormal vascular calcification.

BONES

There are no abnormalities of the imaged thoracic and lumbar spine, or within the pelvis.

SOFT TISSUES

The psoas muscle outline is preserved.

The extraabdominal soft tissues are unremarkable.

OTHER

There are no radiopaque foreign bodies.

There are no vascular lines, drains or surgical clips.

REVIEW AREAS

Gallstones/renal calculi: No radiopaque calculi.
Lung bases: Not fully included.
Spine: Normal.
Femoral heads: Normal.

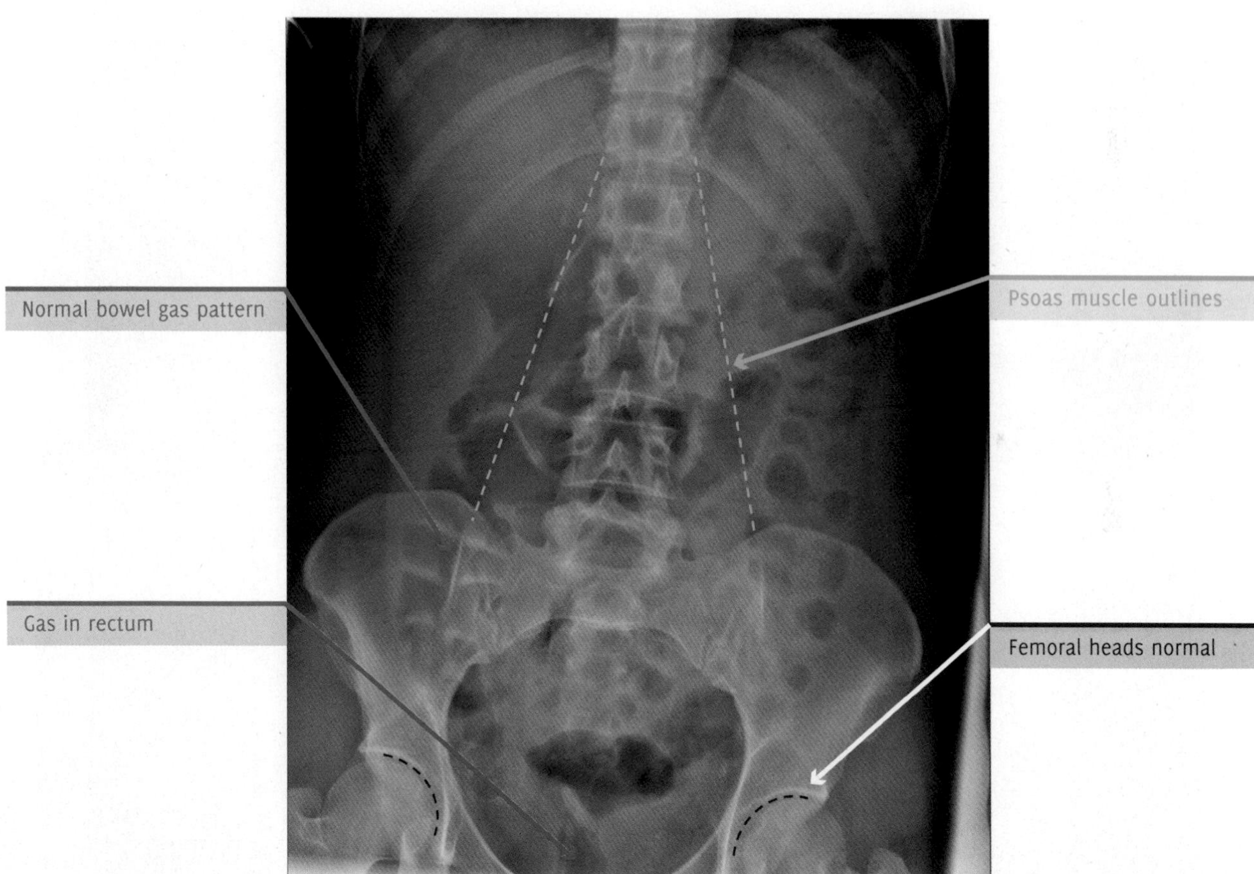

SUMMARY

This X-ray demonstrates a normal appearance with no evidence of bowel obstruction.

INVESTIGATIONS AND MANAGEMENT

Adequate analgesia and hydration should be provided.

Bloods should be taken, including FBC, U&Es, LFTs, amylase, bone profile, blood gas and CRP.

There are no clear findings on the abdominal X-ray to explain the patient's clinical presentation. Surgical input should be sought, and a CT abdomen/pelvis with IV contrast or a sigmoidoscopy considered.

Case

23

A 20-year-old male presents to his doctor with a 3-week history of generalized abdominal pain. He has no significant past medical history and is a nonsmoker. On examination, he has oxygen saturations of 98% in room air and a temperature of 36.6°C. His HR is 65 bpm, RR is 14 and blood pressure is 120/72 mmHg. The abdomen is rigid and there is generalized tenderness with normal bowel sounds. Urine dipstick is unremarkable.

An abdominal X-ray is requested to assess for possible bowel obstruction.

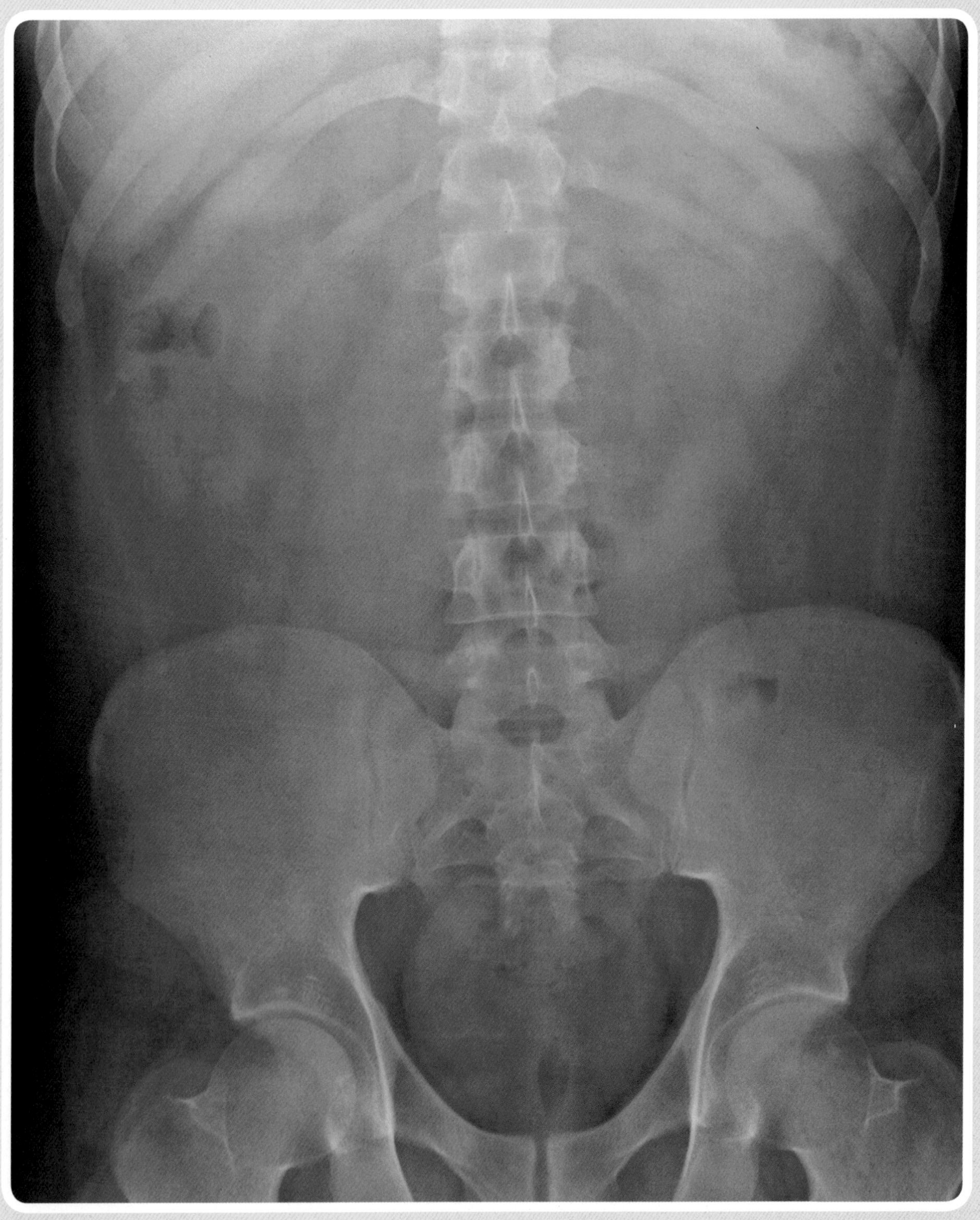

TECHNICAL INFORMATION

Patient ID: Anonymous.
Projection: AP supine.
Rotation: Adequate.
Penetration: Adequate – the spinous processes are visible.
Coverage: Inadequate – the pubic symphysis and inferior pubic rami have not been included.

BOWEL GAS PATTERN

The bowel gas pattern is normal.

BOWEL WALL

There is no evidence of mural thickening or intramural gas within the large or small bowel.

PNEUMOPERITONEUM

There is no evidence of free intraabdominal gas.

SOLID ORGANS

The solid organ contours are within normal limits with no solid organ calcification.

VASCULAR

No abnormal vascular calcification.

BONES

There are no abnormalities of the imaged thoracic and lumbar spine, or within the pelvis.

SOFT TISSUES

The psoas muscle outline is visible bilaterally.

The extraabdominal soft tissues are unremarkable.

OTHER

There are no radiopaque foreign bodies.

There are no vascular lines, drains or surgical clips.

REVIEW AREAS

Gallstones/renal calculi: No radiopaque calculi.
Lung bases: Normal (right lung base not well visualized).
Spine: Normal.
Femoral heads: Normal.

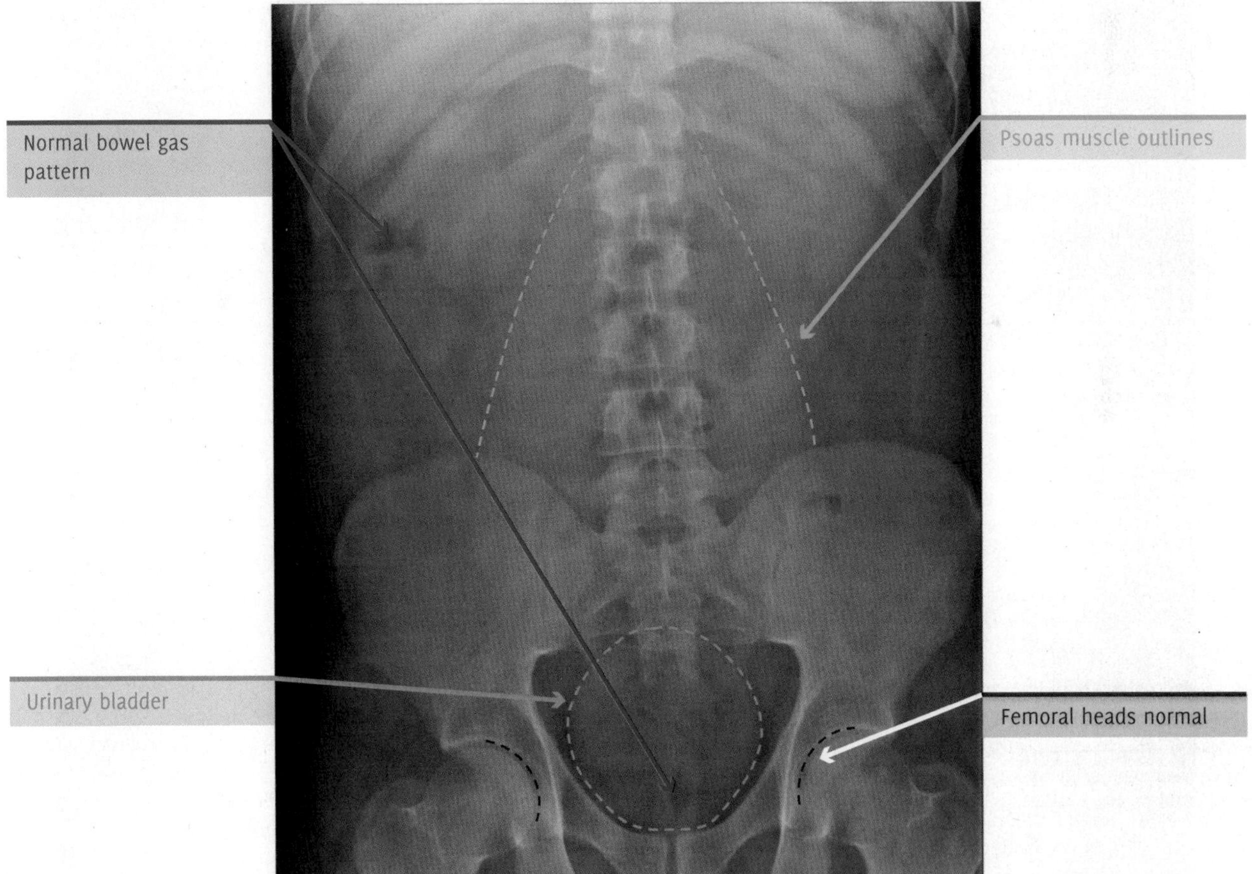

SUMMARY

This X-ray demonstrates normal appearances with no evidence of bowel obstruction.

INVESTIGATIONS AND MANAGEMENT

Adequate analgesia and hydration should be provided.

Bloods should be taken, including FBC, U&Es, LFTs, amylase, bone profile, blood gas and CRP.

There are no clear findings on the abdominal X-ray to explain the patient's clinical presentation. A CT scan of the abdomen/pelvis with IV contrast may be considered for further evaluation of the abdomen and surgical input should be sought.

Case

24

A 17-year-old female presents to her doctor with mild, intermittent left-sided abdominal pain. She has also recently noticed some spotting on her underwear. She has no significant past medical history and is a nonsmoker. She is currently sexually active and has an IUCD in situ. On examination, she has oxygen saturations of 99% in room air and a temperature of 36.8°C. Her HR is 70 bpm, RR is 14 and blood pressure is 115/62 mmHg. The abdomen is soft and there is mild generalized tenderness with normal bowel sounds. Urine dipstick is unremarkable and a pregnancy test is negative.

An abdominal X-ray is requested to assess for possible bowel obstruction.

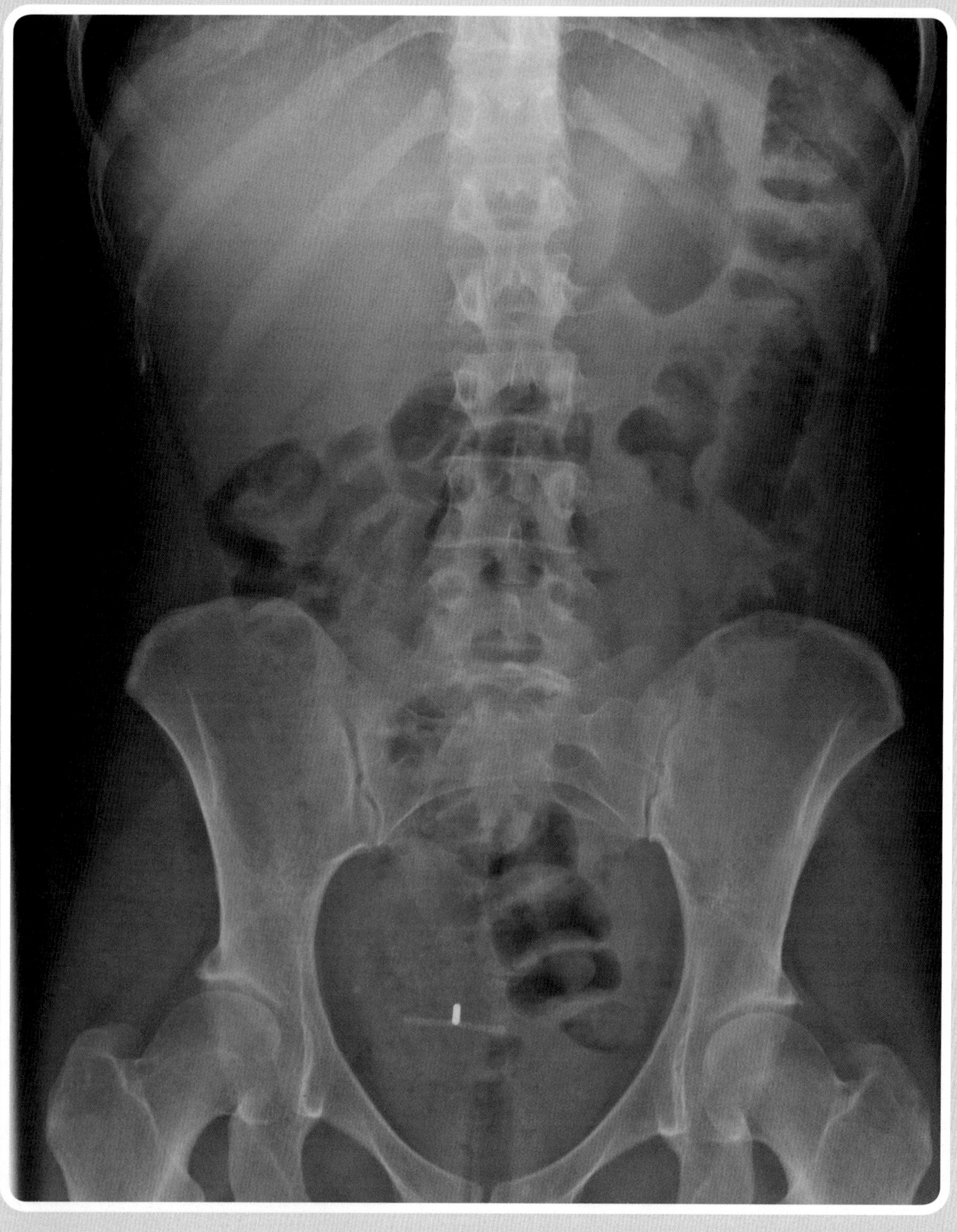

TECHNICAL INFORMATION

Patient ID: Anonymous.
Projection: AP supine.
Rotation: Adequate.
Penetration: Adequate – the spinous processes are visible.
Coverage: Inadequate – the pubic symphysis and inferior pubic rami have not been included.

BOWEL GAS PATTERN

The bowel gas pattern is normal.

BOWEL WALL

There is no evidence of mural thickening or intramural gas within the large or small bowel.

PNEUMOPERITONEUM

There is no evidence of free intraabdominal gas.

SOLID ORGANS

The solid organ contours are within normal limits with no solid organ calcification.

VASCULAR

No abnormal vascular calcification.

BONES

There are no abnormalities of the imaged thoracic and lumbar spine, or within the pelvis.

SOFT TISSUES

The psoas muscle outline is visible bilaterally.

The extraabdominal soft tissues are unremarkable.

OTHER

There is a radiopaque density projected over the region of the pelvis, in keeping with an IUCD. There is a lucency projecting over the region of the lower pelvis in keeping with a tampon in the vagina.

There are no vascular lines, drains or surgical clips.

REVIEW AREAS

Gallstones/renal calculi: No radiopaque calculi.
Lung bases: Normal.
Spine: Normal.
Femoral heads: Normal.

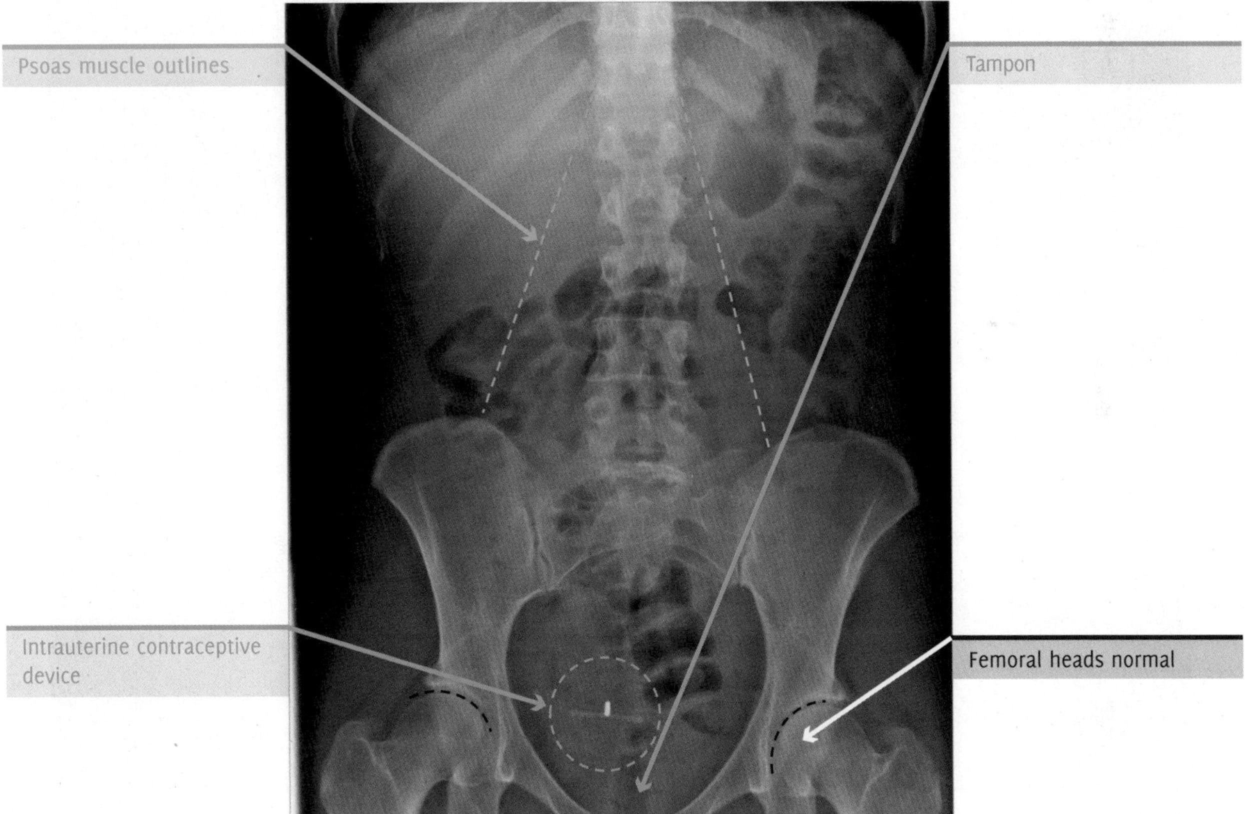

SUMMARY

This X-ray demonstrates a normal abdominal appearance with no evidence of bowel obstruction. The IUCD is projecting within the pelvis. Incidental note is made of a vaginal tampon.

INVESTIGATIONS AND MANAGEMENT

Adequate analgesia and hydration should be provided.

Bloods should be taken, including FBC, U&Es, LFTs, bone profile, amylase, blood gas and CRP.

There are no clear findings on the abdominal X-ray to explain the patient's clinical presentation.

If the patient is otherwise well, and the blood tests are reassuring, the patient should continue to be monitored in the community to assess progression of symptoms.

If the IUCD in situ is a Mirena coil, spotting may be related to this.

An ultrasound scan of the pelvis including a transvaginal scan should be considered if the patient's symptoms fail to resolve. Triple swabs of the vagina should also be considered to further assess for possible pelvic inflammatory disease.

Case

25

A 28-year-old female presents to the renal outpatient clinic with worsening right-sided abdominal pain. Her past medical history is significant for renal failure, and she undergoes peritoneal dialysis. She is a nonsmoker. On examination, she has oxygen saturations of 97% in room air and a temperature of 39°C. Her HR is 109 bpm, RR is 22 and blood pressure is 120/68 mmHg. The abdomen is rigid and there is generalized tenderness with normal bowel sounds. Urine dipstick is unremarkable and a pregnancy test is negative.

An abdominal X-ray is requested to assess for possible bowel obstruction.

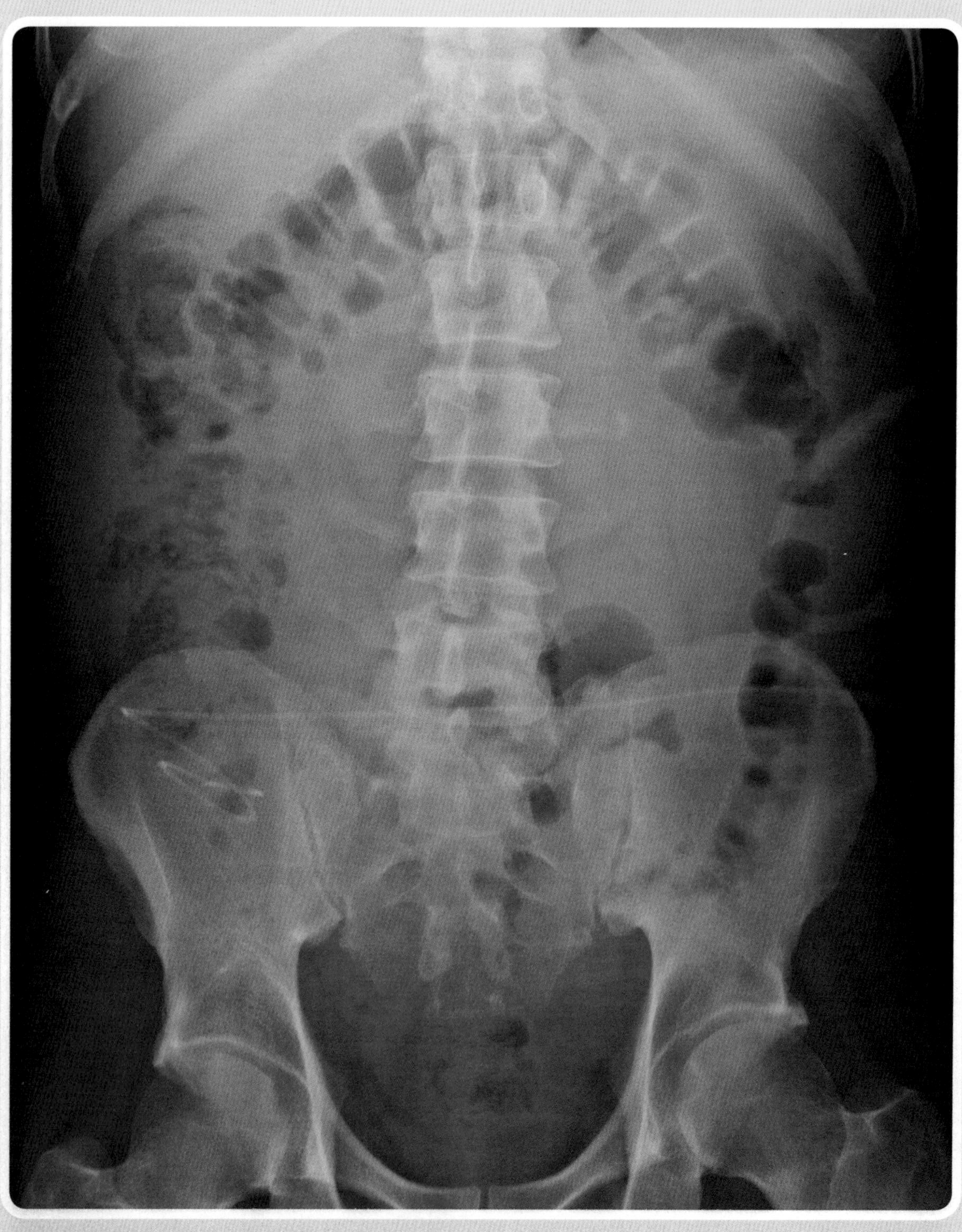

TECHNICAL INFORMATION

Patient ID: Anonymous.
Projection: AP supine.
Rotation: Adequate.
Penetration: Adequate – the spinous processes are visible.
Coverage: Inadequate – the pubic symphysis and inferior pubic rami have not been included.

BOWEL GAS PATTERN

The bowel gas pattern is normal.

There is a mild volume of faecal residue present throughout the ascending colon and within the rectum.

BOWEL WALL

There is no evidence of mural thickening or intramural gas within the large or small bowel.

PNEUMOPERITONEUM

There is no evidence of free intraabdominal gas.

SOLID ORGANS

The solid organ contours are within normal limits with no solid organ calcification.

VASCULAR

No abnormal vascular calcification.

BONES

There are no abnormalities of the imaged thoracic and lumbar spine, or within the pelvis.

SOFT TISSUES

The psoas muscle outline is visible bilaterally.

The extraabdominal soft tissues are unremarkable.

OTHER

There is a radiopaque line projected horizontally across the abdomen from the left side with its tip projecting within the right iliac fossa, in keeping with the known peritoneal dialysis catheter. The continuity of the peritoneal dialysis catheter is interrupted due to being outside the field of view.

There are no vascular lines, drains or surgical clips.

REVIEW AREAS

Gallstones/renal calculi: No radiopaque calculi.
Lung bases: Not fully included.
Spine: Normal.
Femoral heads: Normal.

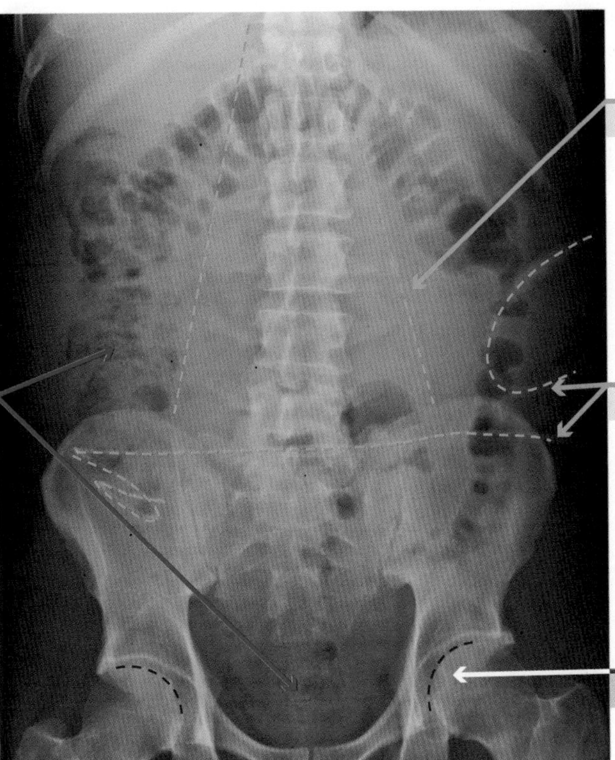

SUMMARY

This X-ray demonstrates a peritoneal dialysis catheter with its tip projecting within the right iliac fossa. There is no evidence of pneumoperitoneum.

INVESTIGATIONS AND MANAGEMENT

The patient should be admitted to hospital and resuscitated using an ABCDE approach.

Adequate analgesia and hydration should be provided.

Urgent bloods should be taken including FBC, U&Es, LFTs, amylase, bone profile, blood culture, blood gas and CRP. Culture of peritoneal fluid should also be sent.

The patient should be made NBM and started on IV fluids and broad-spectrum antibiotics.

There are no clear findings on the abdominal X-ray to explain the patient's clinical presentation. The general surgical team should be involved. The renal team also need to be involved to optimize management of the patient's dialysis.

Case

26

A 13-month-old boy presents to ED with worsening abdominal pain and a 2-day history of diarrhoea and vomiting. He has no significant past medical history. On examination, he has oxygen saturations of 98% in room air and a temperature of 38.3°C. His HR is 150 bpm and RR is 35. The abdomen is soft and there is generalized tenderness with normal bowel sounds. Urine dipstick is unremarkable.

An abdominal X-ray is requested to assess for possible bowel obstruction.

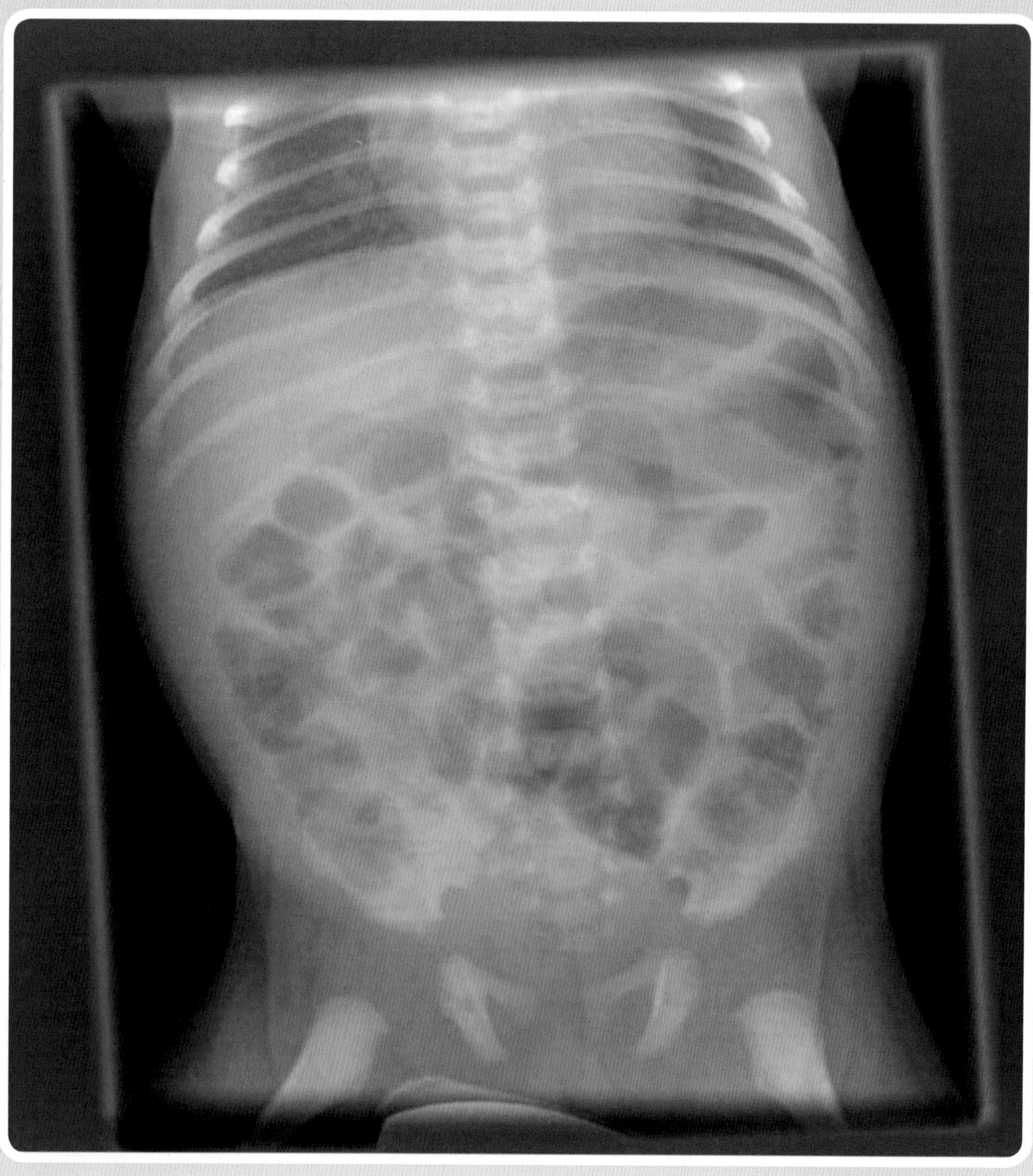

TECHNICAL INFORMATION

Patient ID: Anonymous.
Projection: AP supine.
Rotation: Adequate.
Penetration: Adequate – the spine is visible.
Coverage: Adequate – the anterior ribs are visible superiorly and the inferior pubic rami are visible.

BOWEL GAS PATTERN

The bowel gas pattern is normal.

BOWEL WALL

There is no evidence of mural thickening or intramural gas within the large or small bowel.

PNEUMOPERITONEUM

There is no evidence of free intraabdominal gas.

SOLID ORGANS

The solid organ contours are within normal limits with no solid organ calcification.

VASCULAR

No abnormal vascular calcification.

BONES

There are no abnormalities of the imaged thoracic and lumbar spine, or within the pelvis.

SOFT TISSUES

The psoas muscle outline is not visible bilaterally, which is nonspecific, particularly in a child of this age.

The extraabdominal soft tissues are unremarkable.

OTHER

There is a gonadal shield in situ.

There are no vascular lines, drains or surgical clips.

REVIEW AREAS

Gallstones/renal calculi: No radiopaque calculi.
Lung bases: Normal.
Spine: Normal – cartilage between vertebrae.
Femoral heads: Normal – growth plates present.

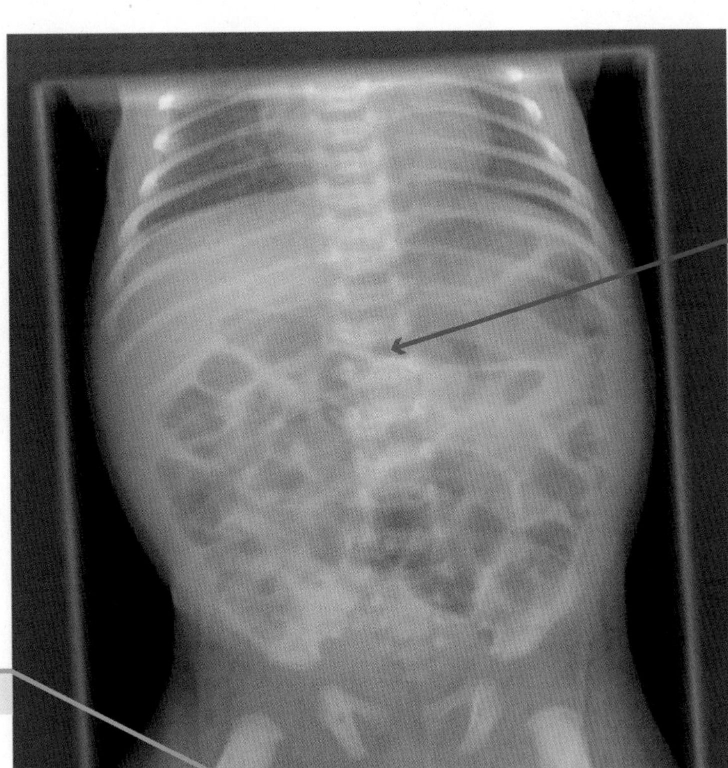

SUMMARY

This X-ray demonstrates a normal abdominal appearance with no evidence of bowel obstruction.

INVESTIGATIONS AND MANAGEMENT

The child should be resuscitated using an ABCDE approach.

Adequate analgesia and hydration should be provided.

Urgent bloods should be taken, including FBC, U&Es, CRP and blood gas.

The most likely diagnosis is gastroenteritis, given the pyrexia, that the child is otherwise well, and the history of diarrhoea and vomiting. Treatment for this would include rehydration (either orally, by NG tube or by IV fluids depending on the clinical picture) and management of the pyrexia if symptomatic.

Case

27

A 40-year-old male presents to ED with worsening abdominal pain. He has no significant past medical history and is a nonsmoker. On examination, he has oxygen saturations of 96% in room air and a temperature of 37.4°C. His HR is 88 bpm, RR is 28 and blood pressure is 128/76 mmHg. The abdomen is rigid and there is generalized tenderness with normal bowel sounds. Urine dipstick is unremarkable.

An abdominal X-ray is requested to assess for possible bowel obstruction.

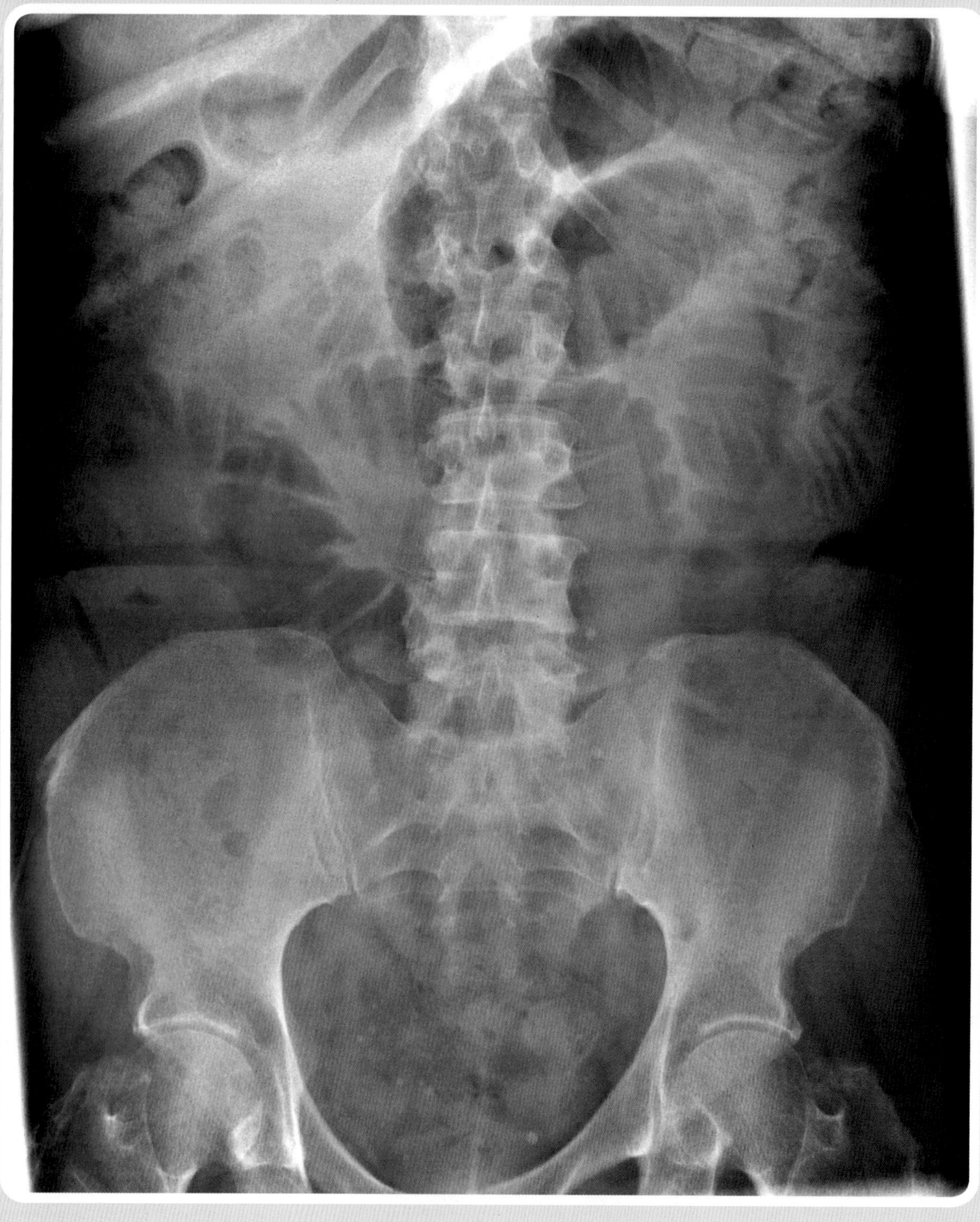

TECHNICAL INFORMATION

Patient ID: Anonymous.
Projection: AP supine.
Rotation: Adequate.
Penetration: Adequate – the spinous processes are visible.
Coverage: Inadequate – the pubic symphysis and inferior pubic rami have not been included.

BOWEL GAS PATTERN

There are multiple loops of dilated bowel seen centrally and in the left upper quadrant within the abdomen demonstrating valvulae conniventes in keeping with small bowel obstruction.

BOWEL WALL

There is no evidence of mural thickening or intramural gas within the large or small bowel.

PNEUMOPERITONEUM

There is no evidence of free intraabdominal gas.

SOLID ORGANS

The solid organ contours are within normal limits with no solid organ calcification.

VASCULAR

No abnormal vascular calcification.

BONES

There is mild degenerative change with osteophyte formation in the lower spine.

SOFT TISSUES

The psoas muscle outline is visible bilaterally.

The extraabdominal soft tissues are unremarkable.

OTHER

There are multiple rounded radiopaque densities projected over the region of the pelvis in keeping with phleboliths.

There are no radiopaque foreign bodies.

There are no vascular lines, drains or surgical clips.

REVIEW AREAS

Gallstones/renal calculi: No radiopaque calculi.
Lung bases: Not fully included.
Spine: Mild degenerative change.
Femoral heads: Normal.

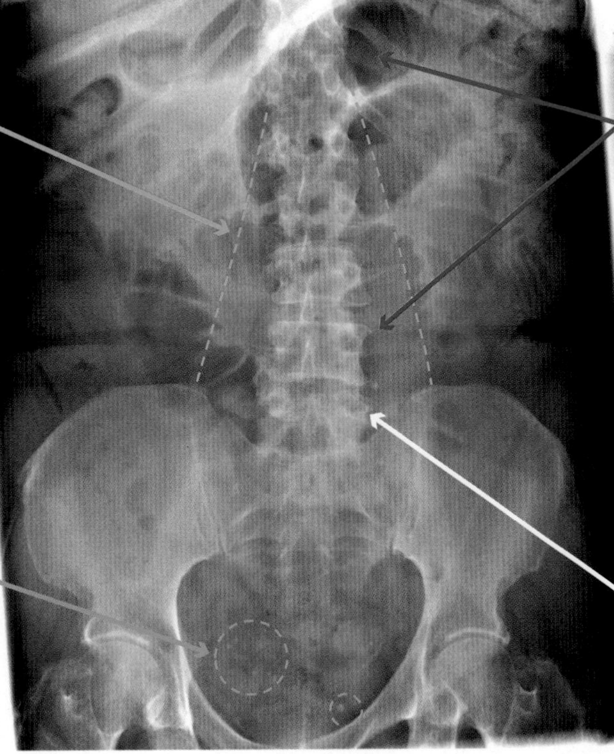

SUMMARY

This X-ray demonstrates multiple loops of dilated bowel centrally and in the left upper quadrant within the abdomen demonstrating valvulae conniventes, in keeping with small bowel obstruction, although the cause of this is not visible on the X-ray. The mild degenerative change in the spine and pelvic phleboliths are incidental findings.

INVESTIGATIONS AND MANAGEMENT

The patient should be resuscitated using an ABCDE approach.

Adequate analgesia and hydration should be provided.

The patient should be kept NBM and have an NG tube inserted on free drainage to relieve the pressure in the small bowel. IV fluids should be commenced.

Urgent bloods should be taken, including FBC, U&Es, CRP, LFTs, coagulation, blood gas, and group and save.

The general surgical team should be contacted urgently and a CT scan of the abdomen/pelvis with IV contrast should be considered for better visualization of the anatomy and further assessment.

Case

28

A 34-year-old female presents to ED with acute generalized abdominal pain. Over the past 3 days she has been experiencing nausea with worsening vomiting which appears bile stained. Her past medical history is significant for an appendicectomy 6 months ago and she is a nonsmoker. On examination, she has oxygen saturations of 99% in room air and a temperature of 36.8°C. Her HR is 94 bpm, RR is 24 and blood pressure is 120/68 mmHg. The abdomen is peritonitic with tinkling bowel sounds. Urine dipstick is unremarkable and a pregnancy test is negative. An abdominal X-ray is requested to assess for possible bowel obstruction.

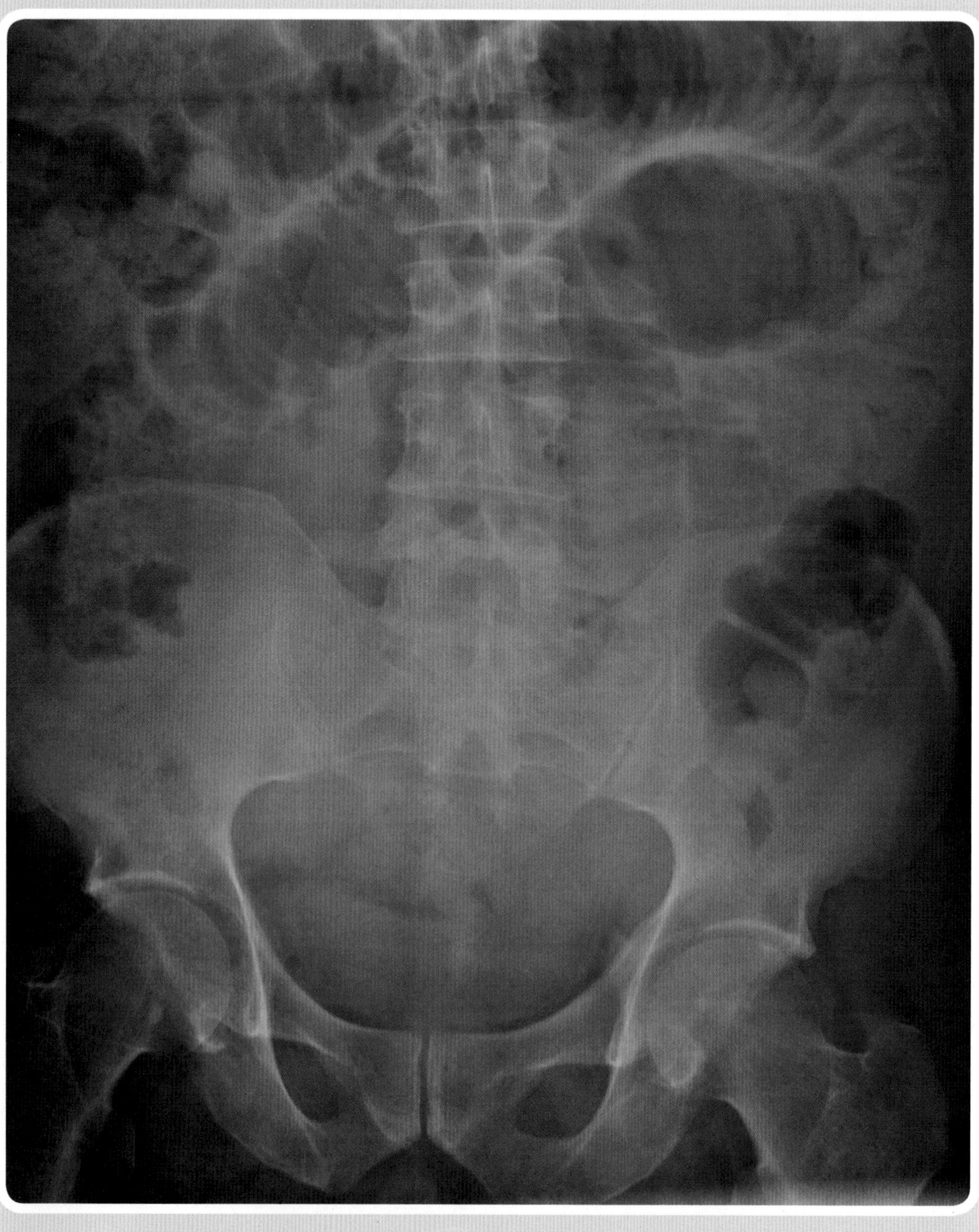

TECHNICAL INFORMATION

Patient ID: Anonymous.
Projection: AP supine.
Rotation: Adequate.
Penetration: Adequate – the spinous processes are visible.
Coverage: Inadequate – the anterior ribs have not been included.

BOWEL GAS PATTERN

There are multiple loops of dilated bowel seen centrally in the abdomen demonstrating valvulae conniventes, in keeping with small bowel obstruction.

There is a small volume of faecal residue throughout the colon.

BOWEL WALL

There is no evidence of mural thickening or intramural gas within the large or small bowel.

PNEUMOPERITONEUM

There is no evidence of free intraabdominal gas.

SOLID ORGANS

The solid organ contours are within normal limits with no solid organ calcification.

VASCULAR

No abnormal vascular calcification.

BONES

There is mild degenerative change seen in the lower lumbar spine.

There is a benign bone island in the right femoral head.

No fractures or destructive bone lesions are visible in the imaged skeleton.

SOFT TISSUES

The psoas muscle outline is visible bilaterally.

The extraabdominal soft tissues are unremarkable.

OTHER

There are no radiopaque foreign bodies.

There are no vascular lines, drains or surgical clips.

REVIEW AREAS

Gallstones/renal calculi: No radiopaque calculi.
Lung bases: Not fully included.
Spine: Mild degenerative change in lower lumbar spine.
Femoral heads: Normal.

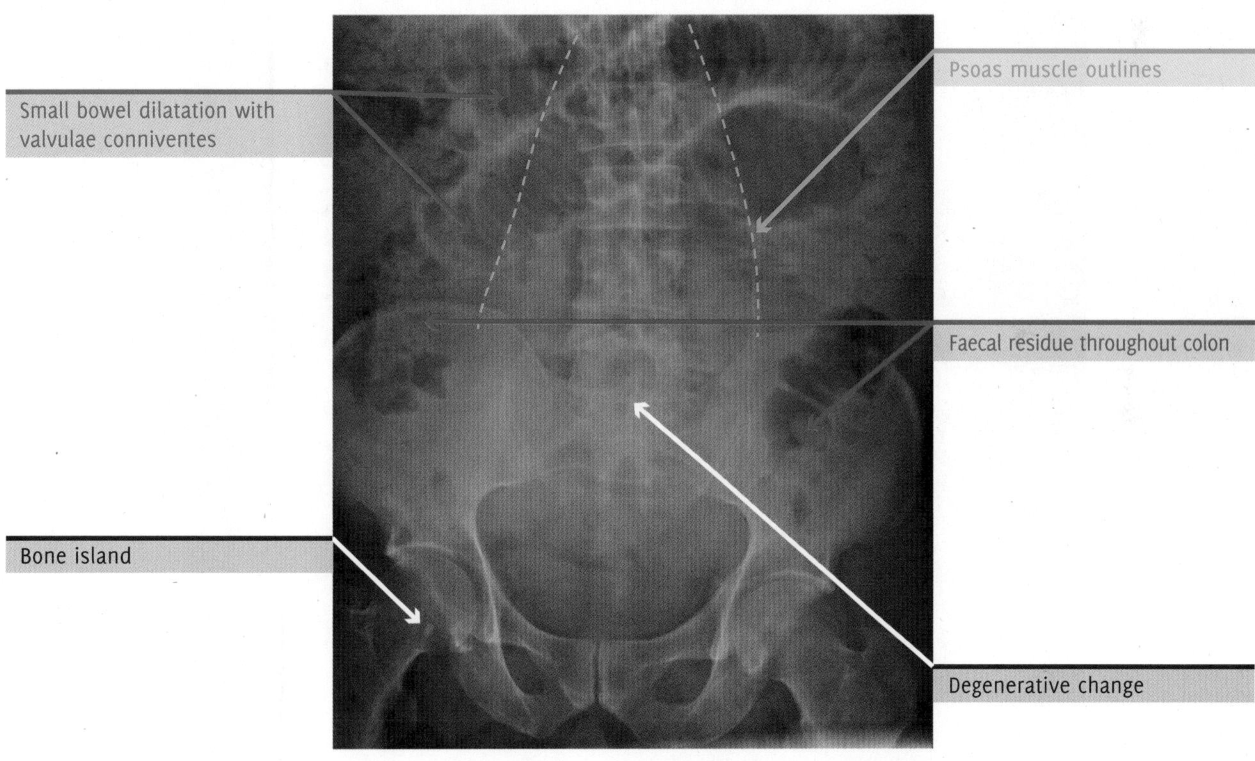

SUMMARY

This X-ray demonstrates multiple loops of dilated bowel seen centrally within the abdomen demonstrating valvulae conniventes, in keeping with small bowel obstruction. The cause of this is not visible on the X-ray, but it may be due to adhesions given the previous surgery. The mild degenerative change in the lower lumbar spine and right femoral head bone island are incidental findings.

INVESTIGATIONS AND MANAGEMENT

The patient should be resuscitated using an ABCDE approach.

Adequate analgesia and hydration should be provided.

The patient should be kept NBM and have an NG tube inserted on free drainage to decompress the small bowel. IV fluids should be commenced.

Urgent bloods should be taken, including FBC, U&Es, bone profile, CRP, LFTs, coagulation, blood gas, and group and save.

The general surgical team should be contacted urgently and a CT scan of the abdomen/pelvis with IV contrast should be considered for better visualization of the anatomy and further assessment.

Arthritic changes in the first instance should be managed with lifestyle changes and analgesia, if they are causing symptoms.

Case

29

A 16-year-old female presents to ED with abdominal and back pain. Her past medical history is significant for sciatica and she is a nonsmoker. On examination, she has oxygen saturations of 97% in room air and a temperature of 36.6°C. Her HR is 84 bpm, RR is 20 and blood pressure is 110/62 mmHg. The abdomen is soft and there is mild generalized tenderness with normal bowel sounds. Urine dipstick is unremarkable and a pregnancy test is negative.

An abdominal X-ray is requested to assess for bowel obstruction.

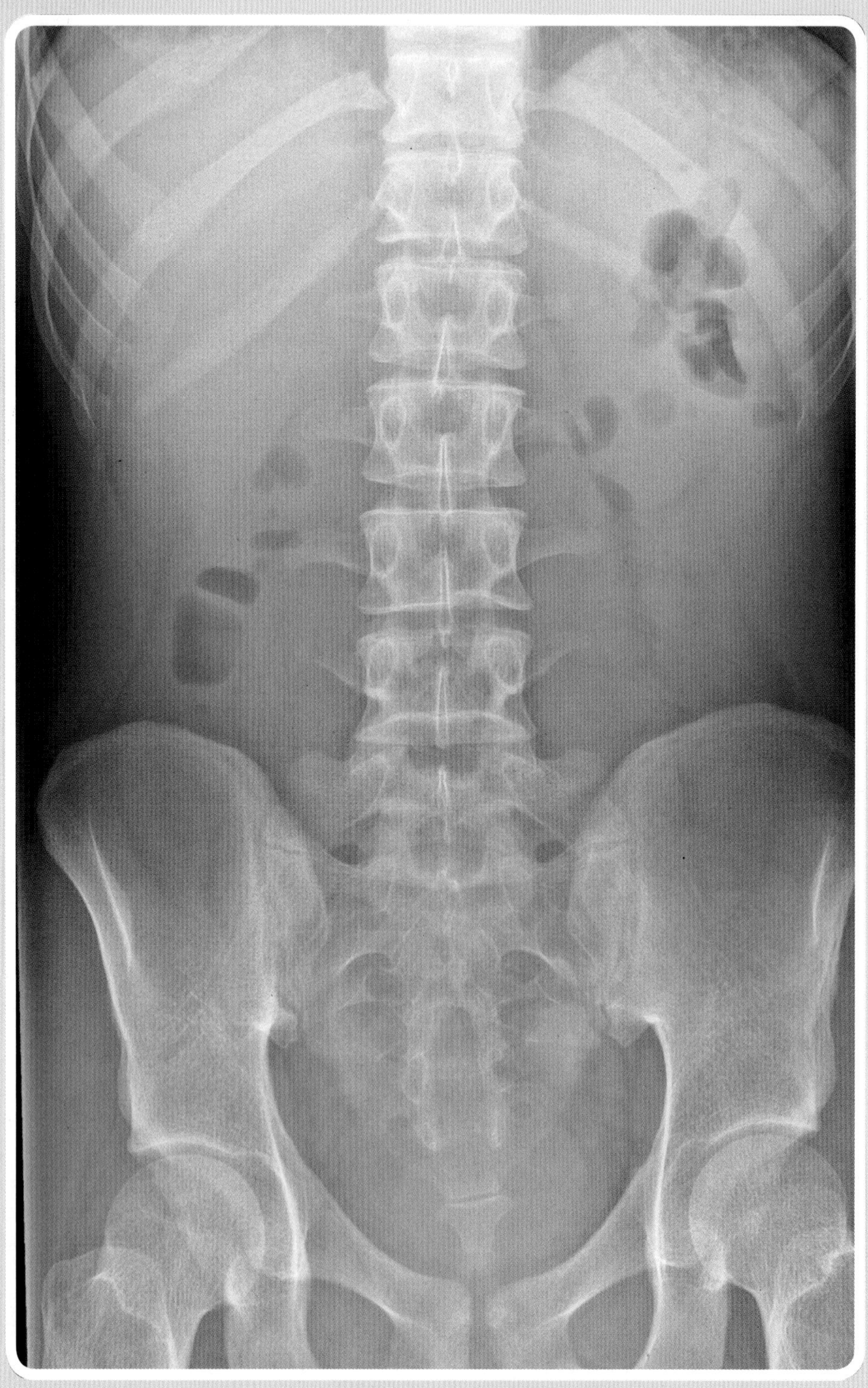

TECHNICAL INFORMATION

Patient ID: Anonymous.
Projection: AP supine.
Rotation: Adequate.
Penetration: Adequate – the spinous processes are visible.
Coverage: Adequate – the anterior ribs are visible superiorly and the pubic rami are visible inferiorly.

BOWEL GAS PATTERN

The bowel gas pattern is normal.

BOWEL WALL

There is no evidence of mural thickening or intramural gas within the large or small bowel.

PNEUMOPERITONEUM

There is no evidence of free intraabdominal gas.

SOLID ORGANS

The solid organ contours are within normal limits with no solid organ calcification.

VASCULAR

No abnormal vascular calcification.

BONES

There is sacralization of the L5 vertebral body, which is a normal anatomical variant.

There are no abnormalities of the imaged thoracic spine.

SOFT TISSUES

The psoas muscle outline is visible bilaterally.

The extraabdominal soft tissues are unremarkable.

OTHER

There are no radiopaque foreign bodies.

There are no vascular lines, drains or surgical clips.

REVIEW AREAS

Gallstones/renal calculi: No radiopaque calculi.
Lung bases: Not fully included.
Spine: Sacralization of the L5 vertebral body.
Femoral heads: Normal.

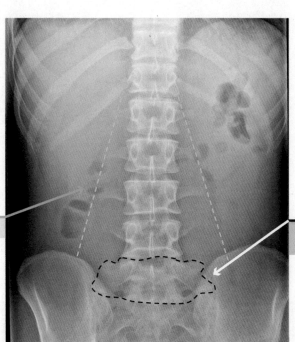

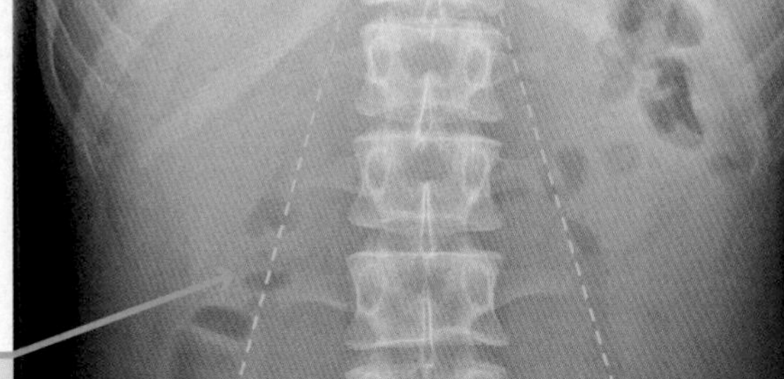

SUMMARY

This X-ray demonstrates no evidence of bowel obstruction with incidental sacralization of the L5 vertebral body.

INVESTIGATIONS AND MANAGEMENT

Adequate analgesia and hydration should be provided.

Further investigation of back and abdominal pain is warranted if symptoms persist.

Case

30

A 30-year-old male presents to ED with generalized abdominal pain and possible foreign body ingestion. His past medical history is significant for schizophrenia and he is a nonsmoker. On examination, he has oxygen saturations of 97% in room air and a temperature of 37.0°C. His HR is 92 bpm, RR is 22 and blood pressure is 125/68 mmHg. The abdomen is soft and there is generalized tenderness with normal bowel sounds. Urine dipstick is unremarkable.

An abdominal X-ray is requested to assess for a possible foreign body.

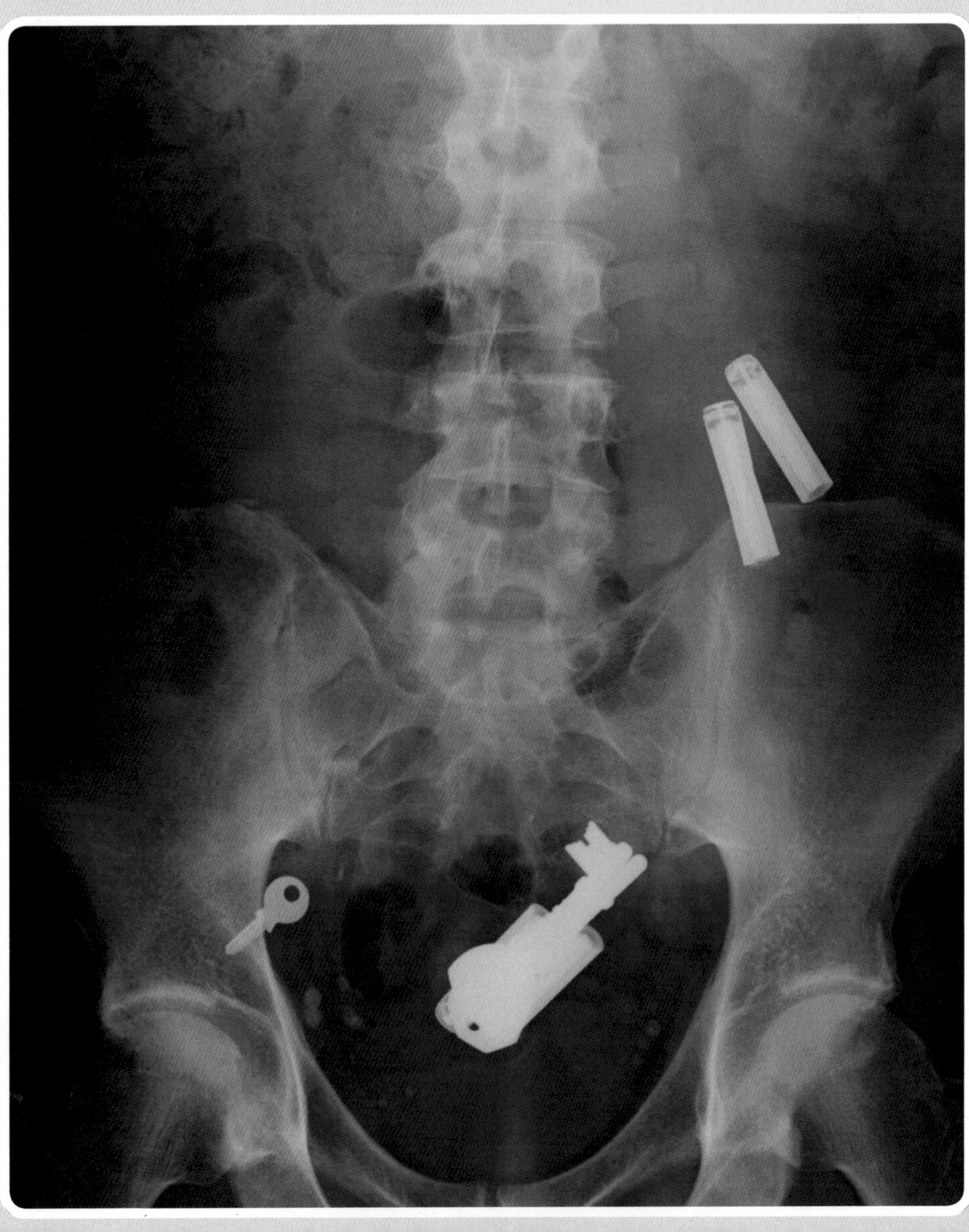

TECHNICAL INFORMATION

Patient ID: Anonymous.
Projection: AP supine.
Rotation: Adequate.
Penetration: Adequate – the spinous processes are visible.
Coverage: Inadequate – the pubic symphysis and inferior pubic rami have not been fully included.

BOWEL GAS PATTERN

The bowel gas pattern is normal.

There is a moderate volume of faecal residue present throughout the ascending colon and hepatic flexure.

BOWEL WALL

There is no evidence of mural thickening or intramural gas within the large or small bowel.

PNEUMOPERITONEUM

There is no evidence of free intraabdominal gas.

SOLID ORGANS

The solid organ contours are within normal limits with no solid organ calcification.

VASCULAR

No abnormal vascular calcification.

BONES

There are no abnormalities of the imaged thoracic and lumbar spine, or within the pelvis.

SOFT TISSUES

The psoas muscle outline is visible bilaterally.

The extraabdominal soft tissues are unremarkable.

OTHER

There are two radiopaque foreign bodies resembling cylindrical cell batteries projected over the left side of the abdomen.

There are several radiopaque foreign bodies projected over the pelvis, resembling two keys, and there are also multiple phleboliths.

There are no vascular lines, drains or surgical clips.

REVIEW AREAS

Gallstones/renal calculi: No radiopaque calculi.
Lung bases: Not fully included.
Spine: Normal.
Femoral heads: Normal.

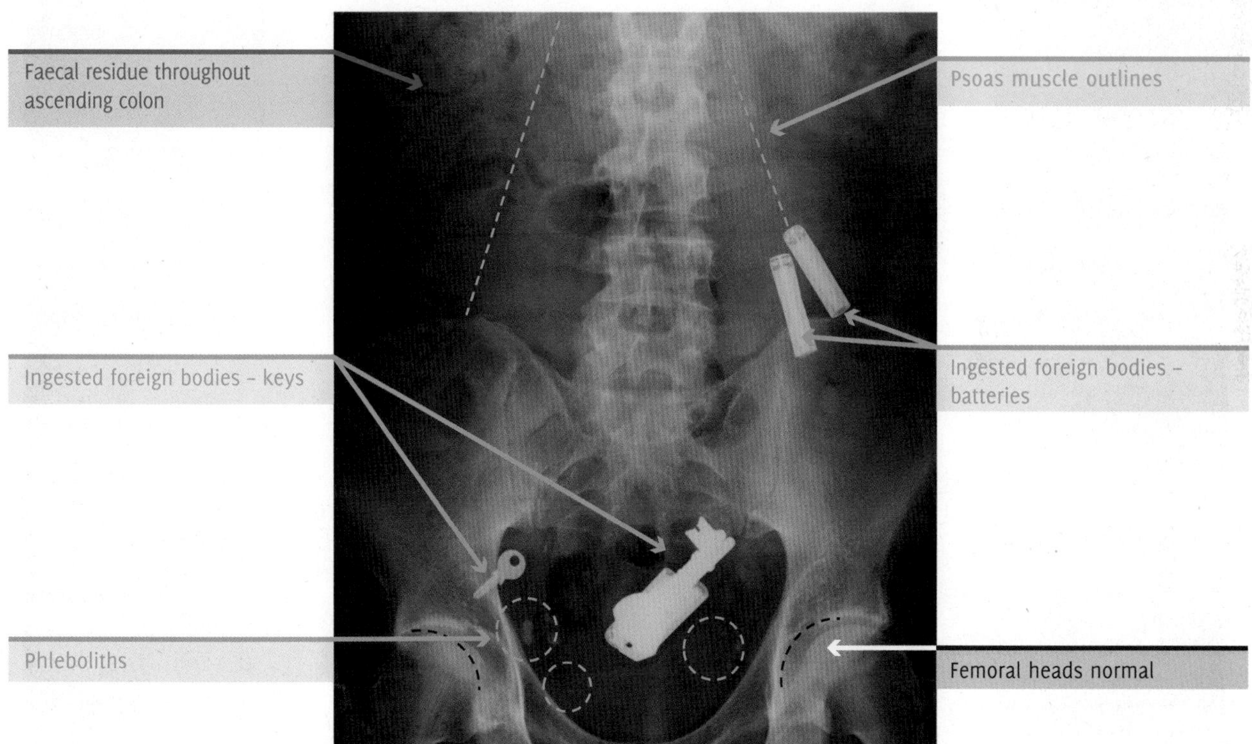

SUMMARY

This X-ray demonstrates multiple radiopaque foreign bodies as described. There is no evidence of pneumoperitoneum. The moderate faecal loading in the ascending colon and hepatic flexure, and pelvic phleboliths are incidental findings.

INVESTIGATIONS AND MANAGEMENT

The patient should be resuscitated using an ABCDE approach.

Adequate analgesia and hydration should be provided.

Urgent bloods should be taken including FBC, U&Es, LFTs, coagulation, blood gas, and group and save.

The patient should be referred urgently to the surgical team for consideration of removal of the foreign bodies. Removal depends on the location, size, shape and duration of ingestion.

Case

31

A 16-year-old male presents to ED with worsening abdominal distension and pain. He has not opened his bowels for more than 24 hours. He has no significant past medical history and is a nonsmoker. On examination, he has oxygen saturations of 98% in room air and a temperature of 36.5°C. His HR is 68 bpm, RR is 16 and blood pressure is 115/65 mmHg. The abdomen is soft and there is generalized tenderness with normal bowel sounds. Urine dipstick is unremarkable.

An abdominal X-ray is requested to assess for possible obstruction.

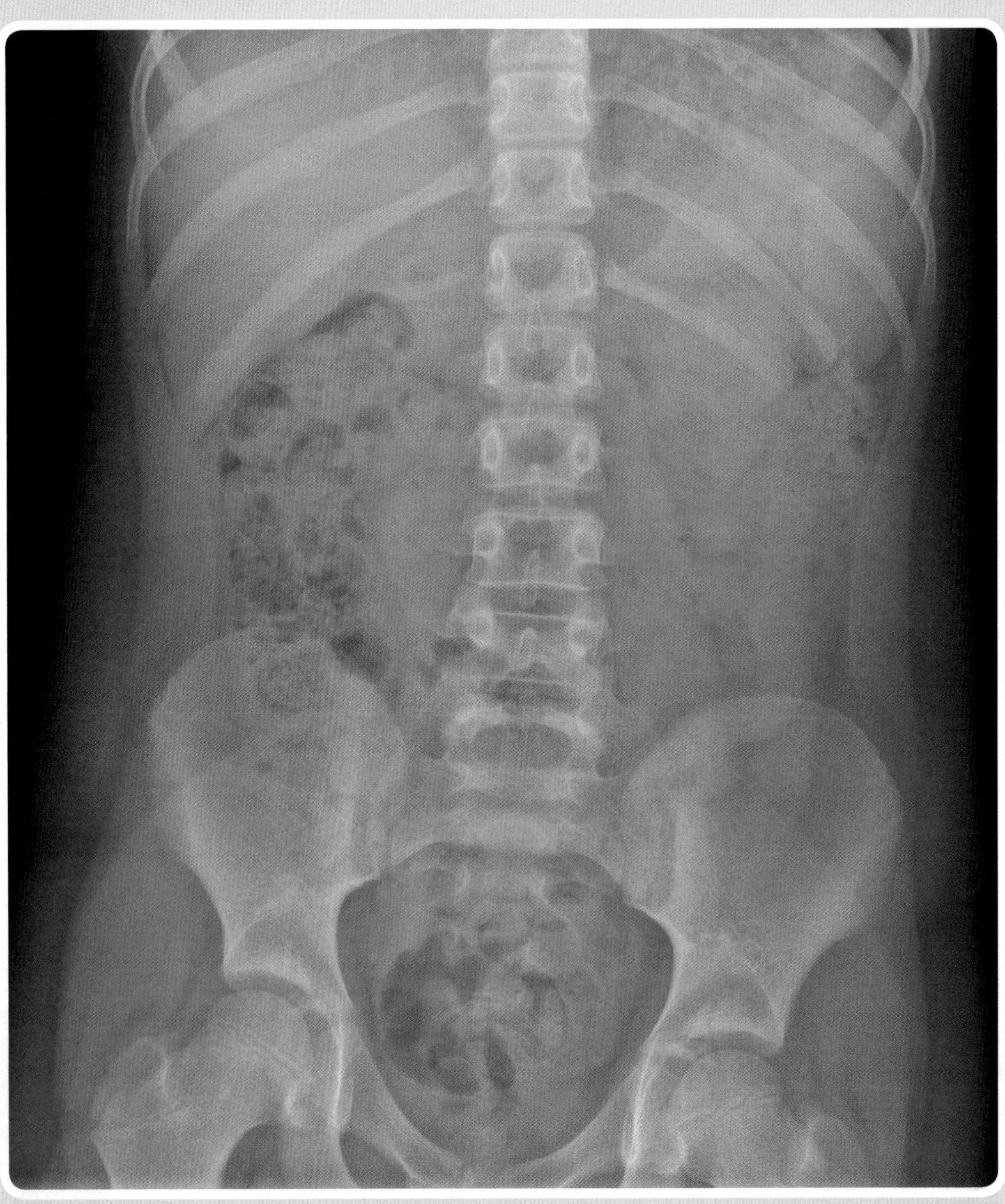

TECHNICAL INFORMATION

Patient ID: Anonymous.
Projection: AP supine.
Rotation: Adequate.
Penetration: Adequate – the spinous processes are visible.
Coverage: Inadequate – the pubic symphysis and inferior pubic rami have not been fully included.

BOWEL GAS PATTERN

The bowel gas pattern is normal.

There is a moderate volume of faecal residue present throughout the large bowel, from the ascending colon to rectum.

BOWEL WALL

There is no evidence of mural thickening or intramural gas within the large or small bowel.

PNEUMOPERITONEUM

There is no evidence of free intraabdominal gas.

SOLID ORGANS

The solid organ contours are within normal limits with no solid organ calcification.

VASCULAR

No abnormal vascular calcification.

BONES

There are no abnormalities of the imaged thoracic and lumbar spine, or within the pelvis.

There are growth plates at the femoral head, greater trochanter and acetabulum as the ossification centres have not yet fused, which is a normal finding in a child of this age.

SOFT TISSUES

The psoas muscle outline is visible bilaterally.

The extraabdominal soft tissues are unremarkable.

OTHER

There are no radiopaque foreign bodies.

There are no vascular lines, drains or surgical clips.

REVIEW AREAS

Gallstones/renal calculi: No radiopaque calculi.
Lung bases: Not fully included.
Spine: Normal.
Femoral heads: Normal – growth plates present.

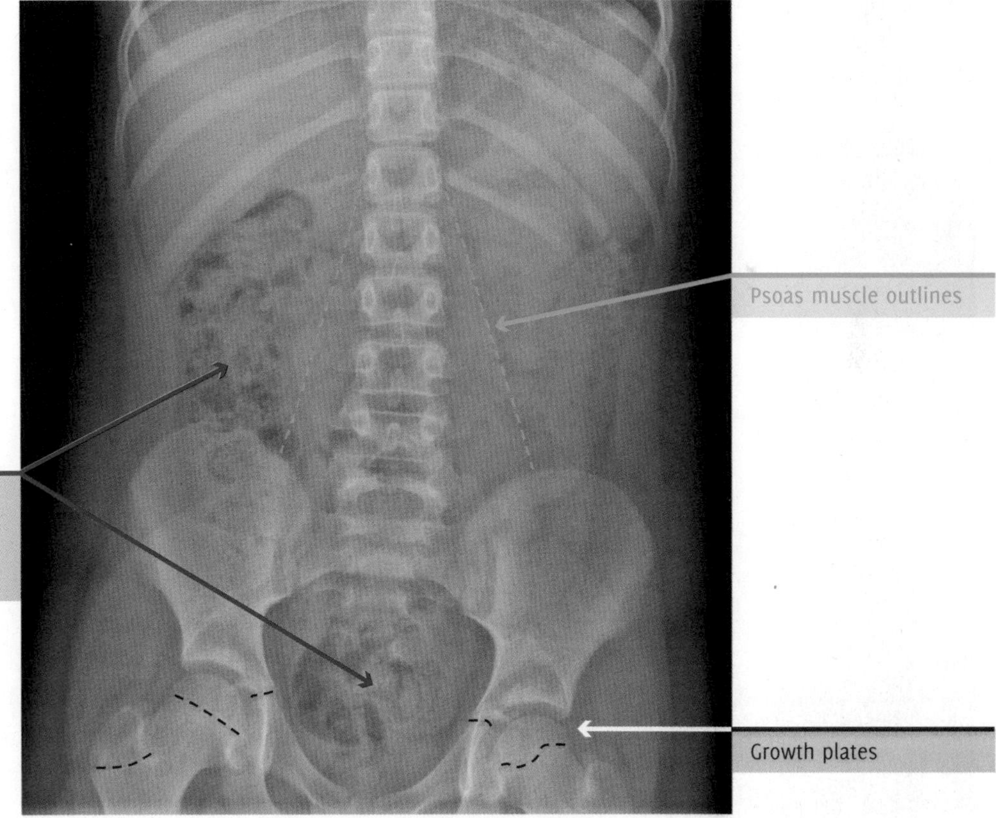

SUMMARY

This X-ray demonstrates a moderate volume of faecal residue throughout the colon and rectum, which is likely within normal limits.

INVESTIGATIONS AND MANAGEMENT

If the patient is otherwise well, no further investigations or imaging is required.

If the patient is clinically constipated, current medications should be reviewed and laxatives considered. Advice should be given regarding lifestyle adjustments, including adequate fluid intake, sufficient dietary fibre and exercise if clinically appropriate.

Case

32

A 2-year-old male presents to ED having swallowed a foreign object. The parents are unsure of what the object is or how many he may have swallowed. He is completely well otherwise. He has no significant past medical history. On examination, he has oxygen saturations of 99% in room air and a temperature of 36.3°C. His HR is 110 bpm and RR is 24. The abdomen is soft and there is no tenderness with normal bowel sounds.

An abdominal X-ray is requested to assess the nature and position of the foreign object.

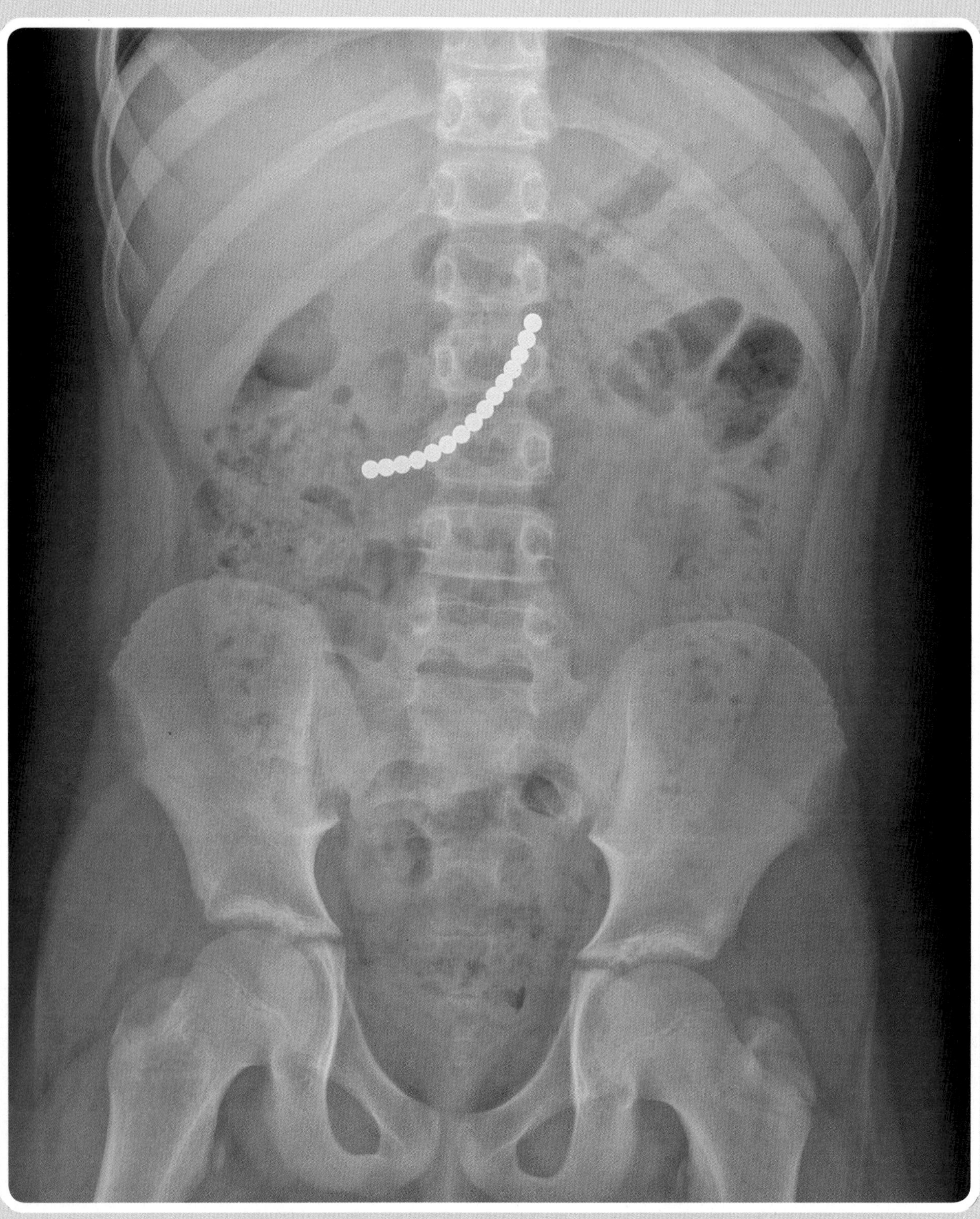

TECHNICAL INFORMATION

Patient ID: Anonymous.
Projection: AP supine.
Rotation: Adequate.
Penetration: Adequate – the spinous processes are visible.
Coverage: Adequate – the anterior ribs are visible superiorly and the pubic rami are visible inferiorly.

BOWEL GAS PATTERN

The bowel gas pattern is normal.

There is a moderate volume of faecal residue present throughout the large bowel.

BOWEL WALL

There is no evidence of mural thickening or intramural gas within the large or small bowel.

PNEUMOPERITONEUM

There is no evidence of free intraabdominal gas.

SOLID ORGANS

The solid organ contours are within normal limits with no solid organ calcification.

VASCULAR

No abnormal vascular calcification.

BONES

There are no abnormalities of the imaged thoracic and lumbar spine, or within the pelvis.

There are growth plates at the femoral head, greater trochanter and acetabulum as the ossification centres have not yet fused, which is a normal finding in a child of this age.

SOFT TISSUES

The right psoas muscle outline is not visible, which is nonspecific.

The extraabdominal soft tissues are unremarkable.

OTHER

There are multiple rounded radiopaque foreign bodies projected over the region of the epigastrium, likely within proximal small bowel, in keeping with ingested magnetic objects that have clumped together.

There are no vascular lines, drains or surgical clips.

REVIEW AREAS

Gallstones/renal calculi: No radiopaque calculi.
Lung bases: Not fully included.
Spine: Normal.
Femoral heads: Normal – growth plates present.

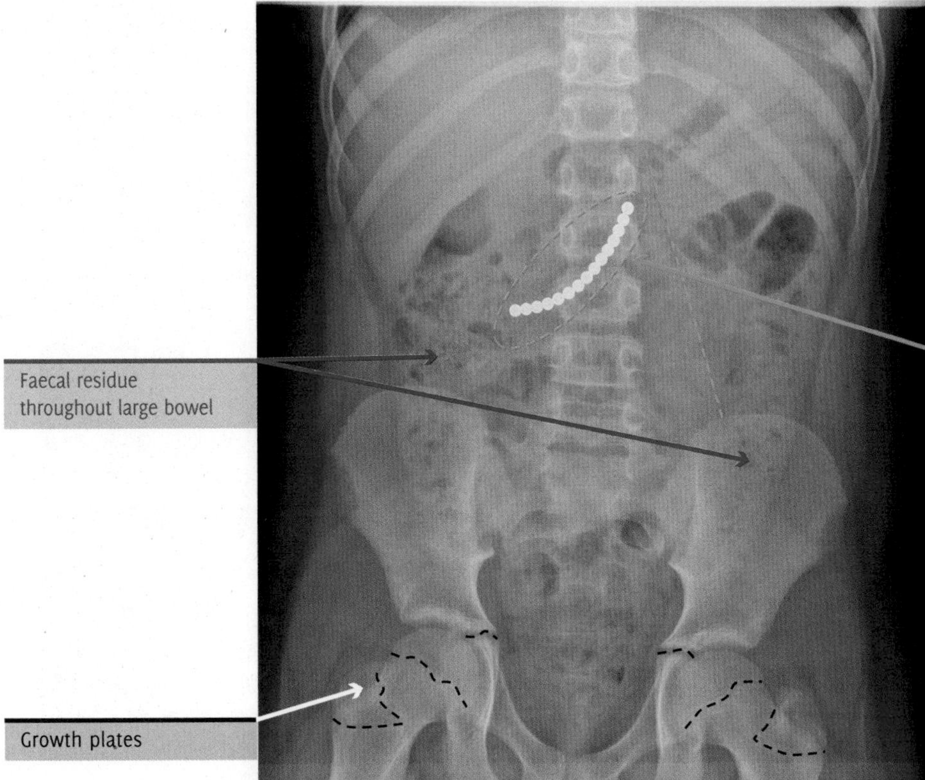

SUMMARY

This X-ray demonstrates multiple rounded radiopaque foreign bodies seen projected over the region of the epigastrium, likely within proximal small bowel, in keeping with ingested magnetic objects that have clumped together.

INVESTIGATIONS AND MANAGEMENT

As there are no signs of bowel perforation and the child appears well, observation with serial X-rays to monitor the progress of the foreign bodies may be appropriate. Laxatives should be considered. The paediatric gastroenterology and paediatric surgery teams should be involved and the patient should be monitored for signs of perforation or abdominal discomfort, in which case surgical intervention to retrieve the magnets will be required.

Case

33

A 3-year-old male presents to ED having swallowed an unknown foreign body. He has no significant past medical history. On examination, he has oxygen saturations of 99% in room air and a temperature of 36.7°C. His HR is 110 bpm and RR is 26. The abdomen is soft and there is no tenderness with normal bowel sounds.

An abdominal X-ray is requested to assess for a possible foreign body.

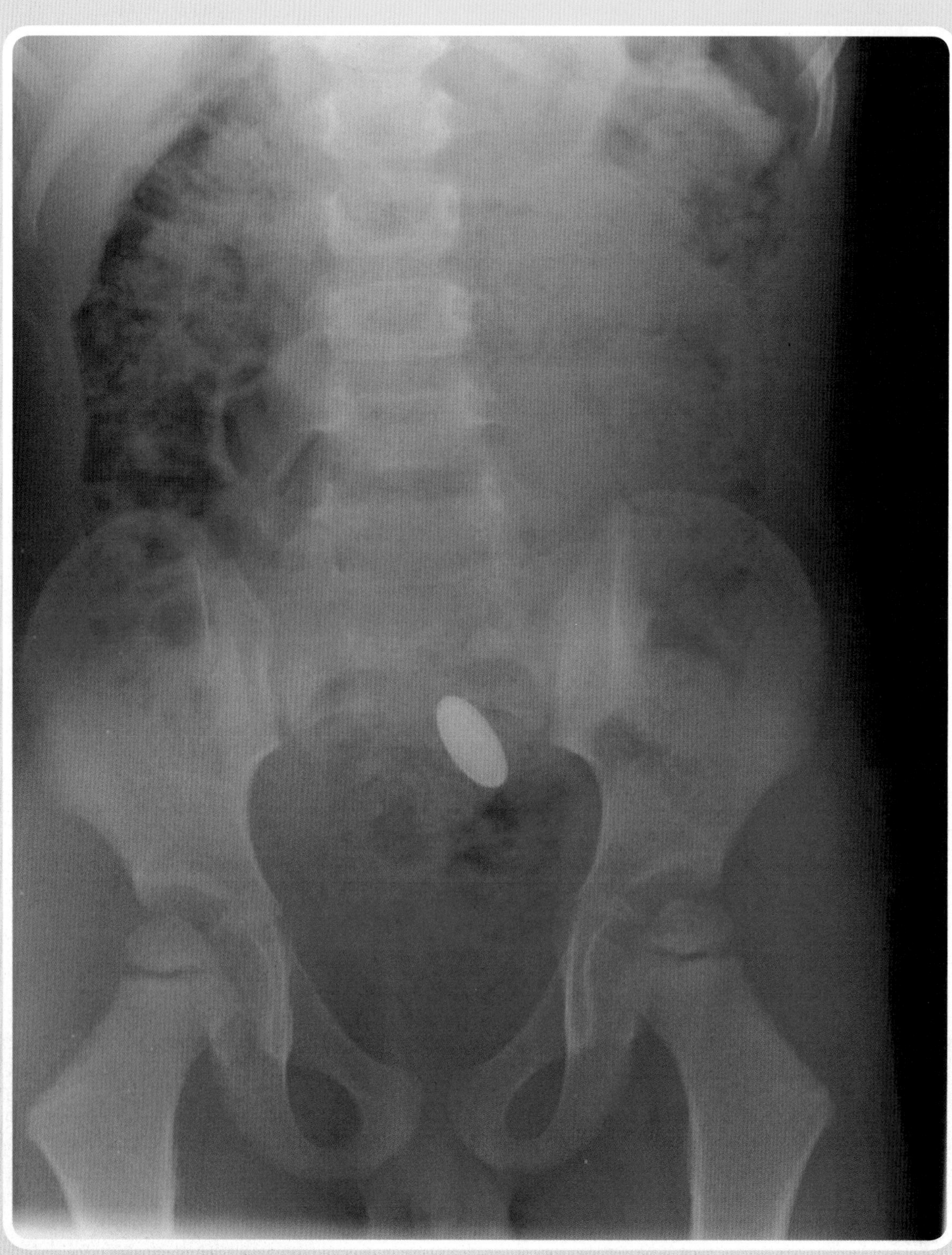

TECHNICAL INFORMATION

Patient ID: Anonymous.
Projection: AP supine.
Rotation: Adequate.
Penetration: Adequate – the spine is visible.
Coverage: Inadequate – the hemidiaphragms have not been included.

BOWEL GAS PATTERN

The bowel gas pattern is normal. There is a moderate volume of faecal residue throughout the colon.

BOWEL WALL

There is no evidence of mural thickening or intramural gas within the large or small bowel.

PNEUMOPERITONEUM

There is no evidence of free intraabdominal gas.

SOLID ORGANS

The solid organ contours are within normal limits with no solid organ calcification.

VASCULAR

No abnormal vascular calcification.

BONES

There are no abnormalities of the imaged thoracic and lumbar spine, or within the pelvis.

There is cartilage present between the pelvic bones and femurs as they have not yet fused, which is a normal finding in a child of this age.

SOFT TISSUES

The psoas muscle outline is not visible bilaterally, which is nonspecific, particularly in a child of this age.

The extraabdominal soft tissues are unremarkable.

OTHER

There is a rounded radiopaque foreign body with a thin peripheral rim of reduced opacification (halo sign), resembling a button battery projecting over the region of the left hemipelvis, likely within distal small bowel or sigmoid colon.

There are no vascular lines, drains or surgical clips.

REVIEW AREAS

Gallstones/renal calculi: No radiopaque calculi.
Lung bases: Not visualized.
Spine: Normal.
Femoral heads: Normal – growth plates present.

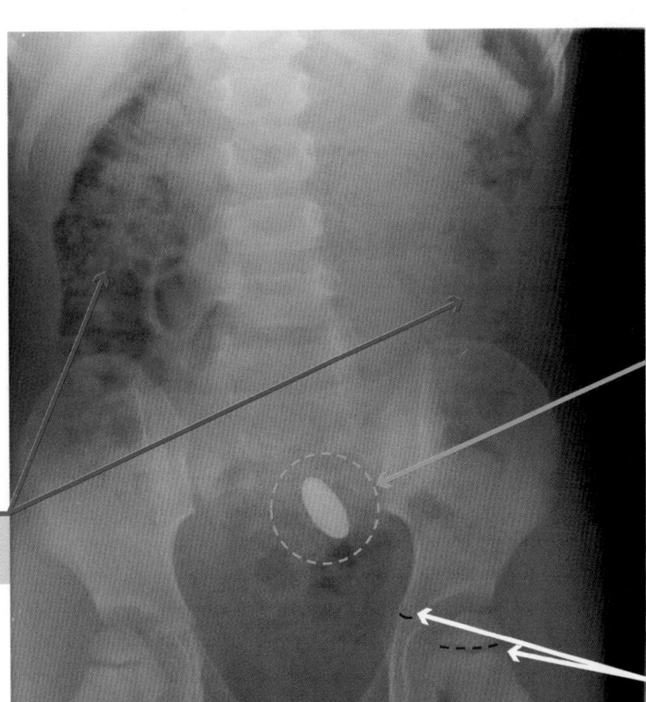

SUMMARY

This X-ray demonstrates a rounded radiopaque foreign body resembling a button battery projecting over the region of the left hemipelvis, likely within distal small bowel or sigmoid colon. The moderate volume of faecal residue throughout the colon is an incidental finding.

INVESTIGATIONS AND MANAGEMENT

Further history should be taken to try and confirm what the foreign body might be. Depending on the size, type and shape of the object, the symptoms and length of time since ingestion, surgical removal may be required. Laxatives should be considered. If it is confirmed that a button battery may have been ingested, urgent surgical intervention is recommended as the patient is at risk from burn injuries to the bowel and resultant serious complications. Otherwise, the patient should have serial repeat abdominal X-rays to follow the foreign body through the gut into the rectum and ensure that it is excreted.

INTERMEDIATE CASES

Case 34

A 75-year-old female presents to ED with generalized abdominal pain and right-sided hip and groin pain radiating to the upper thigh. She is unable to move her right leg due to the pain. She has not opened her bowels in 1 week. Her past medical history is significant for multiple falls and she is a nonsmoker. On examination, she has oxygen saturations of 97% in room air and a temperature of 36.9°C. Her HR is 90 bpm, RR is 20 and blood pressure is 115/65 mmHg. There is pain and bony instability on palpation of the right groin region. There is significant bruising of the groin region and upper thigh.

An abdominal X-ray is requested to assess for possible bowel obstruction.

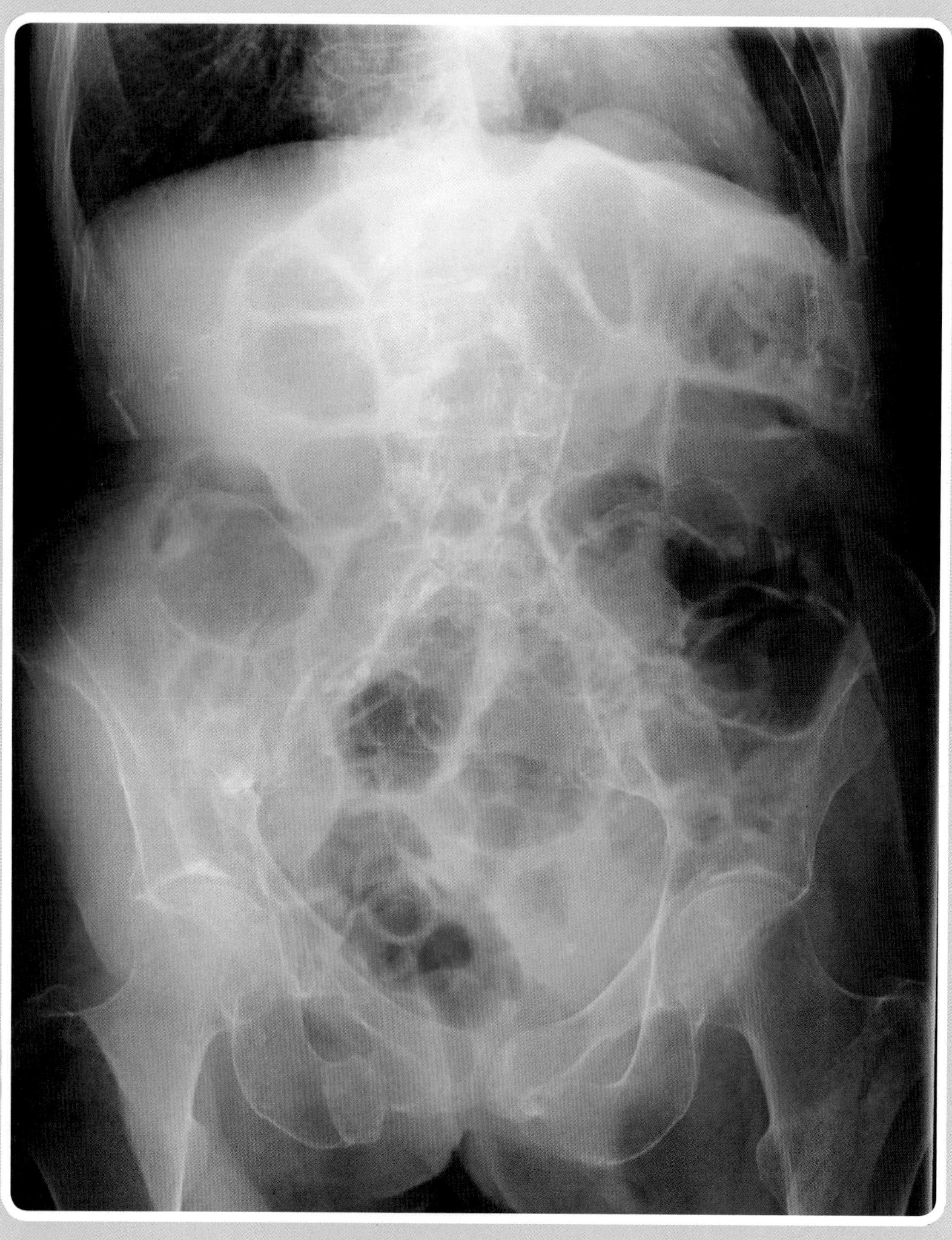

TECHNICAL INFORMATION

Patient ID: Anonymous.
Projection: AP supine.
Rotation: Adequate.
Penetration: Underpenetrated – the spinous processes are not visible.
Coverage: Adequate – the anterior ribs are visible superiorly and the inferior pubic rami are visible.

BOWEL GAS PATTERN

There is a prominence of bowel loops throughout the abdomen, however no dilatation, which may represent a degree of ileus.

BOWEL WALL

There is no evidence of mural thickening or intramural gas within the large or small bowel.

PNEUMOPERITONEUM

There is no evidence of free intraabdominal gas.

SOLID ORGANS

The solid organ contours are within normal limits with no solid organ calcification.

VASCULAR

The abdominal aorta is calcified.

There is calcification of the iliac arteries.

BONES

There are complete moderately displaced fractures of both the right-sided superior and inferior right pubic rami. The superior pubic ramus fracture appears acute. The inferior pubic ramus fracture is well corticated and likely related to an old injury.

There is an area of sclerosis in the right ilium with adjacent disruption of the pelvic ring, which is suspicious for a further old fracture.

The thoracic and lumbar spine are not visible due to poor penetration.

There are no fractures of the femoral heads.

Bone density appears normal.

SOFT TISSUES

The psoas muscle outline is not visible bilaterally, which is nonspecific.

The extraabdominal soft tissues are unremarkable.

OTHER

There are no radiopaque foreign bodies.

There are no vascular lines, drains or surgical clips.

REVIEW AREAS

Gallstones/renal calculi: No radiopaque calculi.
Lung bases: Normal.
Spine: Not visible due to underpenetration.
Femoral heads: Normal.

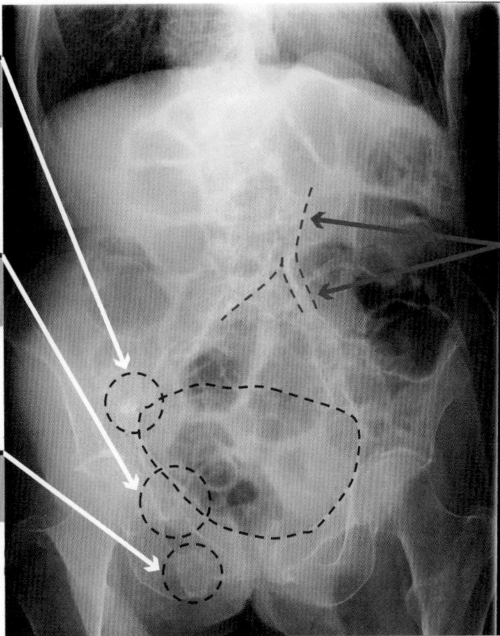

SUMMARY

This X-ray demonstrates prominent bowel loops throughout the abdomen, which may represent a degree of ileus, however no evidence of bowel obstruction. There is a probable acute fracture of the right superior pubic ramus and old fractures of the right ilium and the right inferior pubic ramus. The abdominal aorta is calcified. The iliac vessel calcification is an incidental finding.

INVESTIGATIONS AND MANAGEMENT

The patient should be resuscitated using an ABCDE approach.

Adequate analgesia and hydration should be provided.

Bloods should be taken, including FBC, U&Es, LFTs, bone profile, CRP, TFTs, blood gas, and group and save.

The patient should be referred urgently to the orthopaedic surgical team.

Depending on previous imaging, a CT of the pelvis should be considered to better assess the extent of injury, chronicity of injuries, for any potential operative planning and to assess for potential associated injuries (for example, to the bladder).

Case 35

A 32-year-old male presents to ED with acute abdominal pain and a GCS of 13. He has no significant past medical history and is a nonsmoker. On examination, he has oxygen saturations of 98% in room air and a temperature of 37.6°C. His HR is 75 bpm, RR is 25 and blood pressure is 115/65 mmHg. The abdomen is soft and there is generalized mild tenderness with normal bowel sounds. Urine dipstick is unremarkable.

An abdominal X-ray is requested to look for possible bowel obstruction.

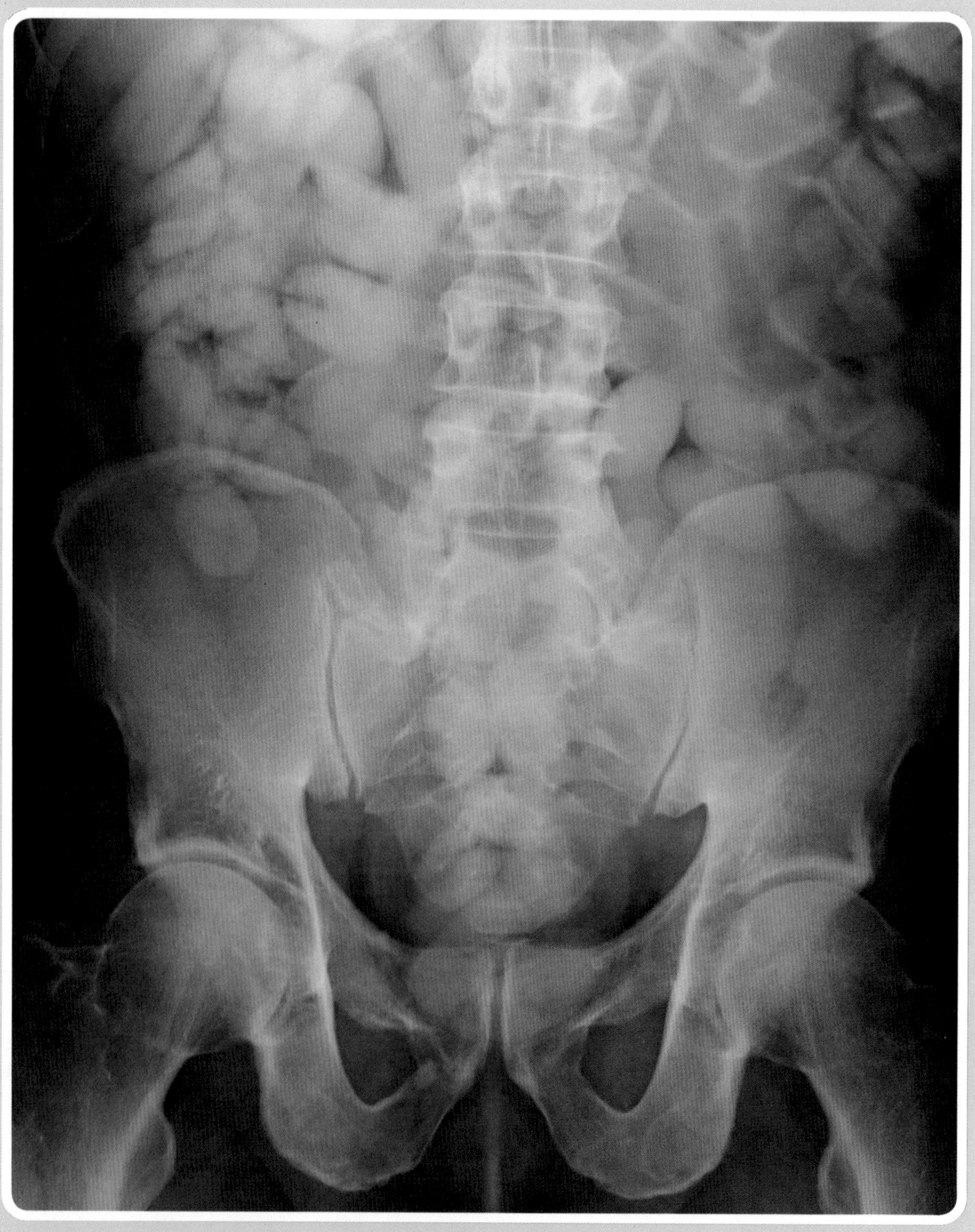

TECHNICAL INFORMATION

Patient ID: Anonymous.
Projection: AP supine.
Rotation: Adequate.
Penetration: Adequate – the spinous processes are visible.
Coverage: Inadequate – the anterior ribs have not been included.

BOWEL GAS PATTERN

There is a prominence of bowel gas; however, there is no bowel dilatation. The bowel gas pattern is partially obscured due to the presence of multiple ovoid radiopaque foreign bodies.

BOWEL WALL

There is no evidence of mural thickening or intramural gas within the large or small bowel.

PNEUMOPERITONEUM

There is no evidence of free intraabdominal gas.

SOLID ORGANS

The solid organ contours are within normal limits with no solid organ calcification.

VASCULAR

No abnormal vascular calcification.

BONES

There is incidental sacralization of L5.

There are no abnormalities of the imaged thoracic and lumbar spine, or within the pelvis.

SOFT TISSUES

The psoas muscle outline is visible bilaterally.

The extraabdominal soft tissues are unremarkable.

OTHER

There are multiple radiopaque densities located predominantly throughout the large bowel and rectum, in keeping with bags of an unknown substance.

There are no vascular lines, drains or surgical clips.

REVIEW AREAS

Gallstones/renal calculi: No radiopaque calculi.
Lung bases: Not fully included.
Spine: Normal.
Femoral heads: Normal.

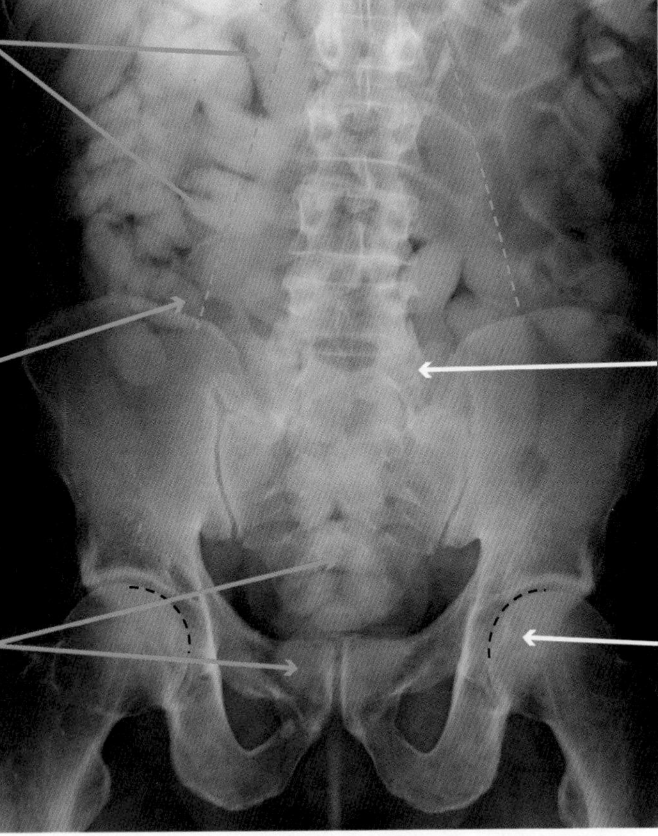

SUMMARY

This X-ray demonstrates multiple radiopaque densities located throughout the abdomen within the colon and rectum, in keeping with a patient who has ingested multiple bags of drugs. The sacralization of L5 is an incidental finding.

INVESTIGATIONS AND MANAGEMENT

The patient should be resuscitated using an ABCDE approach.

Adequate analgesia and hydration should be provided.

Rupture of the drug capsules should be considered and reference to Toxbase for possible overdose management should be sought.

Early surgical referral should be considered, as a laparotomy may be needed.

As this may be associated with possible criminal activity, the police should be involved, although this should be secondary to providing care to the patient.

Case

36

A 24-year-old male presents to ED with worsening abdominal pain and 15 episodes of diarrhoea and passing mucus in the past 24 hours. He has no significant past medical history and is a nonsmoker. On examination, he has oxygen saturations of 97% in room air and a temperature of 38.5°C. His HR is 94 bpm, RR is 22 and blood pressure is 115/65 mmHg. The abdomen is rigid and there is generalized tenderness with normal bowel sounds. Urine dipstick is unremarkable.

An abdominal X-ray is requested to assess for a possible colitis.

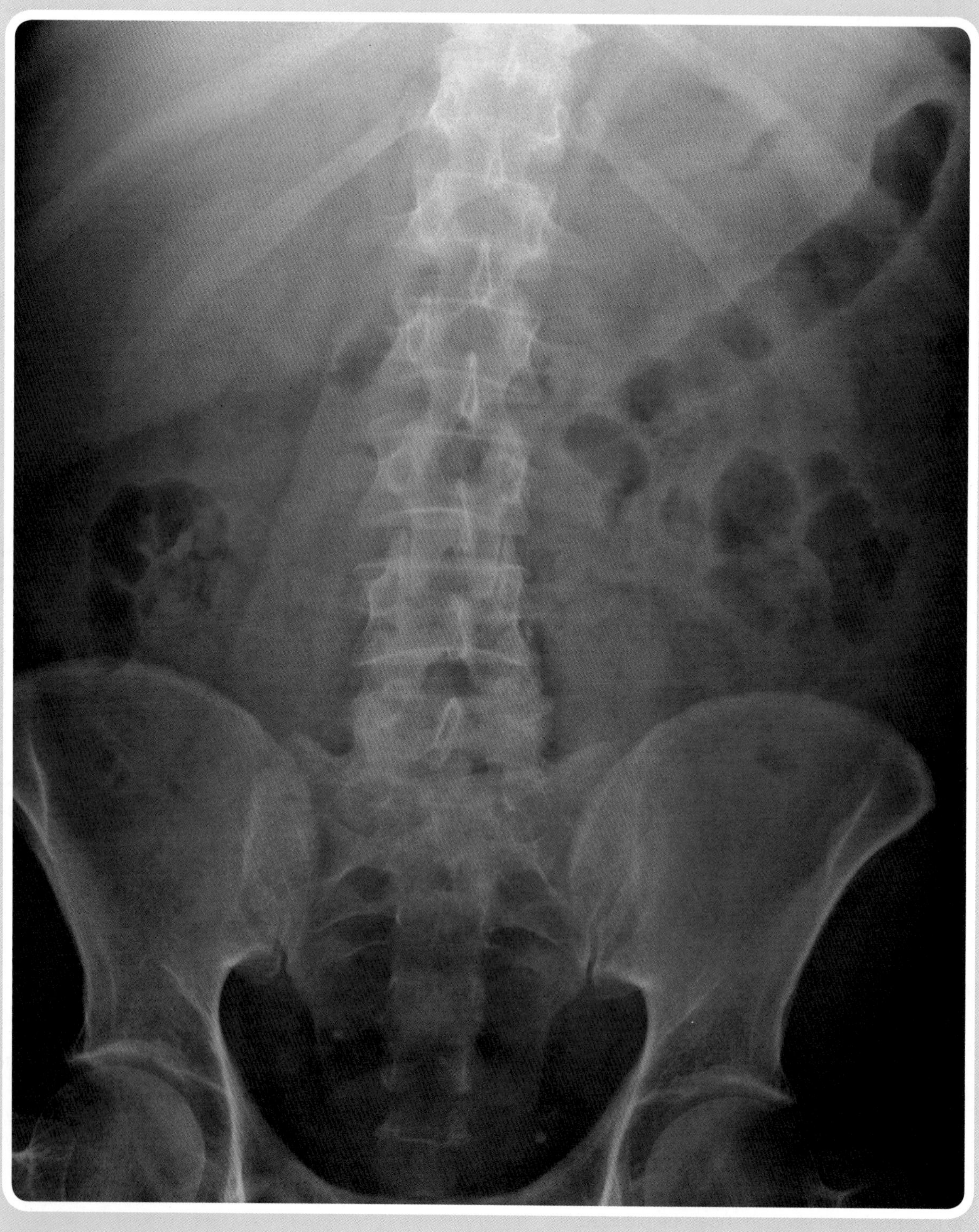

TECHNICAL INFORMATION

Patient ID: Anonymous.
Projection: AP supine.
Rotation: Adequate.
Penetration: Adequate – the spinous processes are visible.
Coverage: Inadequate – the pubic symphysis and inferior pubic rami have not been fully included.

BOWEL GAS PATTERN

The bowel gas pattern is normal.

BOWEL WALL

There is mural thickening of the distal transverse colon up to the splenic flexure in the left upper quadrant, which appears featureless with loss of the normal colonic haustral folds, in keeping with mural oedema. This is termed 'lead pipe colon'.

There is no evidence of intramural gas within the large or small bowel.

PNEUMOPERITONEUM

There is no evidence of free intraabdominal gas.

SOLID ORGANS

The solid organ contours are within normal limits with no solid organ calcification.

VASCULAR

No abnormal vascular calcification.

BONES

There are no abnormalities of the imaged thoracic and lumbar spine, or within the pelvis.

SOFT TISSUES

The psoas muscle outline is visible bilaterally.

The extraabdominal soft tissues are unremarkable.

OTHER

There are no radiopaque foreign bodies.

There are no vascular lines, drains or surgical clips.

There are several rounded radiopaque densities projected over the region of the pelvis in keeping with phleboliths.

REVIEW AREAS

Gallstones/renal calculi: No radiopaque calculi.
Lung bases: Not fully included.
Spine: Normal.
Femoral heads: Normal.

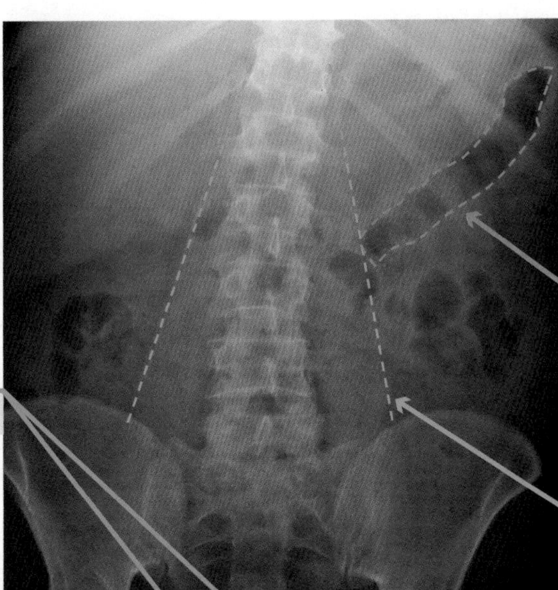

SUMMARY

This X-ray demonstrates mural oedema of the distal transverse colon up to the splenic flexure, which appears featureless with loss of the normal colonic haustral folds. Given the clinical history, this is suggestive of colitis, likely infective or inflammatory in nature. The pelvic phleboliths are an incidental finding.

INVESTIGATIONS AND MANAGEMENT

This patient should be resuscitated using an ABCDE approach.

Adequate analgesia and hydration should be provided.

Urgent bloods should be taken, including FBC, U&Es, LFTs, ESR, CRP, iron studies, folate, blood gas, and group and save. A stool sample should be sent.

Urgent referral to the gastroenterology team should be considered.

A CT scan of the abdomen/pelvis with IV contrast should be considered to better visualize anatomy and to assess for complications such as pneumoperitoneum and abscess formation.

Treatment will depend on the results of further investigations, as well as the clinical condition of the patient.

Case 37

A 60-year-old female is currently admitted to the surgical ward having just had an endovascular aortic stent insertion. Her past medical history is significant for abdominal aortic aneurysm and she is a smoker. On examination, she has oxygen saturations of 98% in room air and a temperature of 36.4°C. Her HR is 68 bpm, RR is 14 and blood pressure is 125/65 mmHg. The abdomen is soft and there is some tenderness centrally with normal bowel sounds. Urine dipstick is unremarkable.

You are asked to review the postoperative abdominal X-ray and comment on the position of the stent.

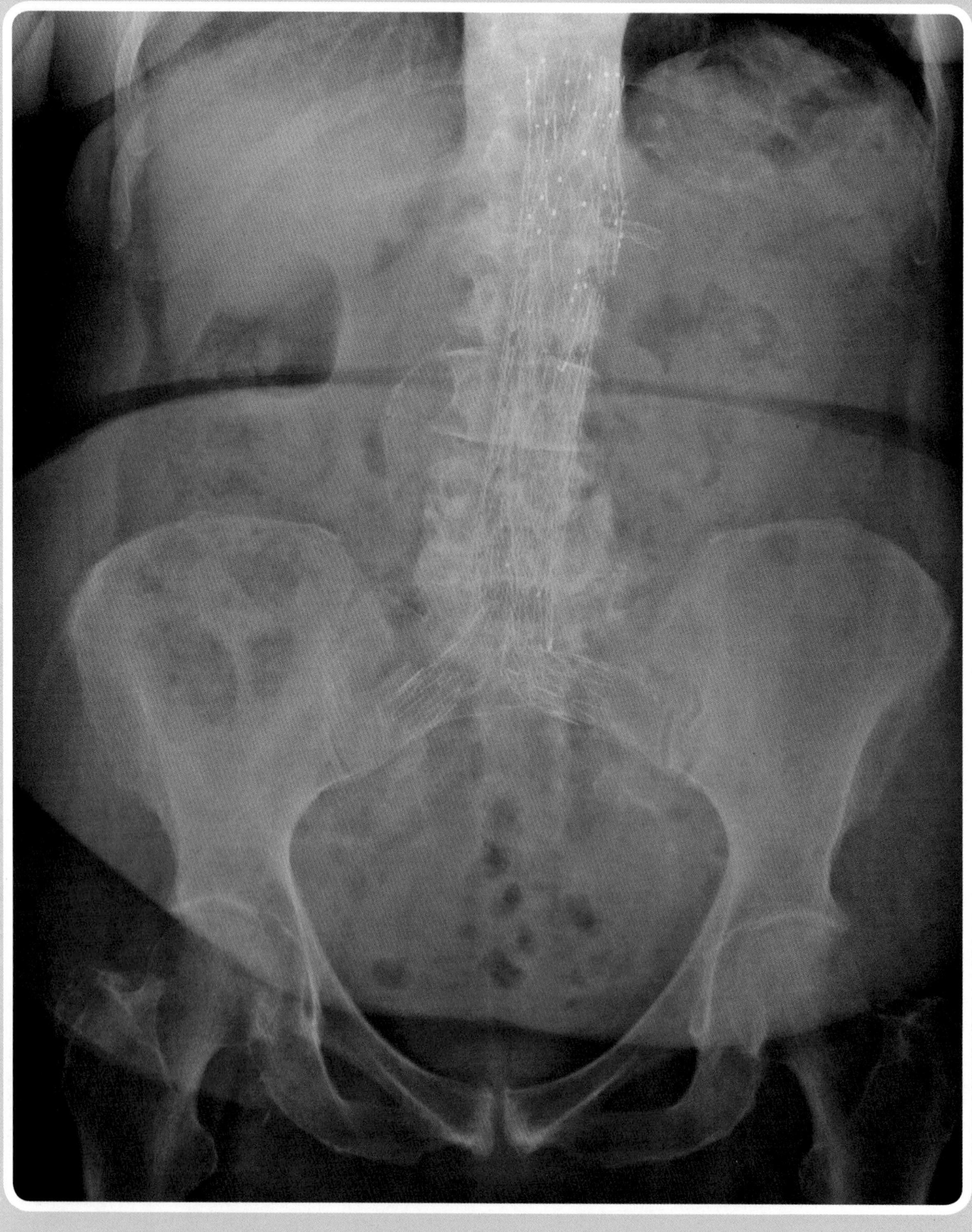

TECHNICAL INFORMATION

Patient ID: Anonymous.
Projection: AP supine.
Rotation: Adequate.
Penetration: Adequate – the spinous processes are visible.
Coverage: Adequate – the anterior ribs are visible superiorly and the pubic rami are visible inferiorly.

BOWEL GAS PATTERN

The bowel gas pattern is normal.

BOWEL WALL

There is no evidence of mural thickening or intramural gas within the large or small bowel.

PNEUMOPERITONEUM

There is no evidence of free intraabdominal gas.

SOLID ORGANS

The solid organ contours are within normal limits with no solid organ calcification.

VASCULAR

There is a fenestrated endovascular iliac branch aortic stent seen within the abdominal aorta, extending into the common iliac arteries bilaterally. There are separate renal artery stents in situ. A partially calcified infrarenal abdominal aortic aneurysm is visible.

BONES

There is minor bilateral degenerative change seen within the hip joints and the pubic symphysis, including narrowing of the joint spaces and sclerosis.

There are no abnormalities of the imaged thoracic and lumbar spine.

SOFT TISSUES

The psoas muscle outline is visible bilaterally.

There are cutaneous fat folds projecting over the region of the abdomen.

OTHER

There are no additional radiopaque foreign bodies.

There are no vascular lines, drains or surgical clips.

REVIEW AREAS

Gallstones/renal calculi: No radiopaque calculi.
Lung bases: Normal.
Spine: Normal.
Femoral heads: Bilateral degenerative change, including narrowing of joint spaces and sclerosis.

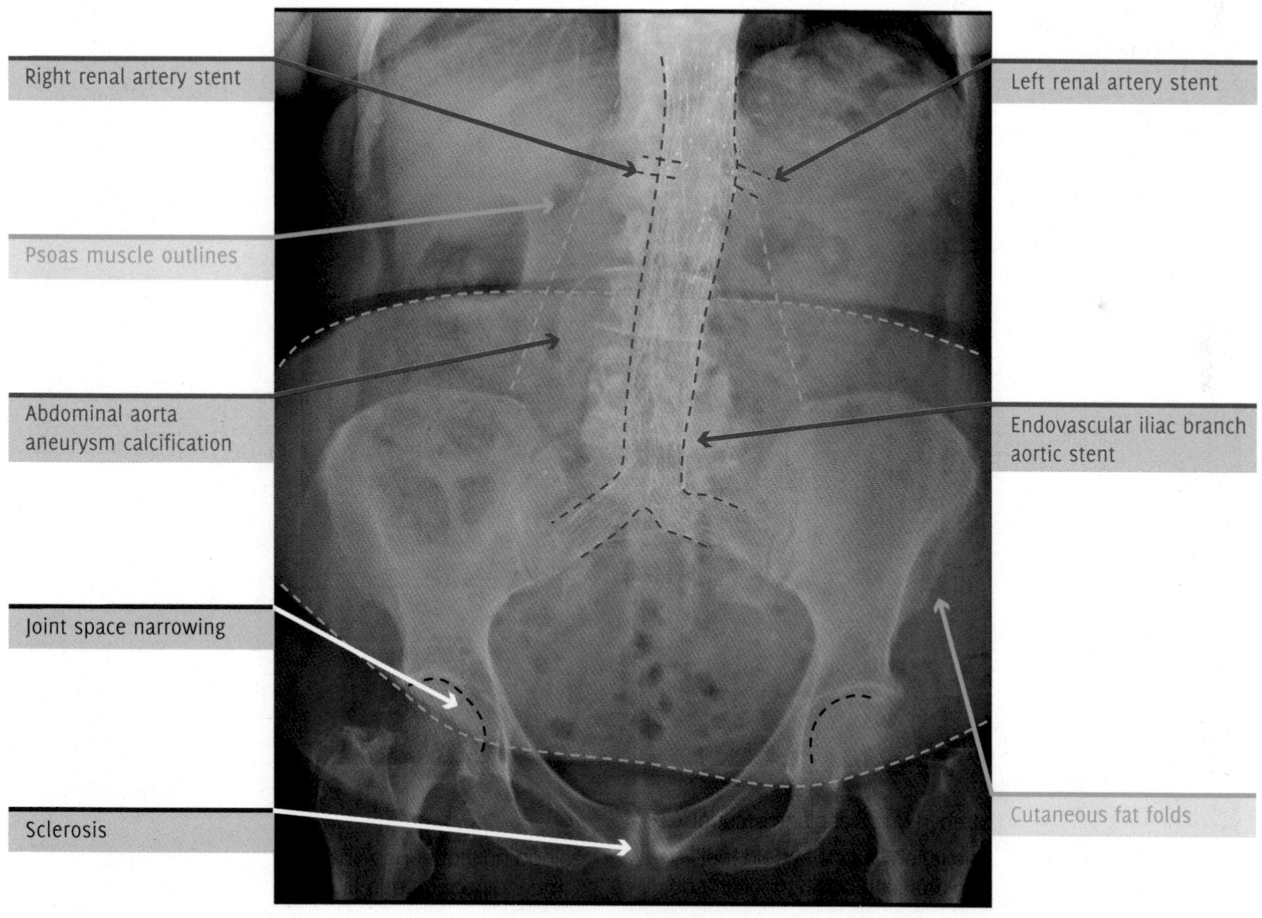

SUMMARY

This X-ray demonstrates a multibranched aortic stent within the abdominal aorta extending into the proximal left renal and bilateral common iliac arteries. The minor degenerative changes seen bilaterally within the hip joints and pubic symphysis are incidental findings.

INVESTIGATIONS AND MANAGEMENT

If the patient is otherwise well, no further investigations or imaging is required. The stents are adequately positioned. Degenerative changes should be correlated with clinical history, and lifestyle advice/analgesia should be considered in the first instance.

Case

38

A 55-year-old male presents to the haematology outpatient clinic as a referral from his primary care physician due to abnormal haematology results with a markedly raised white blood cell (WBC) count. He has no significant past medical history and is a nonsmoker. On examination, he has oxygen saturations of 99% in room air and a temperature of 36.6°C. His HR is 66 bpm, RR is 14 and blood pressure is 120/70 mmHg. The abdomen is soft and there is no tenderness, although massive splenomegaly is detected. Bowel sounds are normal and urine dipstick is unremarkable.

An abdominal X-ray is requested to assess for possible bone abnormalities and organomegaly.

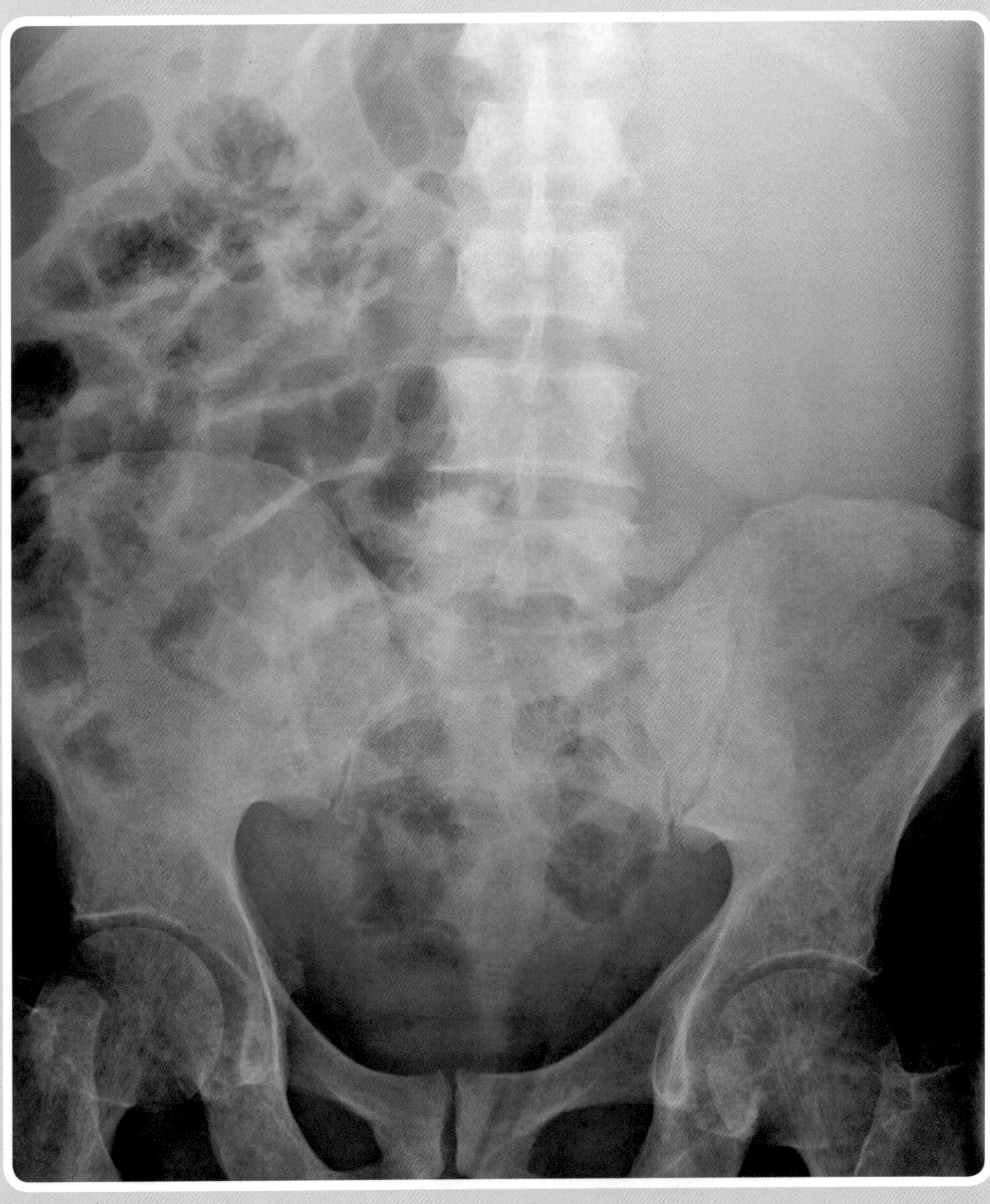

TECHNICAL INFORMATION

Patient ID: Anonymous.
Projection: AP supine.
Rotation: Adequate.
Penetration: Adequate – the spinous processes are visible.
Coverage: Inadequate – the anterior ribs have not been included.

BOWEL GAS PATTERN

The bowel is displaced to the right by a homogeneous opacification in the left upper quadrant of the abdomen.

BOWEL WALL

There is no evidence of mural thickening or intramural gas within the large or small bowel.

PNEUMOPERITONEUM

There is no evidence of free intraabdominal gas.

SOLID ORGANS

There is a large homogeneous opacification within the left upper quadrant of the abdomen, in keeping with an enlarged spleen.

VASCULAR

No abnormal vascular calcification.

BONES

There is a mottled appearance of the bones of the pelvis and the imaged femur.

There are no abnormalities of the imaged thoracic and lumbar spine.

SOFT TISSUES

The psoas muscle outline is visible bilaterally.

The extraabdominal soft tissues are unremarkable.

OTHER

There are no radiopaque foreign bodies.

There are no vascular lines, drains or surgical clips.

REVIEW AREAS

Gallstones/renal calculi: No radiopaque calculi.
Lung bases: Not fully included.
Spine: Normal.
Femoral heads: Mottled appearance of bones.

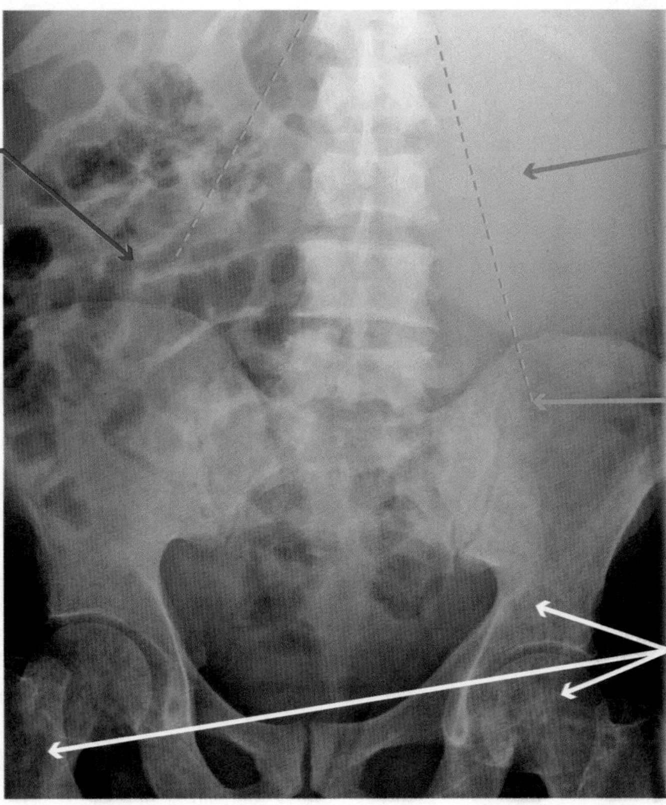

SUMMARY

This X-ray demonstrates splenomegaly with displacement of the bowel to the right. It also demonstrates an associated mottled appearance of the bones of the pelvis and femurs. Given the clinical history, these findings are suggestive of a myeloproliferative disorder.

INVESTIGATIONS AND MANAGEMENT

Bloods should be taken, including FBC, U&Es, LFTs, CRP, ESR, bone profile, LDH, coagulation, hepatitis screening, cytomegalovirus (CMV) and Epstein–Barr virus (EBV) screening, ESR, blood gas and blood film. Additional tests such as flow cytometry, FISH and PCR testing for BCR-ABL/JAK2 gene should be considered, as well as a bone marrow biopsy. An abdominal USS should be performed to confirm splenomegaly and further evaluate the abdominal solid organs.

The patient should be followed up by haematology. Diagnosis and treatment will depend on the results of the tests and the patient's wishes. Treatment options potentially include observation, chemotherapy, radiation therapy, biological therapies or stem cell transplantation.

Case

39

A 35-year-old female presents to ED with worsening back pain and pyrexia of unknown origin. She has no significant past medical history but has recently travelled to Thailand. She is a nonsmoker. On examination, she has oxygen saturations of 98% in room air and a temperature of 38.6°C. Her HR is 96 bpm, RR is 20 and blood pressure is 105/62 mmHg. The abdomen is rigid and there is generalized tenderness with normal bowel sounds. Urine dipstick is unremarkable and a pregnancy test is negative.

An abdominal X-ray is requested to assess for possible bowel obstruction.

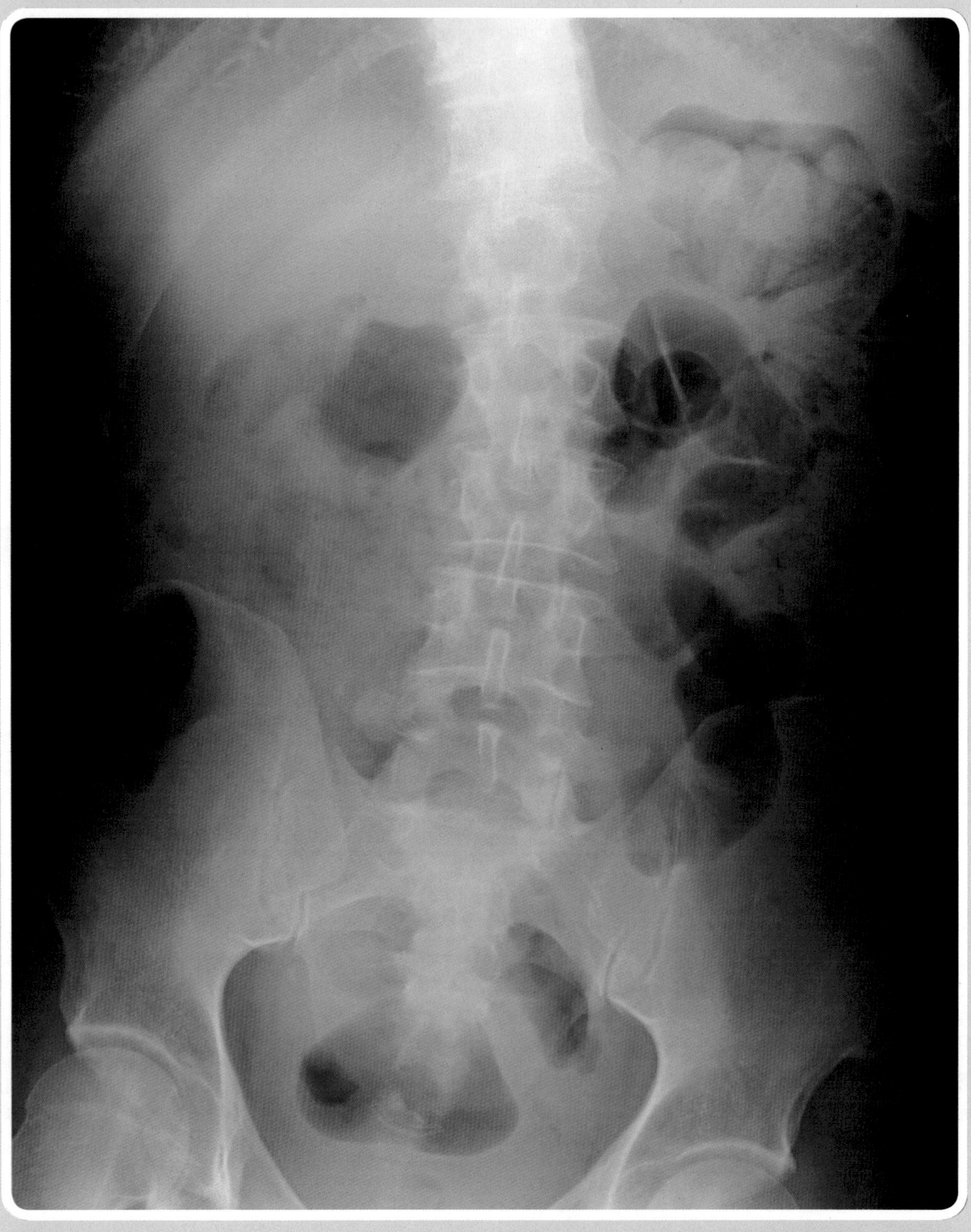

TECHNICAL INFORMATION

Patient ID: Anonymous.
Projection: AP supine.
Rotation: Adequate.
Penetration: Adequate – the spinous processes are visible.
Coverage: Inadequate – the pubic symphysis, inferior pubic rami and hip joints have not been fully included.

BOWEL GAS PATTERN

The bowel gas pattern is normal.

There are hard faeces in the distal transverse colon and a small volume of faecal material present throughout the descending colon.

BOWEL WALL

There is no evidence of mural thickening or intramural gas within the large or small bowel.

PNEUMOPERITONEUM

There is no evidence of free intraabdominal gas.

SOLID ORGANS

The solid organ contours are within normal limits with no solid organ calcification.

VASCULAR

No abnormal vascular calcification.

BONES

There is thoracolumbar scoliosis seen convex to the left, centred at the L1/L2 level. No fractures or destructive bone lesions are visible in the imaged skeleton.

SOFT TISSUES

There is a mottled appearance projecting over the right psoas muscle outline and the left psoas muscle outline is not visible.

The extraabdominal soft tissues are unremarkable.

OTHER

There are no radiopaque foreign bodies.

There are no vascular lines, drains or surgical clips.

REVIEW AREAS

Gallstones/renal calculi: No radiopaque calculi.
Lung bases: Not fully included.
Spine: Thoracolumbar scoliosis convex to the left, centred at the L1/L2 level.
Femoral heads: Not fully included.

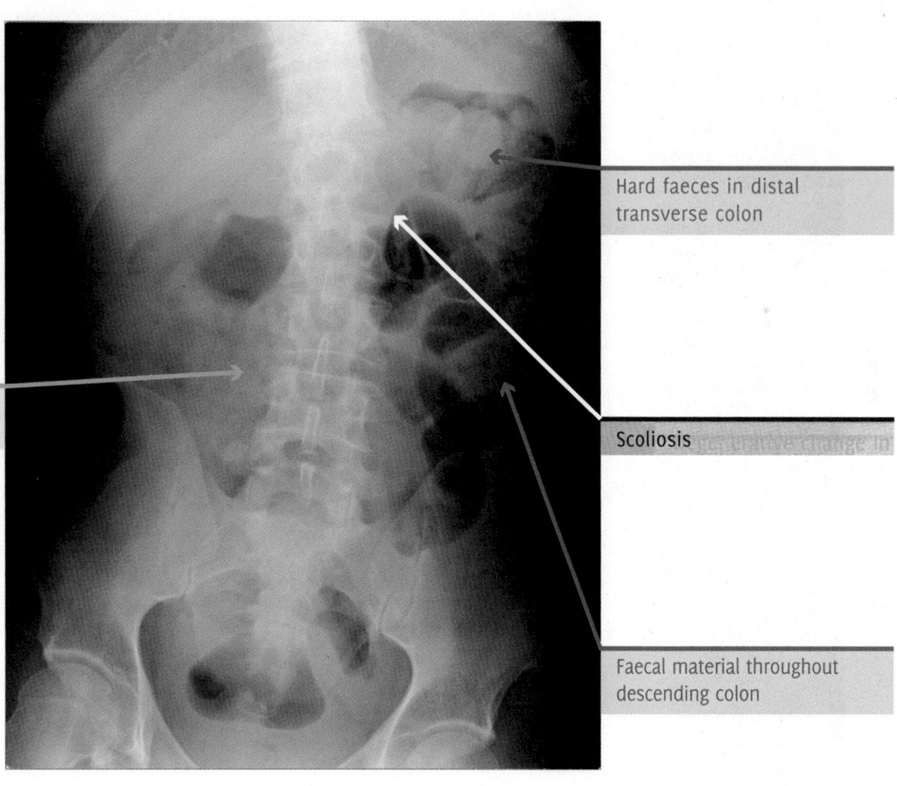

SUMMARY

This X-ray demonstrates a mottled appearance overlying the right psoas muscle outline. Given the clinical history, this is likely to represent a psoas abscess. The lumbar scoliosis is an incidental finding but may be secondary to the abscess.

INVESTIGATIONS AND MANAGEMENT

The patient should be resuscitated using an ABCDE approach.

Adequate analgesia and hydration should be provided.

Urgent bloods should be taken, including FBC, U&Es, CRP, bone profile, LFTs, clotting, blood cultures, a blood gas, and group and save.

Broad-spectrum antibiotics should be prescribed. The patient should be made NBM and started on IV fluids.

The Sepsis 6 pathway should be started immediately, including administration of oxygen, IV antibiotics and consideration of a fluid bolus as well as measurement of lactate, monitoring urine output and taking blood cultures.

A CT scan of the abdomen/pelvis with IV contrast should be considered for further evaluation of the possible abscess, and the general surgical team should be involved for consideration of possible percutaneous drainage or surgical management.

Case

40

A 63-year-old female presents to ED with an increasing sensation of fullness of the abdomen and worsening bilateral pedal oedema. She has no significant past medical history and is a nonsmoker. On examination, she has oxygen saturations of 97% in room air and a temperature of 36.6°C. Her HR is 72 bpm, RR is 14 and blood pressure is 122/76 mmHg. The abdomen is distended and soft with no tenderness and normal bowel sounds. Urine dipstick is unremarkable.

An abdominal X-ray is requested to assess for possible bowel obstruction.

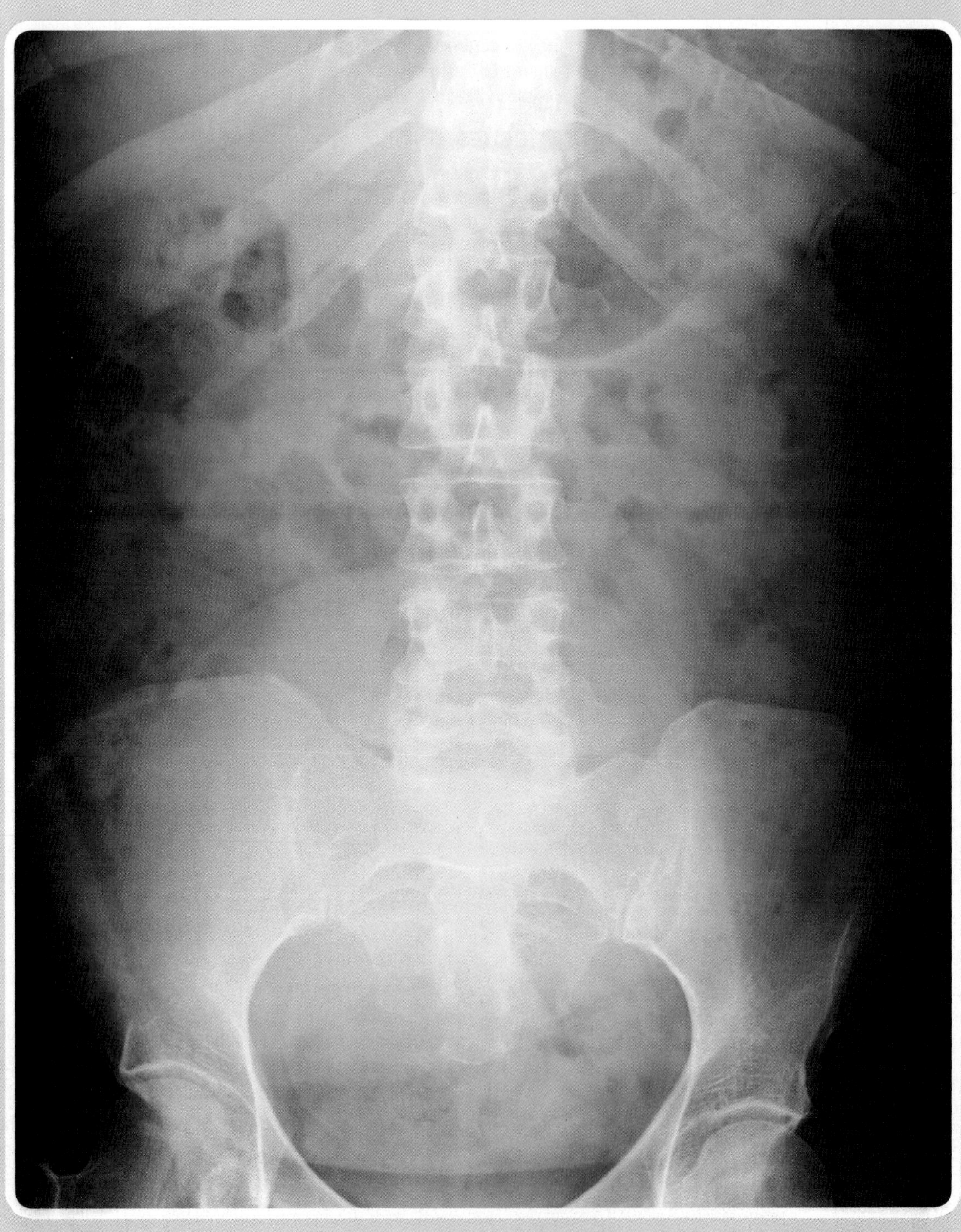

TECHNICAL INFORMATION

Patient ID: Anonymous.
Projection: AP supine.
Rotation: Adequate.
Penetration: Adequate – the spinous processes are visible.
Coverage: Inadequate – the pubic symphysis, inferior pubic rami and hip joints have not been included.

BOWEL GAS PATTERN

The bowel gas pattern is normal.

BOWEL WALL

There is no evidence of mural thickening or intramural gas within the large or small bowel.

PNEUMOPERITONEUM

There is no evidence of free intraabdominal gas.

SOLID ORGANS

The solid organ contours are within normal limits with no solid organ calcification.

VASCULAR

No abnormal vascular calcification.

BONES

There are no abnormalities of the imaged thoracic and lumbar spine, or within the pelvis.

SOFT TISSUES

The psoas muscle outline is not visible bilaterally, which is nonspecific.

There is a large, rounded, well-circumscribed soft-tissue density mass centred around the right sacrum projecting over the lower abdomen and pelvis with a smaller well-circumscribed soft-tissue density mass centred projecting over the right pelvis.

The urinary bladder is visualized separate to these two masses.

The extraabdominal soft tissues are unremarkable.

OTHER

There are no radiopaque foreign bodies.

There are no vascular lines, drains or surgical clips.

REVIEW AREAS

Gallstones/renal calculi: No radiopaque calculi.
Lung bases: Not fully included.
Spine: Normal.
Femoral heads: Not visible.

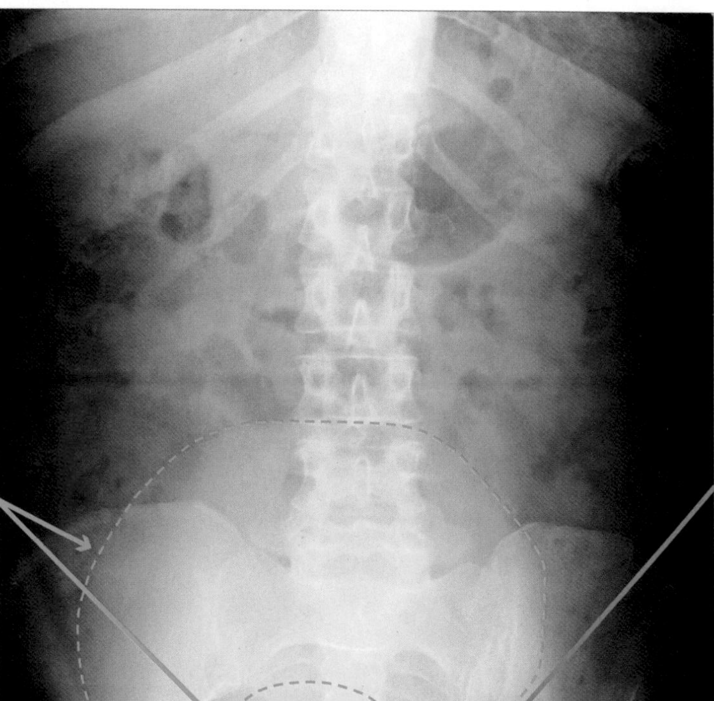

SUMMARY

This X-ray demonstrates two rounded, well-circumscribed masses of soft-tissue density projecting over the pelvis and lower abdomen, which appear separate from the urinary bladder. Differentials include fibroids and ovarian masses, both malignant and benign.

INVESTIGATIONS AND MANAGEMENT

Adequate analgesia and hydration should be provided.

Urgent bloods should be taken, including FBC, U&Es, CRP, LFTs, bone profile, blood gas and tumour markers (including CA-125).

The patient should be referred to gynaecology. An ultrasound scan of the abdomen and pelvis may be helpful to better assess the masses with a view to a CT or MRI scan of the abdomen and pelvis for further assessment.

Case

41

A 4-year-old boy presents to ED with right iliac fossa pain, nausea, vomiting and pyrexia. He has no significant past medical history. On examination, he has oxygen saturations of 99% in room air and a temperature of 38.6°C. His HR is 120 bpm, RR is 28 and blood pressure is 90/50 mmHg. The abdomen is soft and there is tenderness in the right iliac fossa with normal bowel sounds. Urine dipstick is unremarkable.

An abdominal X-ray is requested to assess for possible bowel obstruction.

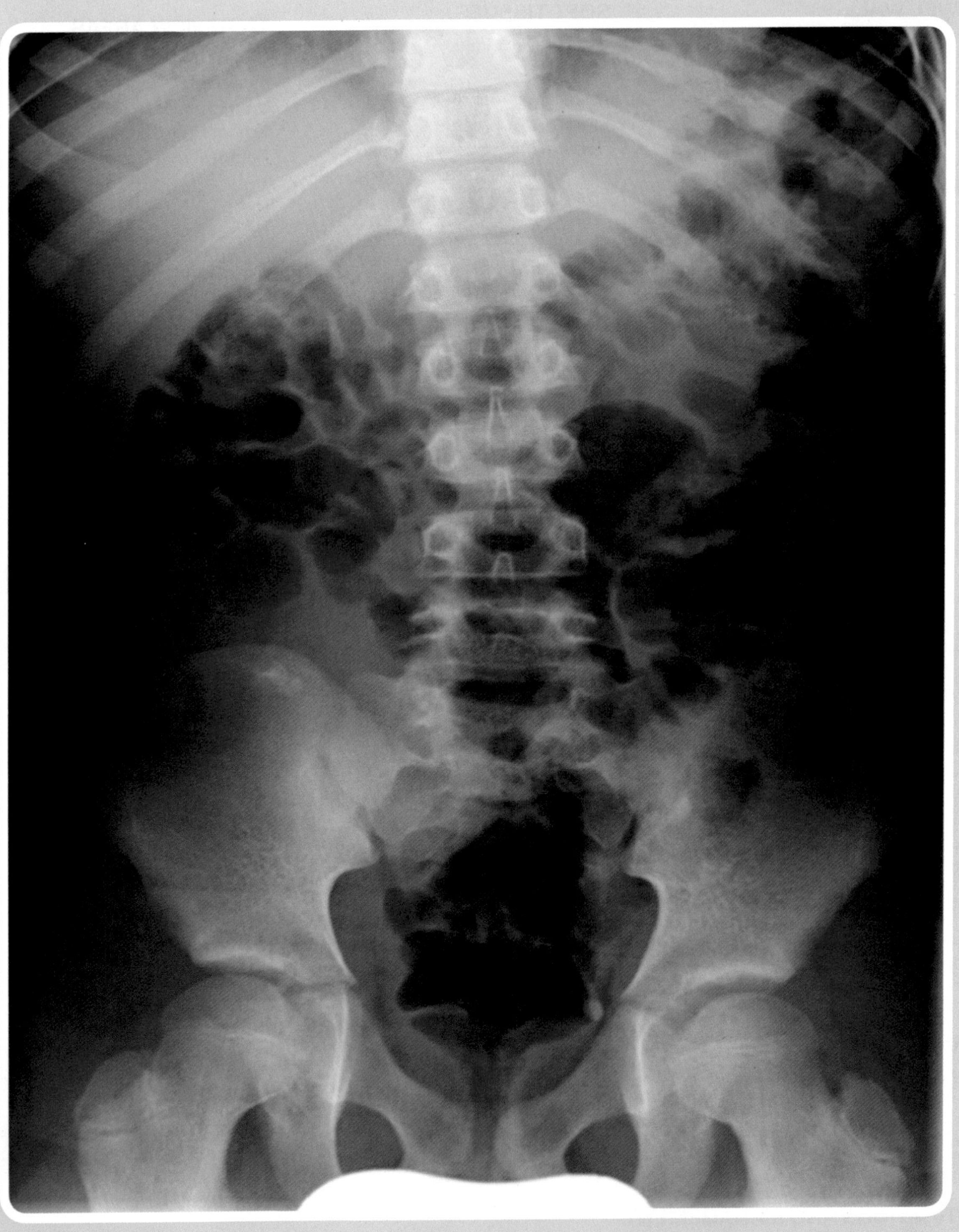

TECHNICAL INFORMATION

Patient ID: Anonymous.
Projection: AP supine.
Rotation: Adequate.
Penetration: Adequate – the spinous processes are visible.
Coverage: Adequate – the anterior ribs are visible superiorly and the inferior pubic rami are visible.

BOWEL GAS PATTERN

The bowel gas pattern is normal.

BOWEL WALL

There is no evidence of mural thickening or intramural gas within the large or small bowel.

PNEUMOPERITONEUM

There is no evidence of free intraabdominal gas.

SOLID ORGANS

The solid organ contours are within normal limits with no solid organ calcification.

VASCULAR

No abnormal vascular calcification.

BONES

There are no abnormalities of the imaged thoracic and lumbar spine, or within the pelvis.

There are growth plates at the femoral head, greater trochanter and acetabulum as the ossification centres have not yet fused, which is a normal finding in a child of this age.

SOFT TISSUES

The psoas muscle outline is visible bilaterally.

The extraabdominal soft tissues are unremarkable.

OTHER

There is a radiopaque density projected over the region of the right iliac fossa.

There is a gonadal shield in situ.

There are no vascular lines, drains or surgical clips.

REVIEW AREAS

Gallstones/renal calculi: No radiopaque calculi.
Lung bases: Normal.
Spine: Normal.
Femoral heads: Normal – growth plates present.

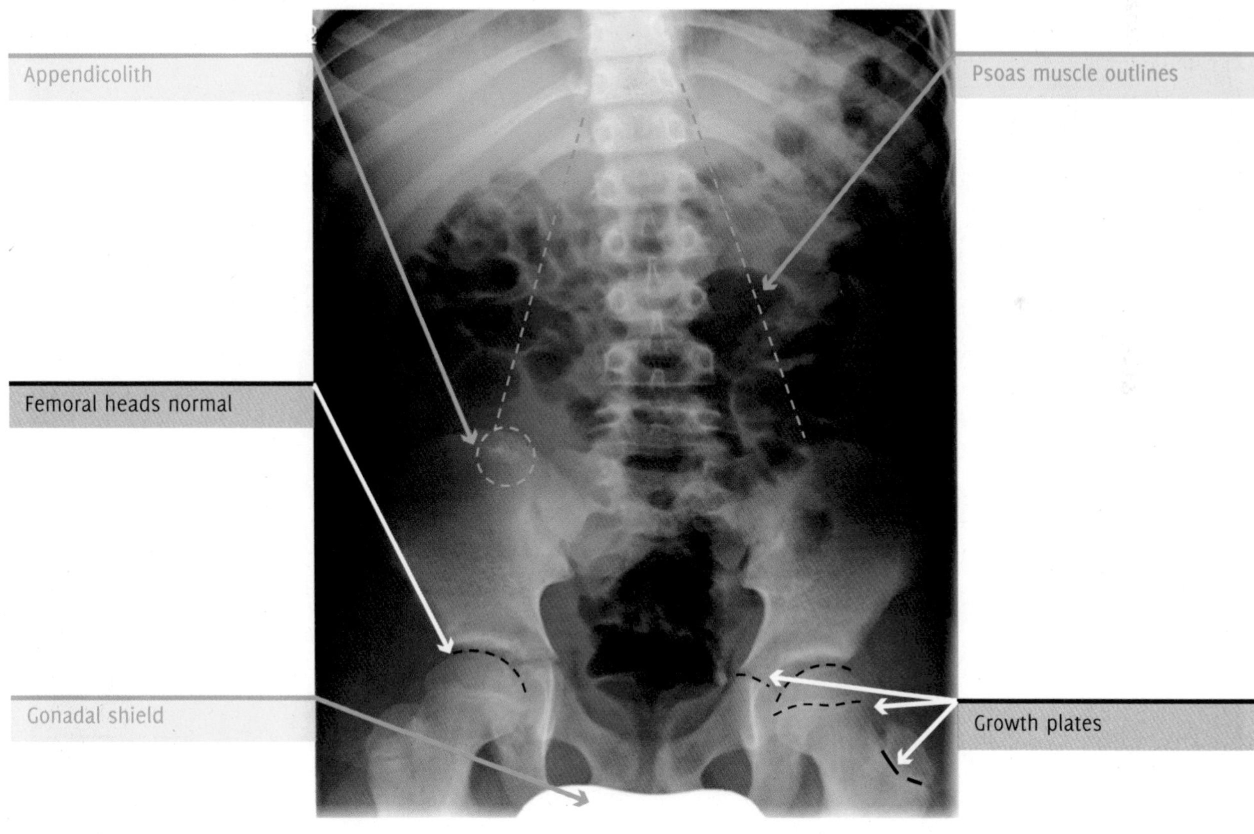

SUMMARY

This X-ray demonstrates a radiopaque density projected over the region of the right iliac fossa, in keeping with an appendicolith within the appendix. There is no evidence of bowel obstruction or pneumoperitoneum.

INVESTIGATIONS AND MANAGEMENT

The patient should be resuscitated using an ABCDE approach.

Adequate analgesia and hydration should be provided.

The patient should be made NBM and started on IV fluids.

Urgent bloods should be taken, including FBC, U&Es, blood culture, blood gas, coagulation, group and save and CRP.

The patient should be commenced on broad-spectrum antibiotics.

The patient should be referred urgently to the paediatric surgeons for consideration of an appendicectomy.

Case

42

A 1-week-old baby boy, currently admitted to SCBU, is acutely unwell and deteriorating rapidly. He was born prematurely at 32 weeks but has been progressing well up until this point. On examination, he has oxygen saturations of 96% in room air and a temperature of 38.5°C. His HR is 245 bpm and RR is 68. The abdomen is rigid with tinkling bowel sounds.

An abdominal X-ray is requested to assess for possible necrotizing enterocolitis.

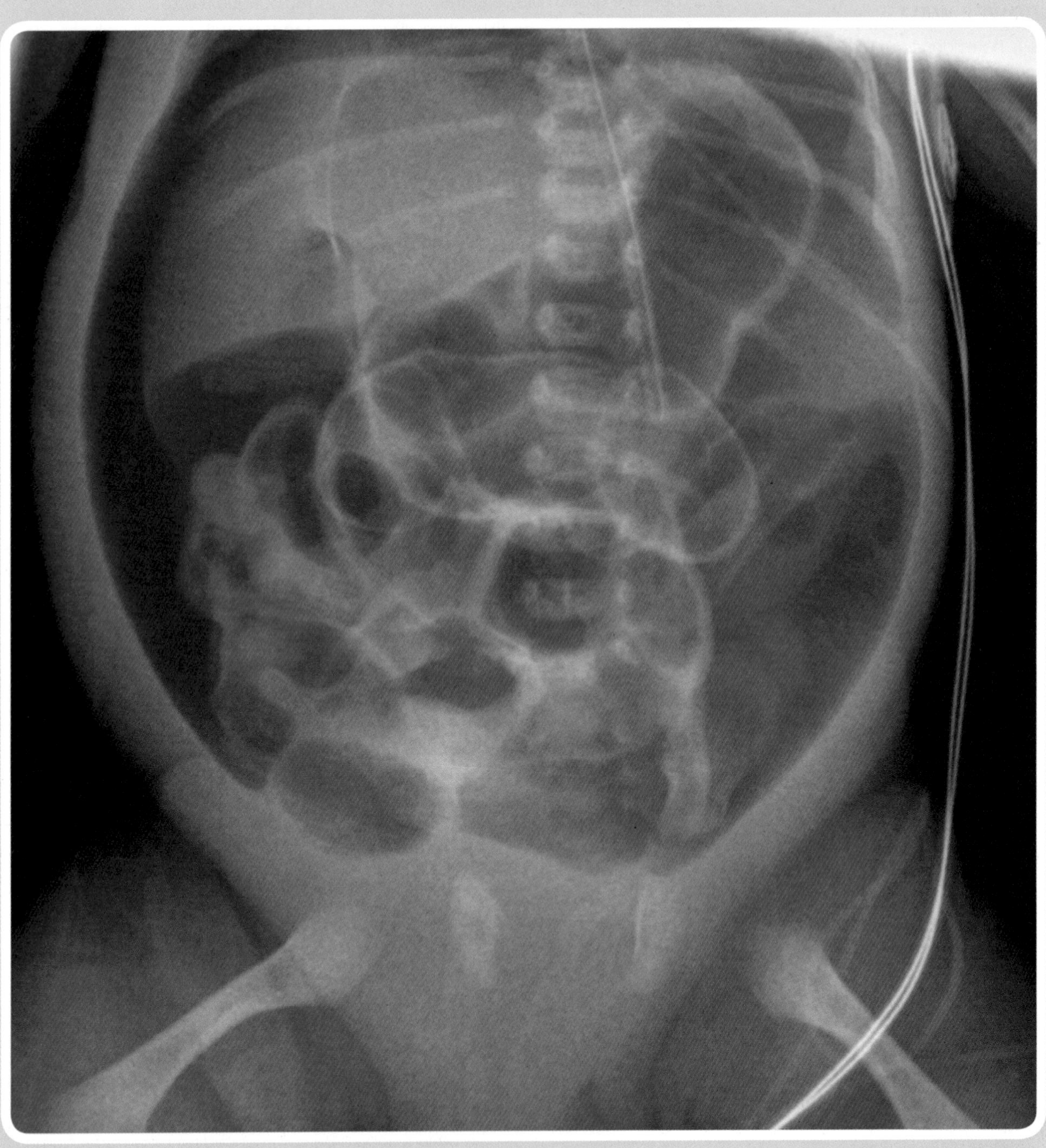

TECHNICAL INFORMATION

Patient ID: Anonymous.
Projection: AP supine.
Rotation: Asymmetrical appearances of the pelvis with deviation of the spine to the left in keeping with patient rotation to the right.
Penetration: Adequate – the spine is visible.
Coverage: Inadequate – the hemidiaphragms have not been included.

BOWEL GAS PATTERN

There are multiple loops of dilated bowel seen centrally within the abdomen. There is no gas within the rectum.

BOWEL WALL

There is no evidence of mural thickening or intramural gas within the large or small bowel.

PNEUMOPERITONEUM

There is evidence of free intraabdominal gas, in keeping with pneumoperitoneum.

Rigler's sign (double-wall sign) can be seen, in keeping with air present on both the luminal and peritoneal sides of the bowel wall.

The falciform ligament sign can be seen, in keeping with a large amount of air present within the abdomen outlining the falciform ligament.

The football sign can be seen, in keeping with a large amount of air present within the abdomen outlining the entire abdominal cavity.

SOLID ORGANS

The liver and falciform ligament are well outlined by free gas in the abdomen.

VASCULAR

No abnormal vascular calcification.

BONES

There are no abnormalities of the imaged thoracic and lumbar spine, or within the pelvis.

There is cartilage present between the pelvic bones and femurs as they have not yet fused, which is a normal finding in a child of this age.

There is cartilage seen between the vertebrae, which is a normal finding in a child of this age.

SOFT TISSUES

The psoas muscle outline is not seen bilaterally, which is nonspecific, particularly in a child of this age.

The extraabdominal soft tissues are unremarkable.

OTHER

There is an NG tube in situ, although given how straight it is, there is a possibility it has perforated the oesophagus.

There is an electrode and lead external to the patient on the left, in keeping with cardiopulmonary monitoring.

There are no vascular lines, drains or surgical clips.

REVIEW AREAS

Gallstones/renal calculi: No radiopaque calculi.
Lung bases: Not fully included.
Spine: Normal – cartilage between vertebrae.
Femoral heads: Normal – growth plates present.

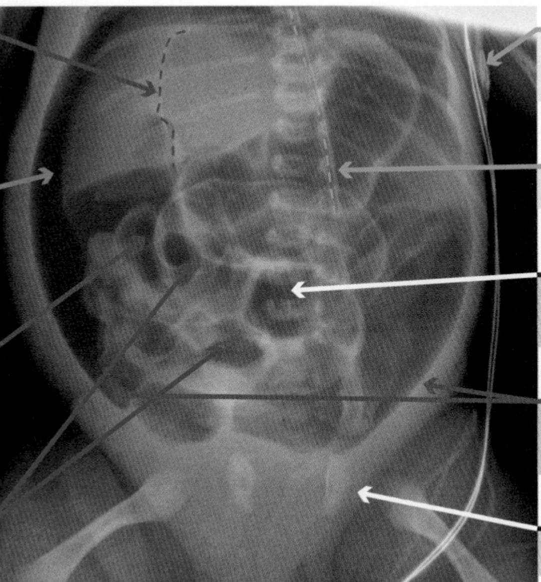

SUMMARY

This X-ray demonstrates multiple loops of dilated bowel throughout the abdomen with evidence of pneumoperitoneum. There is no gas within the rectum. Given the clinical history, the most likely diagnosis is bowel perforation, which may be due to necrotizing enterocolitis. The NG tube should be checked to ensure there is a gastric aspirate.

INVESTIGATIONS AND MANAGEMENT

The baby should be resuscitated using an ABCDE approach.

The baby should be started on broad-spectrum antibiotics, made NBM and started on IV fluids.

The baby needs to be intubated given the perforation.

Urgent bloods should be taken, including FBC, U&Es, CRP, bone profile, LFTs, coagulation, blood cultures, blood gas, and group and save. A lateral shoot-through AXR would be helpful to confirm perforation and NG position.

The patient should be referred urgently to the neonatal surgeons for ongoing management.

Case

43

A 14-year-old male attends the spinal outpatient clinic for a routine follow-up appointment but is noted to be vomiting. His past medical history is significant for spina bifida occulta. On examination, he has oxygen saturations of 99% in room air and a temperature of 37.0°C. His HR is 80 bpm, RR is 15 and blood pressure is 120/72 mmHg. The abdomen is soft but mildly tender with normal bowel sounds.

An abdominal X-ray is requested to assess for possible bowel obstruction.

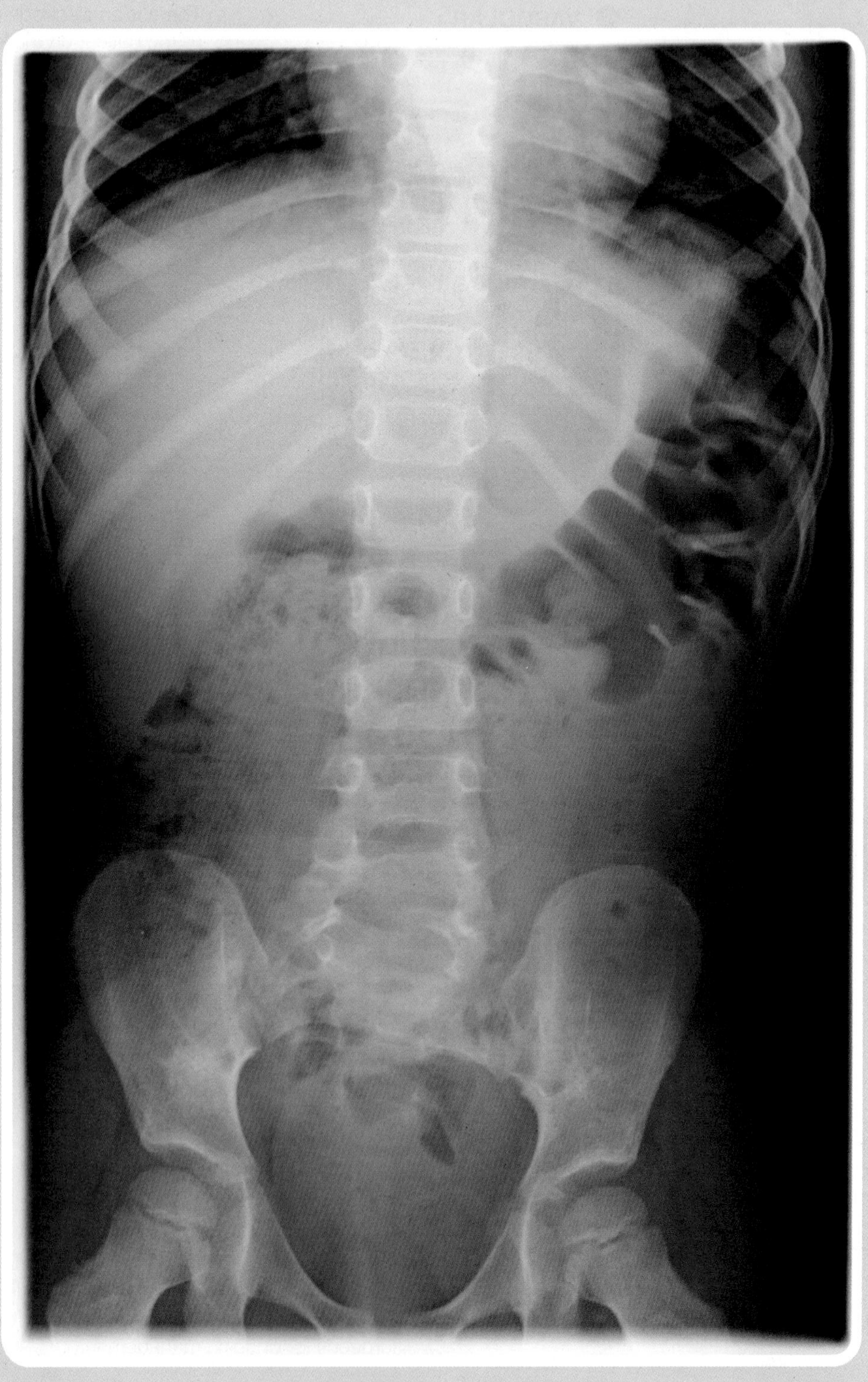

TECHNICAL INFORMATION

Patient ID: Anonymous.
Projection: AP supine.
Rotation: Adequate.
Penetration: Adequate – the spine is visible.
Coverage: Inadequate – the pubic symphysis and inferior pubic rami are not fully included.

BOWEL GAS PATTERN

There is a mild to moderate volume of faecal residue present in the ascending and proximal transverse colon.

BOWEL WALL

There is no evidence of mural thickening or intramural gas within the large or small bowel.

PNEUMOPERITONEUM

There is no evidence of free intraabdominal gas.

SOLID ORGANS

The solid organ contours are within normal limits with no solid organ calcification.

VASCULAR

No abnormal vascular calcification.

BONES

There is a lateral hemivertebra segmentation anomaly present at the level of L5, however no associated scoliosis.

There is lumbarization of S1.

There are growth plates at the femoral head and acetabulum (triradiate cartilage) as the ossification centres have not yet fused, which is a normal finding in a child of this age.

SOFT TISSUES

The psoas muscle outline is visible bilaterally.

The extraabdominal soft tissues are unremarkable.

OTHER

There are no radiopaque foreign bodies.

There are no vascular lines, drains or surgical clips.

REVIEW AREAS

Gallstones/renal calculi: No radiopaque calculi.
Lung bases: Normal.
Spine: Normal.
Femoral heads: Normal – growth plates present.

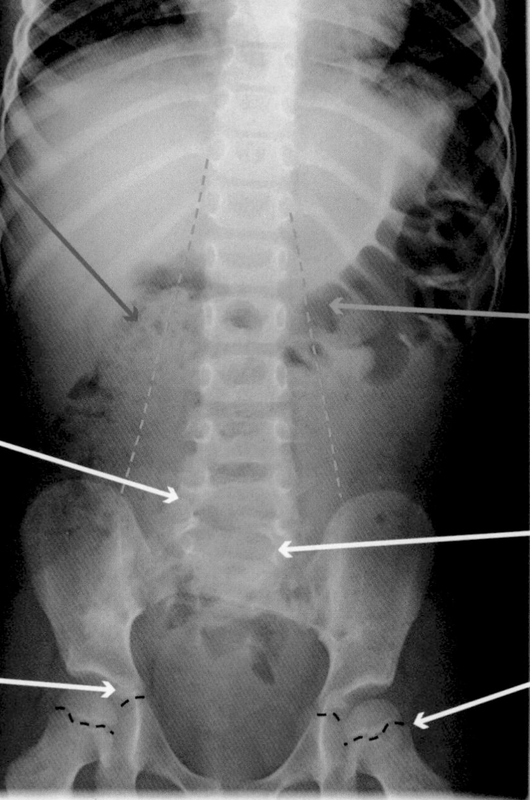

SUMMARY

This X-ray demonstrates mild to moderate volume of faecal residue in the ascending and proximal transverse colon. There is an L5 hemivertebra, in keeping with the patient's background history of spina bifida occulta, and lumbarization of S1.

INVESTIGATIONS AND MANAGEMENT

If the patient is otherwise well, no further investigation or imaging is required at present. If the patient is clinically constipated, current medications should be reviewed and laxatives considered. Advice should be given regarding lifestyle adjustments, including adequate fluid intake, sufficient dietary fibre and exercise if clinically appropriate.

Case

44

A 70-year-old male has recently had an AAA repaired but is otherwise well and is a nonsmoker. On examination, he has oxygen saturations of 99% in room air and a temperature of 37.0°C. His HR is 70 bpm, RR is 18 and blood pressure is 120/72 mmHg. The abdomen is soft but mildly tender with normal bowel sounds.

You are given his postoperative X-ray to review.

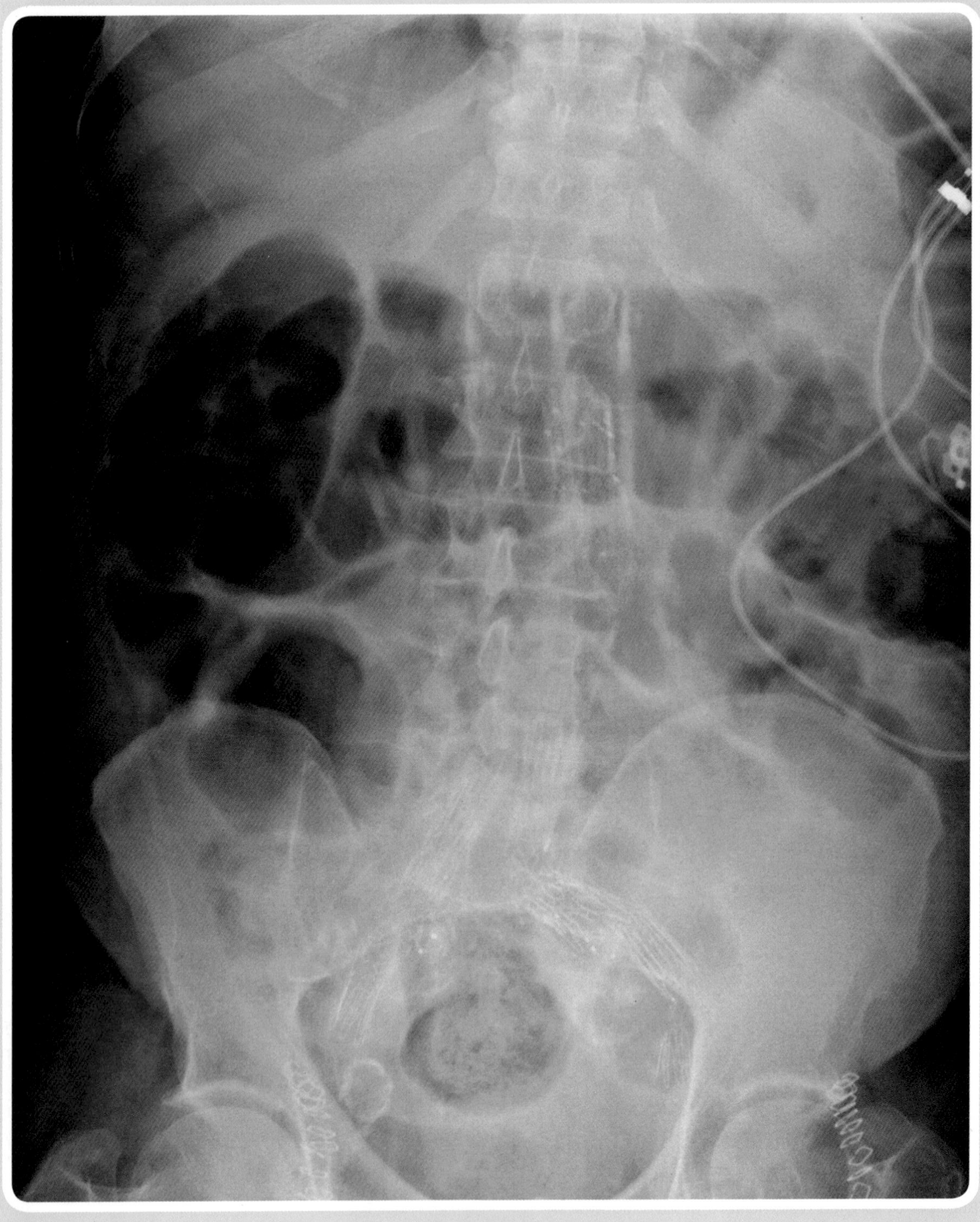

TECHNICAL INFORMATION

Patient ID: Anonymous.
Projection: AP supine.
Rotation: Asymmetrical appearances of the pelvis in keeping with mild patient rotation.
Penetration: Adequate.
Coverage: Inadequate – inferior pubic rami not included.

BOWEL GAS PATTERN

There is a prominent transverse colon loop, however no significant dilatation.

BOWEL WALL

There is no evidence of mural thickening or intramural gas within the large or small bowel.

PNEUMOPERITONEUM

There is no evidence of free intraabdominal gas.

SOLID ORGANS

The solid organ contours are within normal limits with no solid organ calcification.

VASCULAR

There is a fenestrated endovascular iliac branch aortic stent seen within the abdominal aorta, extending into the common iliac arteries bilaterally.

BONES

There are osteophytes in the spine in keeping with mild degenerative changes.

SOFT TISSUES

The psoas muscle outline is visible bilaterally.

Extraabdominal soft tissues are unremarkable.

OTHER

There is a radiopaque ECG lead seen external to the patient on the left side.

There are surgical clips projecting over the femoral regions bilaterally.

There are no vascular lines or drains.

REVIEW AREAS

Gallstones/renal calculi: No radiopaque calculi.
Lung bases: Not fully included.
Spine: Mild degenerative changes.
Femoral heads: Normal.

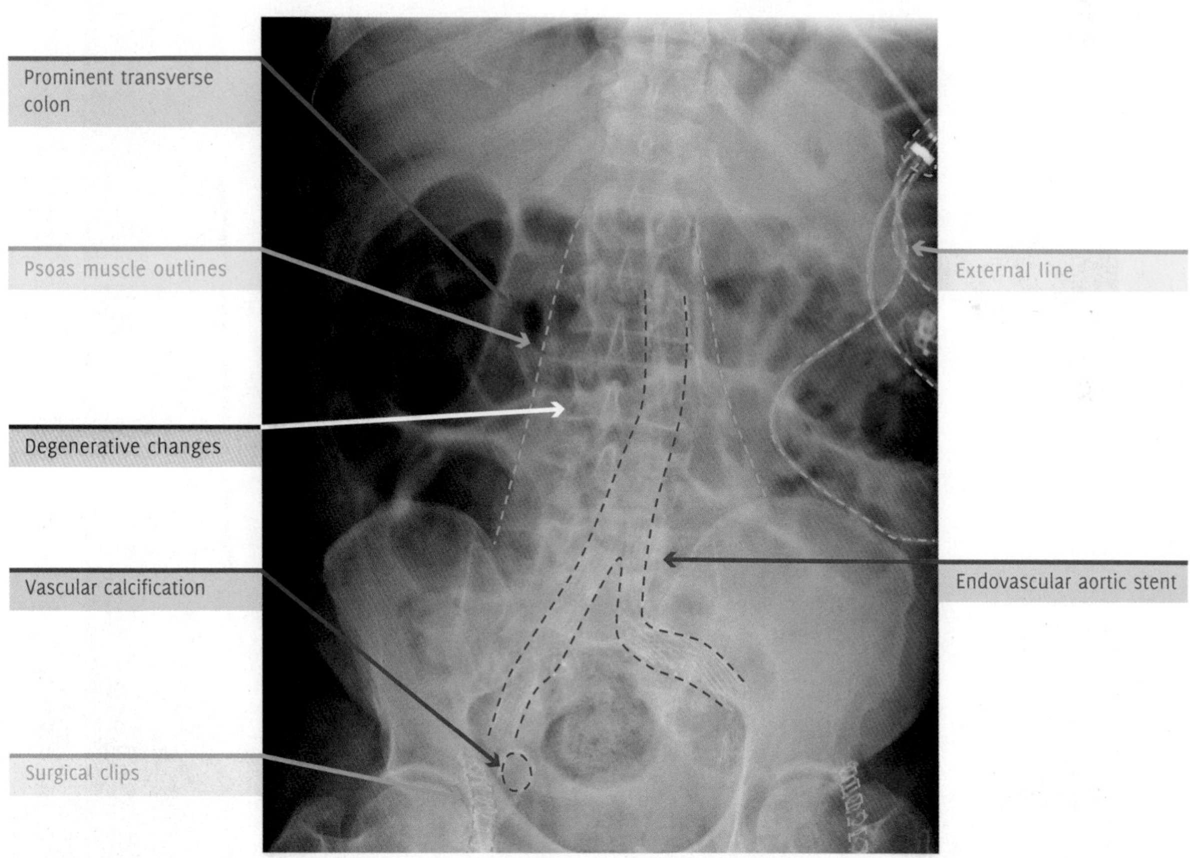

SUMMARY

There is a fenestrated endovascular iliac branch aortic stent seen within the abdominal aorta, extending into the common iliac arteries bilaterally. The surgical clips projecting over the femoral regions bilaterally are in keeping with the recent endovascular aneurysm repair (EVAR).

INVESTIGATIONS AND MANAGEMENT

The iliac branch aortic stent is appropriately sited, and there are no other abnormalities to report on the AXR. Patients with ruptured AAA should initially be cared for in ICU/HDU, but elective patients may be suitable for ward-level care. It is important to ensure that adequate maintenance fluids are prescribed to limit renal damage following CT contrast. Long-term follow-up includes monitoring for signs of AAA increasing in size, and ensuring of compliance with medications and optimal lifestyle strategies to minimize cardiovascular risk.

Case

45

A 64-year-old male presents to ED with right iliac fossa pain and lethargy. His past medical history is significant for type II diabetes mellitus and he is a nonsmoker. On examination, he has oxygen saturations of 95% in air and a temperature of 38.6°C. His HR is 80 bpm, RR is 18 and blood pressure is 120/85 mmHg. The abdomen is soft and there is tenderness in the right iliac fossa with tinkling bowel sounds. Urine dipstick is unremarkable.

An abdominal X-ray is requested to assess for possible bowel obstruction.

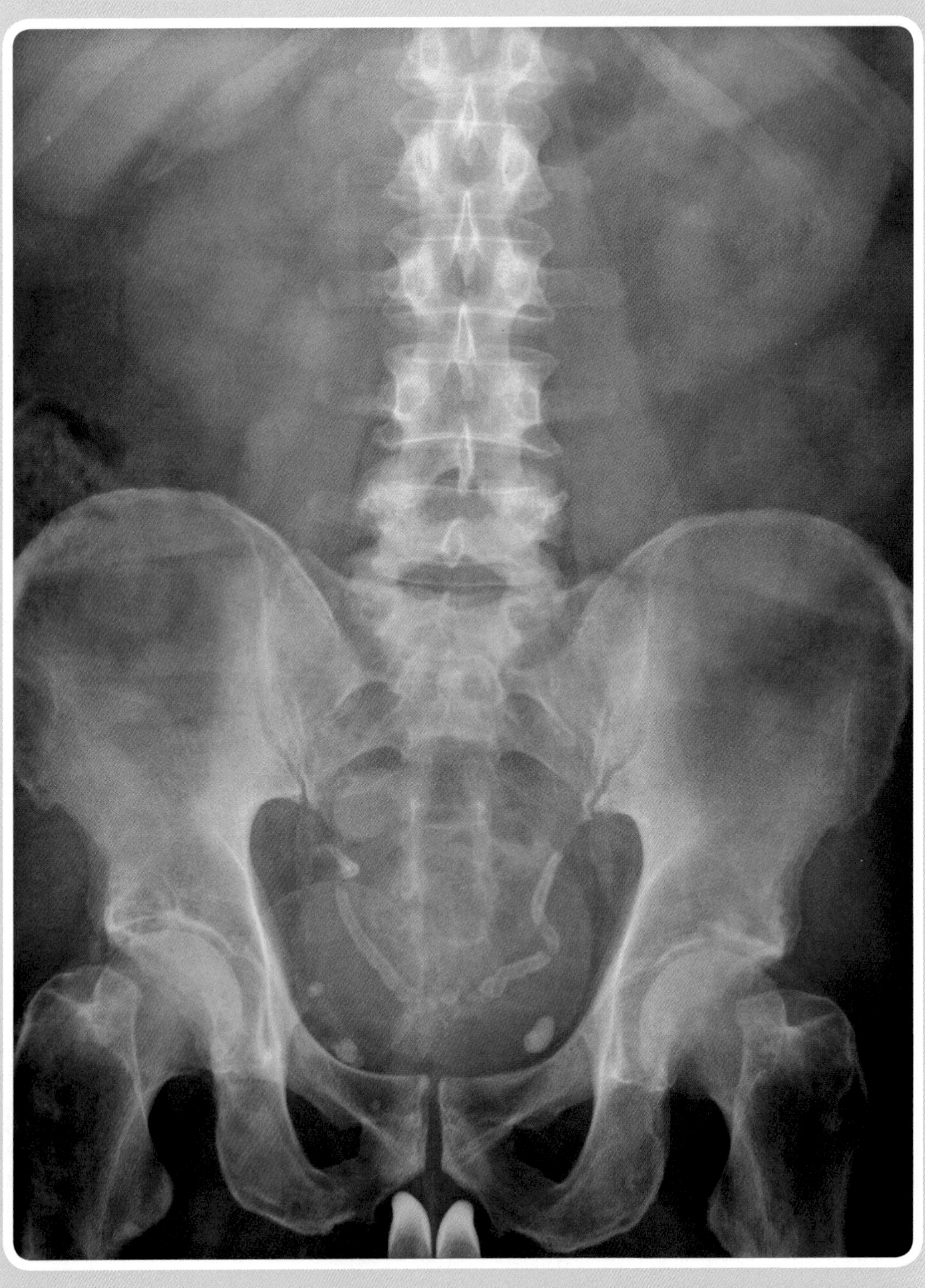

TECHNICAL INFORMATION

Patient ID: Anonymous.
Projection: AP supine.
Rotation: Adequate.
Penetration: Adequate – the spinous processes are visible.
Coverage: Adequate – the anterior ribs are visible superiorly and the inferior pubic rami are visible.

BOWEL GAS PATTERN

The bowel gas pattern is normal.

There is a small volume of faecal residue present in the ascending colon.

BOWEL WALL

There is no evidence of mural thickening or intramural gas within the large or small bowel.

PNEUMOPERITONEUM

There is no evidence of free intraabdominal gas.

SOLID ORGANS

The solid organ contours are within normal limits with no solid organ calcification.

VASCULAR

No abnormal vascular calcification.

BONES

There are no abnormalities of the imaged lumbar spine, or within the pelvis.

SOFT TISSUES

The psoas muscle outline is visible bilaterally.

The extraabdominal soft tissues are unremarkable.

OTHER

There are bilateral serpiginous radiopacities projected over the region of the pelvis, which most likely represents vas deferens calcification.

There are several rounded radiopaque densities projected over the region of the pelvis, which most likely represent phleboliths.

There is a penile implant in situ and a penile implant reservoir projecting over the right hemipelvis.

There are no vascular lines, drains or surgical clips.

REVIEW AREAS

Gallstones/renal calculi: No radiopaque calculi.
Lung bases: Not fully included.
Spine: Normal.
Femoral heads: Normal.

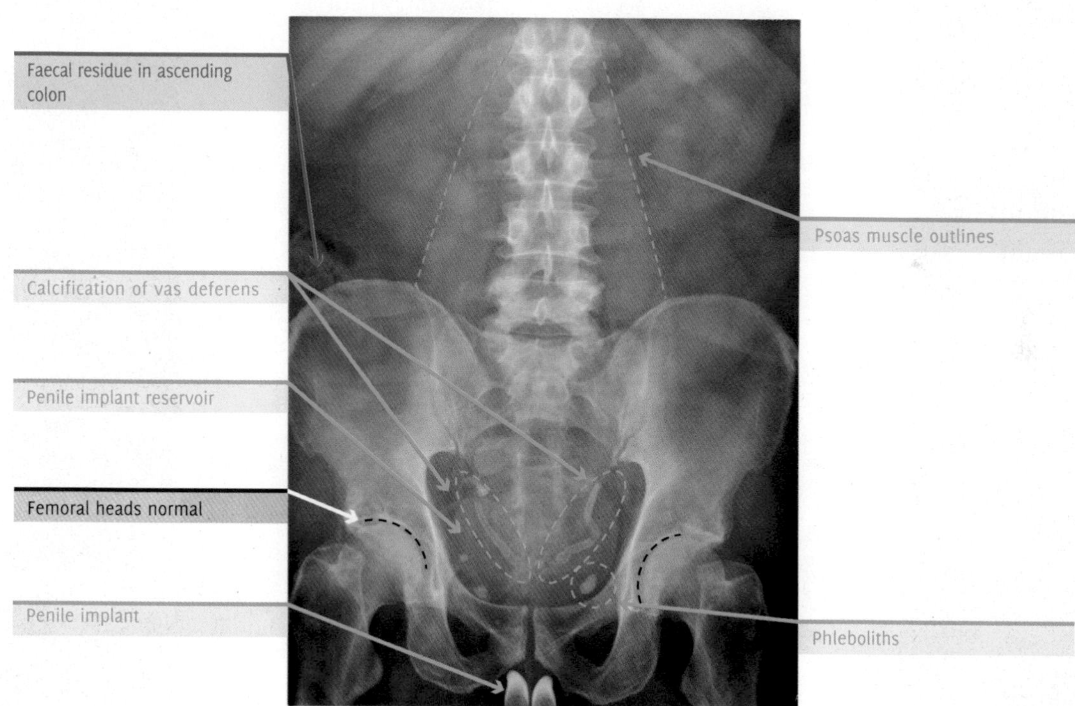

SUMMARY

This X-ray demonstrates serpiginous calcification bilaterally within the pelvis, in keeping with calcification of the vas deferens. It also demonstrates several rounded calcific densities projected over the region of the pelvis, in keeping with phleboliths (areas of calcification within a vein). The penile implant is an incidental finding, likely related to the patient's diabetes resulting in erectile dysfunction. There is no evidence of bowel obstruction or pneumoperitoneum.

INVESTIGATIONS AND MANAGEMENT

The patient should be resuscitated using an ABCDE approach.

Adequate analgesia and hydration should be provided.

Bloods should be taken, including FBC, U&Es, LFTs, amylase, bone profile, CRP, coagulation, blood gas, blood cultures, and group and save.

A CT scan of the abdomen/pelvis with IV contrast may be considered for further evaluation of the abdomen and surgical input should be sought.

Case

46

A 21-year-old female presents to ED with worsening, repeated episodes of bloody diarrhoea for the past 48 hours. She has no significant past medical history and is a nonsmoker. On examination, she has oxygen saturations of 98% in room air and a temperature of 37.9°C. Her HR is 104 bpm, RR is 21 and blood pressure is 128/72 mmHg. The abdomen is soft with generalized tenderness and normal bowel sounds. Urine dipstick is unremarkable and a pregnancy test is negative.

An abdominal X-ray is requested to assess for possible colitis.

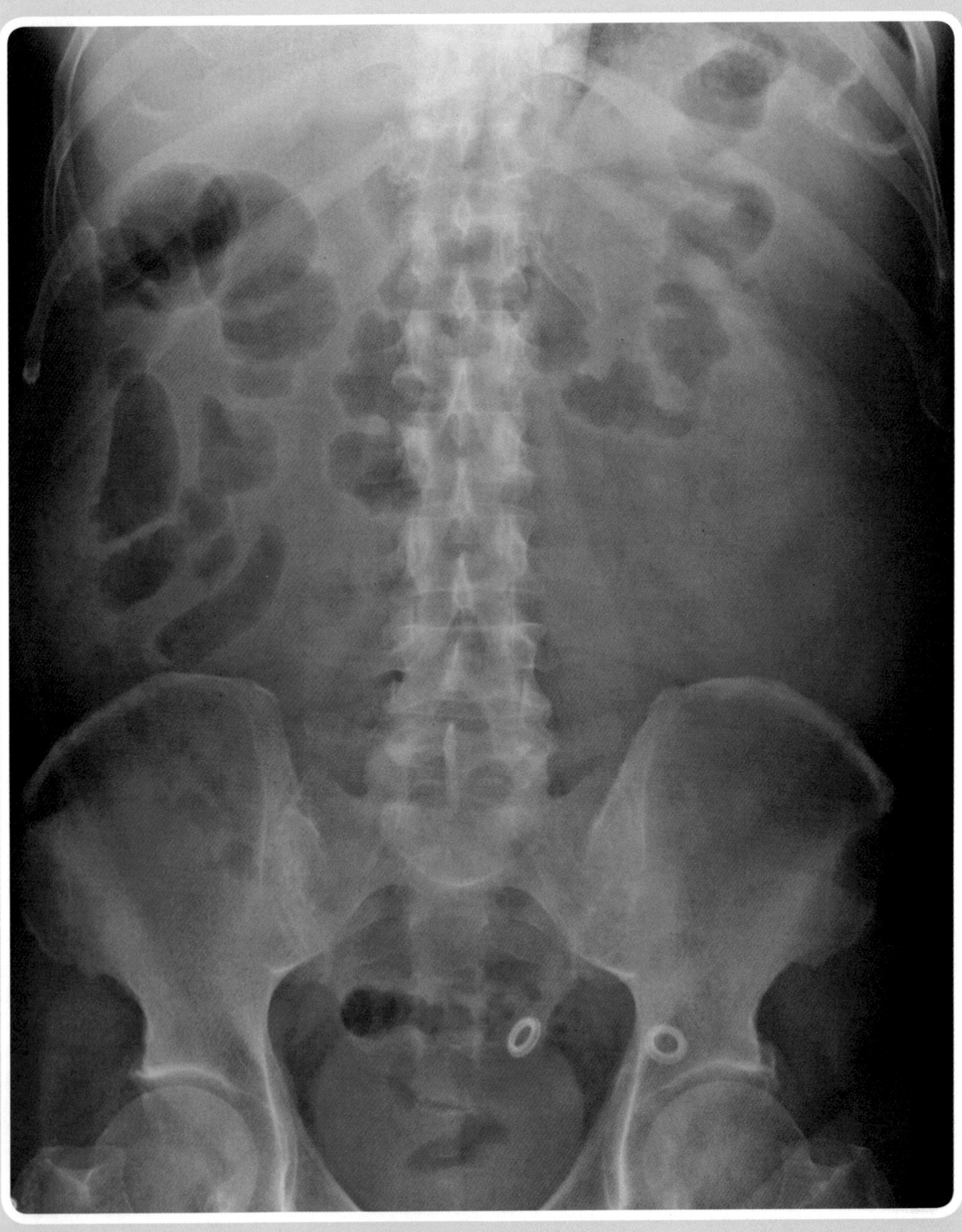

TECHNICAL INFORMATION

Patient ID: Anonymous.
Projection: AP supine.
Rotation: Adequate.
Penetration: Adequate – the spinous processes are visible.
Coverage: Inadequate – the pubic symphysis and inferior pubic rami have not been included.

BOWEL GAS PATTERN

The bowel gas pattern is normal.

BOWEL WALL

There is mural thickening of the transverse colon in the left upper quadrant, with loss of the normal colonic haustral folds and evidence of 'thumbprinting', in keeping with mural oedema.

There is no evidence of intramural gas within the large or small bowel.

PNEUMOPERITONEUM

There is no evidence of free intraabdominal gas.

SOLID ORGANS

The solid organ contours are within normal limits with no solid organ calcification.

VASCULAR

No abnormal vascular calcification.

BONES

There are no abnormalities of the imaged thoracic and lumbar spine, or within the pelvis.

SOFT TISSUES

The psoas muscle outline is visible bilaterally.

The extraabdominal soft tissues are unremarkable.

OTHER

There are two rounded radiopaque bodies seen projected over the left hemipelvis in keeping with clothing artefact.

There are no vascular lines, drains or surgical clips.

REVIEW AREAS

Gallstones/renal calculi: No radiopaque calculi.
Lung bases: Not fully included.
Spine: Normal.
Femoral heads: Normal.

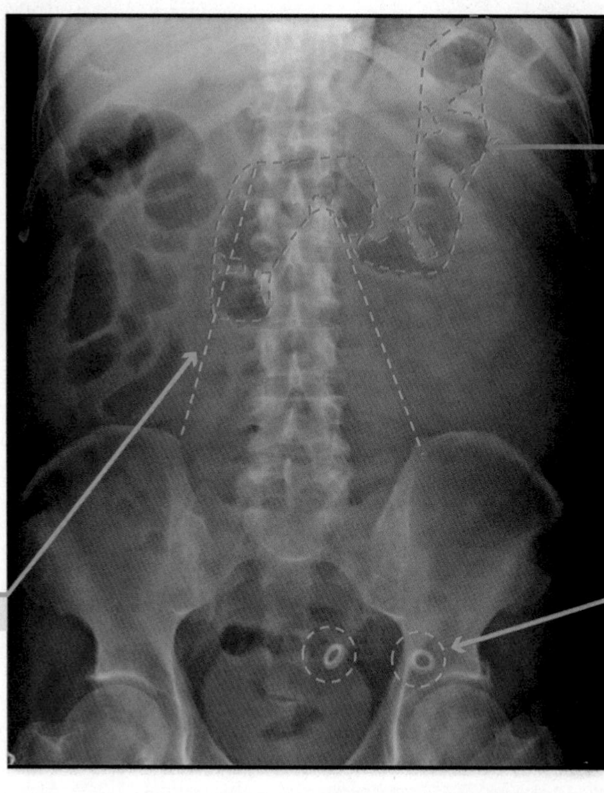

SUMMARY

This X-ray demonstrates mural oedema of the transverse colon, with loss of the normal colonic haustral folds and evidence of thumbprinting, suggestive of colitis. Given the clinical history, this is likely infective or inflammatory in nature.

INVESTIGATIONS AND MANAGEMENT

This patient should be resuscitated using an ABCDE approach.

Adequate analgesia and hydration should be provided.

Urgent bloods should be taken, including FBC, U&Es, LFTs, ESR, CRP, iron studies, folate, blood gas, and group and save. A stool sample should be sent.

Urgent referral to the gastroenterology team should be considered.

A CT scan of the abdomen/pelvis with IV contrast should be considered for better visualization of the anatomy and to assess for complications.

Treatment will depend on the results of further investigations, as well as the clinical state of the patient.

Case

47

A 20-year-old female presents to ED with repeated episodes of bloody diarrhoea that have been getting worse over the past 24 hours. She has no significant past medical history and is a nonsmoker. On examination, she has oxygen saturations of 98% in room air and a temperature of 39.2°C. Her HR is 88 bpm, RR is 20 and blood pressure is 120/68 mmHg. The abdomen is rigid and there is generalized tenderness with normal bowel sounds. Urine dipstick is unremarkable and a pregnancy test is negative.

An abdominal X-ray is requested as assess for possible bowel obstruction.

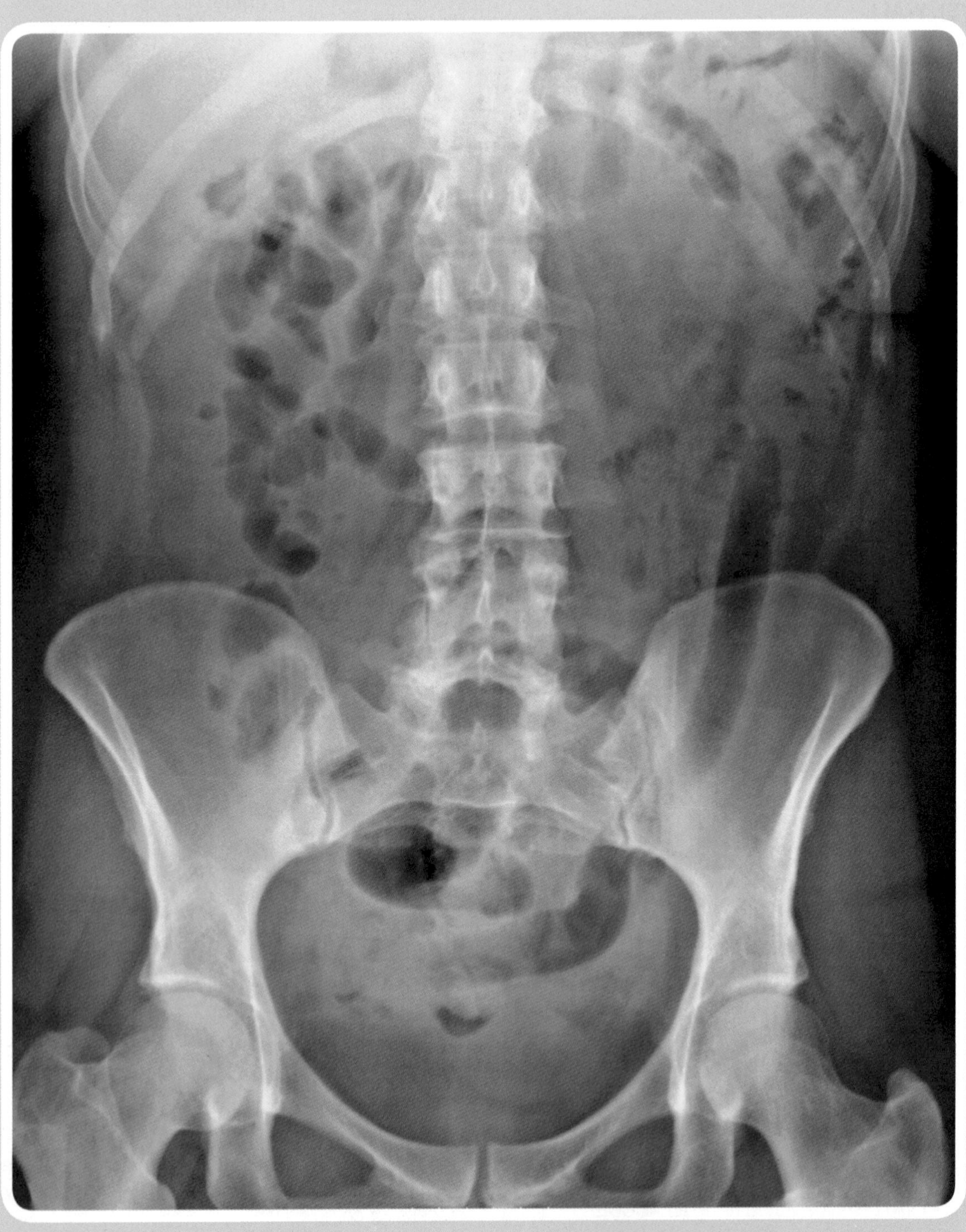

TECHNICAL INFORMATION

Patient ID: Anonymous.
Projection: AP supine.
Rotation: Adequate.
Penetration: Adequate – the spinous processes are visible.
Coverage: Adequate – the anterior ribs are visible superiorly and the pubic rami are visible inferiorly.

BOWEL GAS PATTERN

The bowel gas pattern is normal.

BOWEL WALL

There is evidence of mural thickening within the distal descending and sigmoid colon in the left lower quadrant, with loss of the normal colonic haustral folds, in keeping with mural oedema. This is termed 'lead pipe colon'.

There is no evidence of intramural gas within the large or small bowel.

PNEUMOPERITONEUM

There is no evidence of free intraabdominal gas.

SOLID ORGANS

The solid organ contours are within normal limits with no solid organ calcification.

VASCULAR

No abnormal vascular calcification.

BONES

There is lumbarization of S1, which is a normal anatomical variant. There are no other abnormalities of the imaged thoracic and lumbar spine, or within the pelvis.

SOFT TISSUES

The psoas muscle outline is visible bilaterally.

The extraabdominal soft tissues are unremarkable.

OTHER

There are no radiopaque foreign bodies.

There are no vascular lines, drains or surgical clips.

REVIEW AREAS

Gallstones/renal calculi: No radiopaque calculi.
Lung bases: Not fully included.
Spine: Normal.
Femoral heads: Normal.

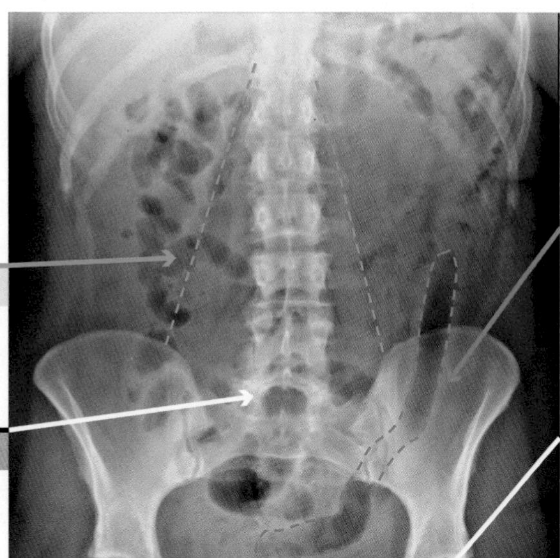

SUMMARY

This X-ray demonstrates mural oedema of the distal descending and sigmoid colon, with loss of the normal colonic haustral folds. Given the clinical history, these findings are likely secondary to acute colitis which is infective or inflammatory in nature.

INVESTIGATIONS AND MANAGEMENT

This patient should be resuscitated using an ABCDE approach.

Adequate analgesia and hydration should be provided.

Urgent bloods should be taken, including FBC, U&Es, LFTs, ESR, CRP, iron studies, folate, blood gas, and group and save. A stool sample should be sent.

Urgent referral to the gastroenterology team should be considered.

A CT scan of the abdomen/pelvis with IV contrast should be considered for better visualization of the anatomy and to assess for complications.

Treatment will depend on the results of further investigations as well as the clinical state of the patient.

Case

48

A 17-year-old male presents to ED with abdominal pain, vomiting and an inability to bear weight on his left leg. His past medical history is significant for congenital spinal problems and he is a nonsmoker. He has a VP shunt in situ and is awaiting a PEG-J tube due to severe reflux. On examination, he has oxygen saturations of 99% in room air and a temperature of 36.4°C. His HR is 95 bpm, RR is 23 and blood pressure is 126/69 mmHg. The abdomen is soft with generalized mild tenderness and normal bowel sounds. He is unable to perform any voluntary movements of the back or left hip due to pain.

An abdominal X-ray is requested to assess for the position of the VP shunt, and for possible bowel obstruction.

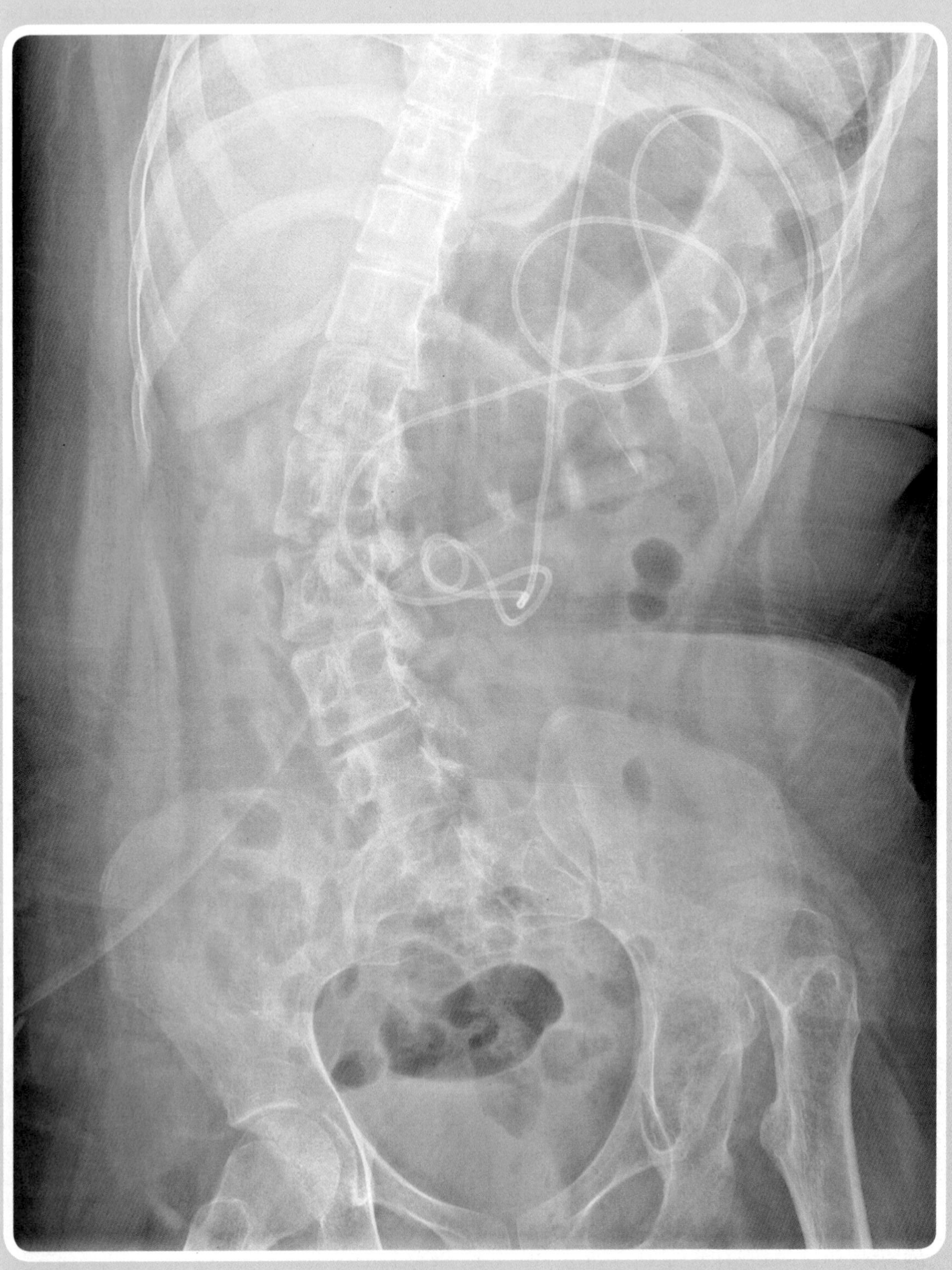

TECHNICAL INFORMATION

Patient ID: Anonymous.
Projection: AP supine.
Rotation: Adequate.
Penetration: Adequate – the spinous processes are visible.
Coverage: Inadequate – the pubic symphysis and inferior pubic rami have not been fully included.

BOWEL GAS PATTERN

The bowel gas pattern is normal.

BOWEL WALL

There is no evidence of mural thickening or intramural gas within the large or small bowel.

PNEUMOPERITONEUM

There is no evidence of free intraabdominal gas.

SOLID ORGANS

The solid organ contours are within normal limits with no solid organ calcification.

VASCULAR

No abnormal vascular calcification.

BONES

There is a moderate thoracolumbar scoliosis seen convex to the right, centred on the L2 vertebral body.

There are osteophytes in the lower thoracic and upper lumbar spine with left-sided bridging osteophyte formation.

The left femoral head is abnormally positioned superolaterally to the acetabulum in keeping with a posterior hip dislocation. There is no associated fracture.

SOFT TISSUES

The psoas muscle outline is visible bilaterally.

The extraabdominal soft tissues are unremarkable.

OTHER

There is a VP shunt in situ, which appears intact with its tip projecting over the left upper quadrant.

There is a radiopaque line seen, which is likely external to the patient, projected across the abdomen of indeterminate significance.

There are no vascular lines, drains or surgical clips.

REVIEW AREAS

Gallstones/renal calculi: No radiopaque calculi.
Lung bases: Right lung base not fully included.
Spine: Thoracolumbar scoliosis convex to the right, centred on the L2 vertebral body with osteophyte formation and bridging osteophytes on the left.
Femoral heads: The contours of the left hip are abnormal. The acetabulum is shallow and there is superolateral displacement of the left femoral head consistent with a posterior hip dislocation. The femoral head is also dysplastic.

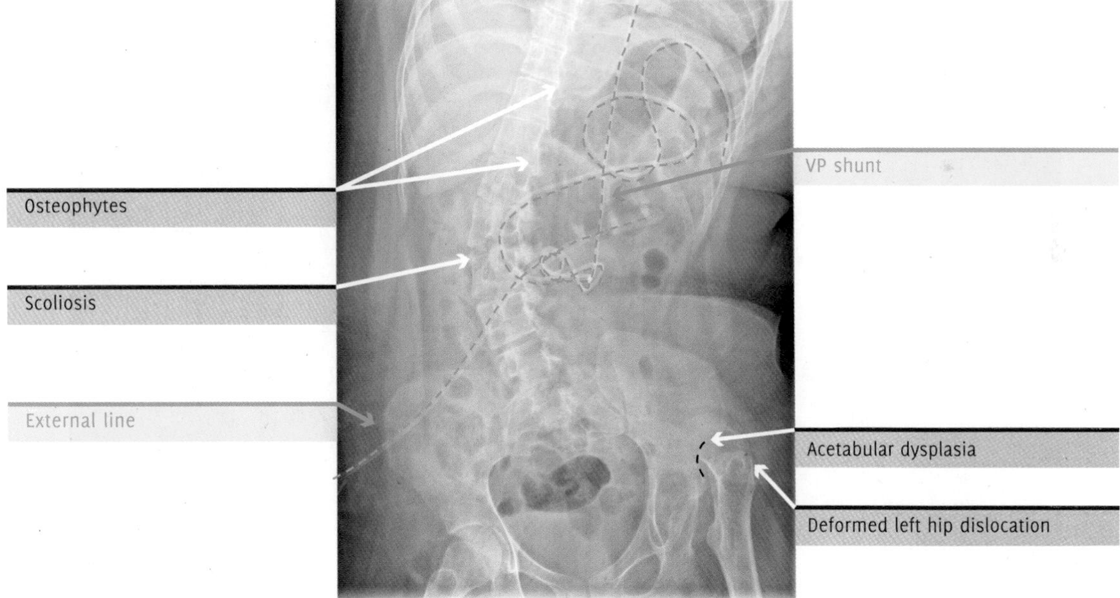

SUMMARY

This X-ray demonstrates a moderate thoracolumbar scoliosis convex to the right, centred on the L2 vertebral body, bridging osteophyte formation in the lower thoracic and upper lumbar spine, and an associated left hip posterior dislocation, which is likely to be chronic given the dysplasia of the acetabulum and femoral head. There is no evidence of any other significant abnormalities. Note is made of the VP shunt with its tip projecting over the left upper quadrant.

INVESTIGATIONS AND MANAGEMENT

This patient should be resuscitated using an ABCDE approach.

Adequate analgesia should be provided.

Bloods should be taken, including FBC, U&Es, bone profile, LFTs, CRP, coagulation, and group and save.

Previous imaging should be reviewed to confirm the age of the hip dislocation, which appears chronic, as well as the scoliosis, and should be discussed with the orthopaedic team.

The patient should be referred to the paediatric team with input from neurosurgery to exclude VP shunt dysfunction.

Case 49

A 2-year-old male presents to ED with worsening abdominal pain. His past medical history is significant for faltering growth, for which he is requiring PEG feeding. On examination, he has oxygen saturations of 97% in room air and a temperature of 37.2°C. His HR is 152 bpm and RR is 40. The abdomen is soft and there is generalized tenderness with normal bowel sounds. Urine dipstick is unremarkable.

An abdominal X-ray is requested to assess for possible bowel obstruction.

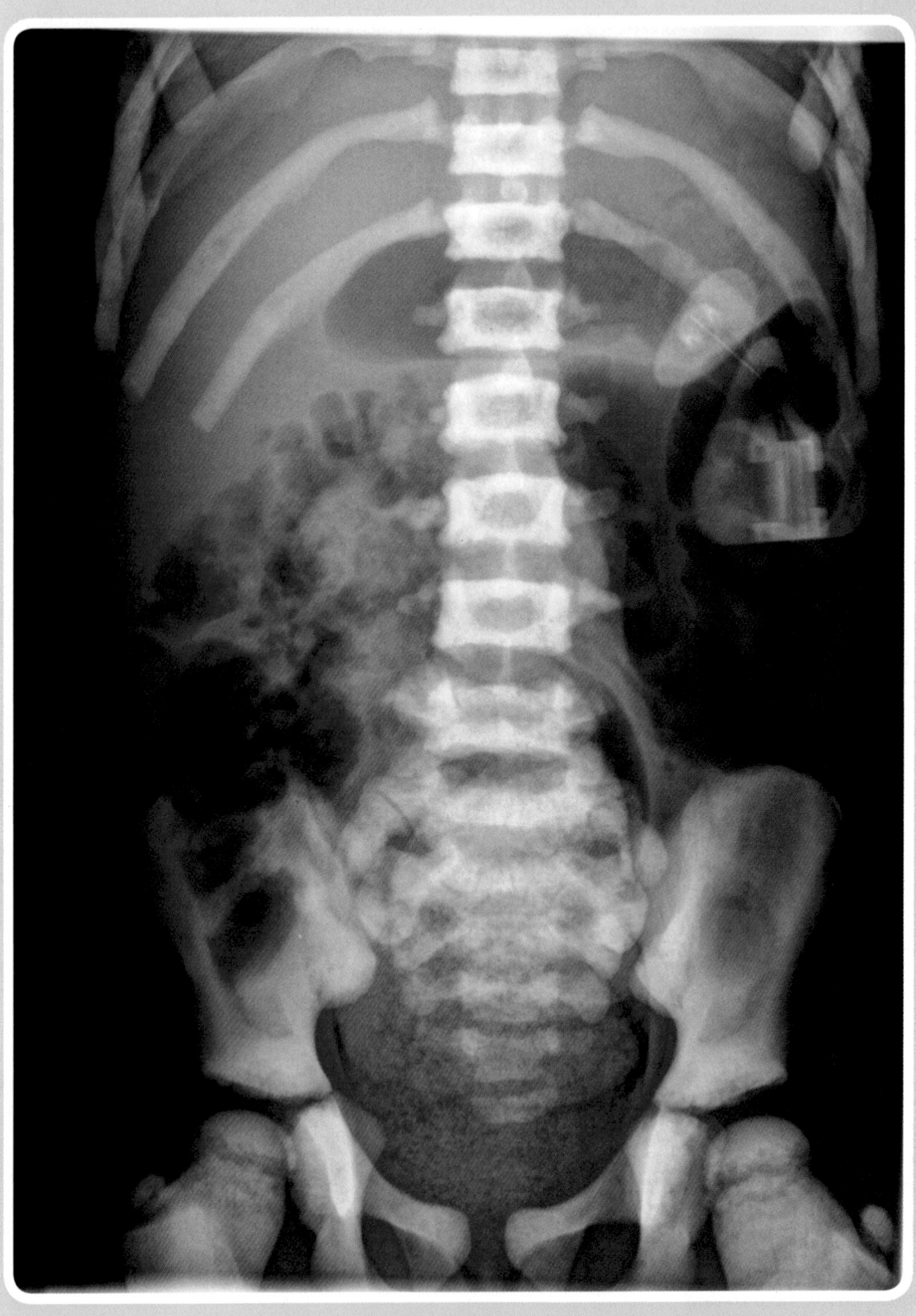

TECHNICAL INFORMATION

Patient ID: Anonymous.
Projection: AP supine.
Rotation: Adequate.
Penetration: Adequate – the spinous processes are visible.
Coverage: Inadequate – the inferior pubic rami have not been fully included.

BOWEL GAS PATTERN

There is a significant volume of faecal residue in the rectum. There is no bowel dilatation.

BOWEL WALL

There is no evidence of mural thickening or intramural gas within the large or small bowel.

PNEUMOPERITONEUM

There is no evidence of free intraabdominal gas.

SOLID ORGANS

The solid organ contours are within normal limits with no solid organ calcification.

VASCULAR

No abnormal vascular calcification.

BONES

There is homogeneous sclerosis and increased density of the bones diffusely.

The vertebrae demonstrate multilevel sub-endplate densities with relative central vertebral lucencies in keeping with 'rugger-jersey spine' appearance.

There is metaphyseal splaying of the femoral necks bilaterally.

There are growth plates at the femoral head, greater trochanter and acetabulum as the ossification centres have not yet fused, which is a normal finding in a child of this age.

SOFT TISSUES

The psoas muscle outline is not visible bilaterally, which is nonspecific, particularly in a child of this age.

The extraabdominal soft tissues are unremarkable.

OTHER

There is a port and radiopaque tube projecting over the left upper quadrant, in keeping with a PEG.

There are no vascular lines, drains or surgical clips.

REVIEW AREAS

Gallstones/renal calculi: No radiopaque calculi.
Lung bases: Not fully included.
Spine: Rugger-jersey appearance.
Femoral heads: Metaphyseal splaying of femoral necks bilaterally and growth plates present.

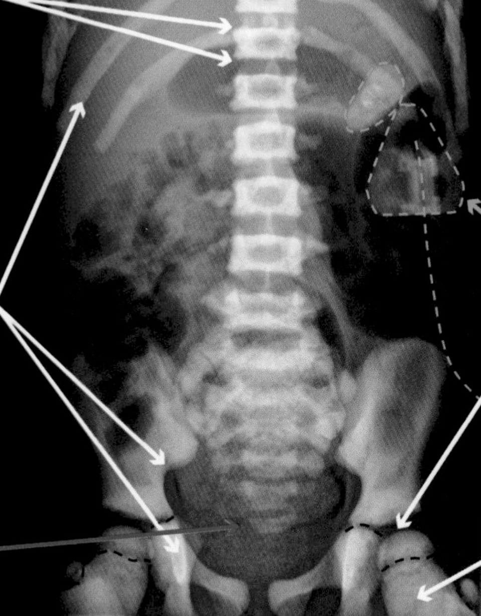

SUMMARY

This X-ray demonstrates diffuse increased bone density, a 'rugger-jersey' spine appearance and metaphyseal splaying of the femoral necks bilaterally. Given the clinical history, the most likely diagnosis is osteopetrosis. Note is made of the PEG gastrostomy in the left upper quadrant. There is a significant volume of faecal residue in the rectum, however no evidence of bowel obstruction.

INVESTIGATIONS AND MANAGEMENT

Adequate analgesia and hydration should be provided.

Bloods should be taken, including FBC, U&Es, bone profile, LFTs, CRP, blood gas, and group and save.

There are no clear findings on the abdominal X-ray to explain the patient's abdominal pain. Surgical input should be sought.

The patient should be referred on to a specialist for further assessment and management of possible osteopetrosis.

Given the complex needs including faltering growth and PEG feeding, the patient is likely to require multidisciplinary team input.

Case

50

An 80-year-old female presents to ED with worsening abdominal distension, nausea and bilious vomiting. Her past medical history is significant for hypertension, osteoarthritis and type II diabetes mellitus. She is a smoker. On examination, she has oxygen saturations of 100% in room air and a temperature of 37.2°C. Her HR is 100 bpm, RR is 22 and blood pressure is 145/90 mmHg. The abdomen is rigid with generalized tenderness and tinkling bowel sounds. Urine dipstick is unremarkable.

An abdominal X-ray is requested to assess for possible bowel obstruction.

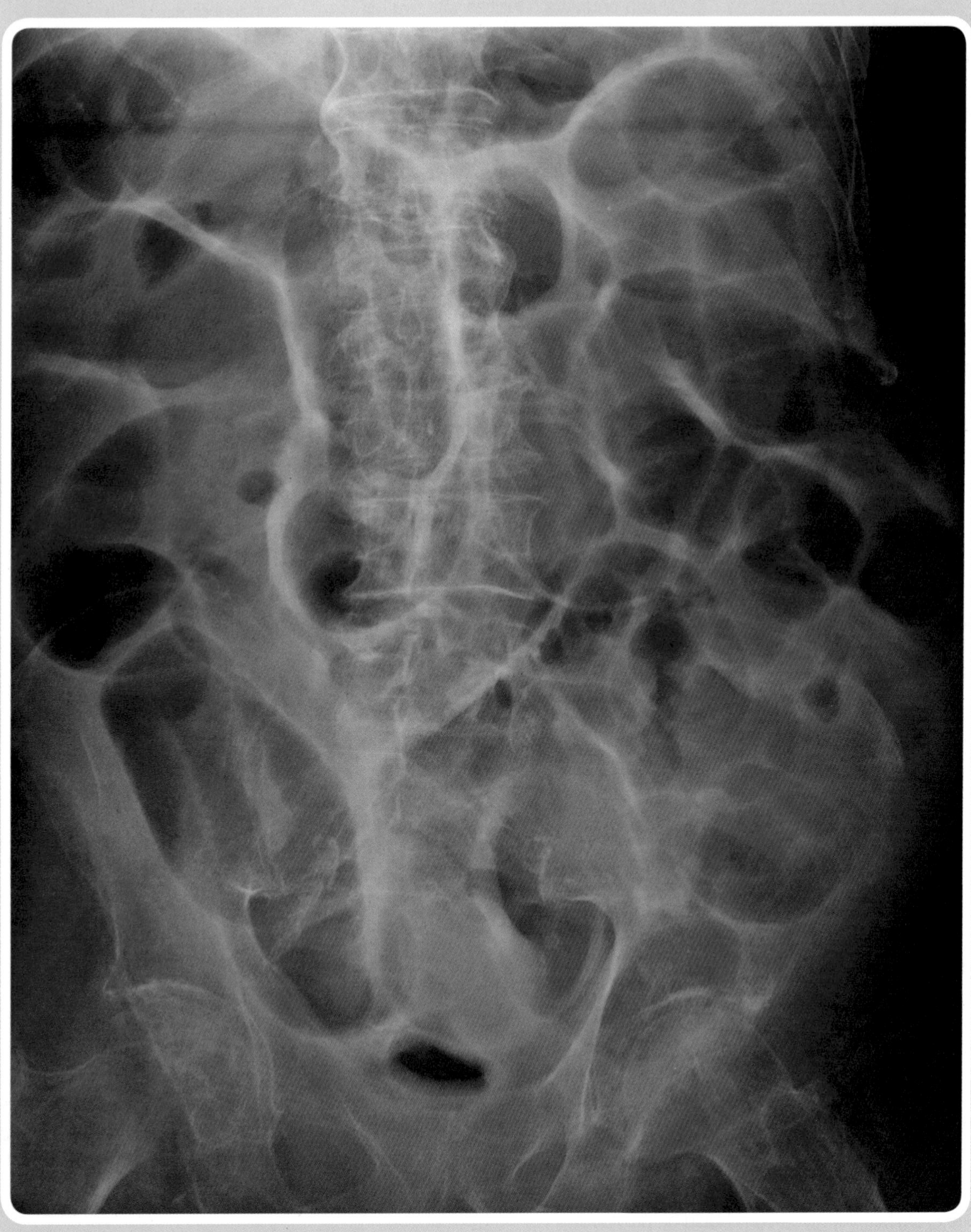

TECHNICAL INFORMATION

Patient ID: Anonymous.
Projection: AP supine.
Rotation: Adequate.
Penetration: Adequate – the spinous processes are visible.
Coverage: Adequate – the anterior ribs are visible superiorly and the inferior pubic rami are visible.

BOWEL GAS PATTERN

There are multiple loops of dilated small and large bowel seen centrally and peripherally within the abdomen, in keeping with bowel obstruction.

BOWEL WALL

There is no evidence of mural thickening or intramural gas within the large or small bowel.

PNEUMOPERITONEUM

There is no evidence of free intraabdominal gas.

SOLID ORGANS

The solid organ contours are within normal limits with no solid organ calcification.

VASCULAR

There is calcification of the right femoral artery and iliac arteries bilaterally.

BONES

There is moderate to severe degenerative change with osteophyte formation and intervertebral disc space narrowing seen throughout the spine.

There is moderate osteoarthritic change seen within both hip joints, including subchondral sclerosis and narrowing of the joint spaces.

There is diffuse osteopenia of the bones.

SOFT TISSUES

The psoas muscle outline is not visible bilaterally, which is nonspecific.

The extraabdominal soft tissues are unremarkable.

OTHER

There are no radiopaque foreign bodies.

There are no vascular lines, drains or surgical clips.

REVIEW AREAS

Gallstones/renal calculi: No radiopaque calculi.
Lung bases: Not fully included.
Spine: Moderate to severe degenerative change.
Femoral heads: Moderate degenerative change.

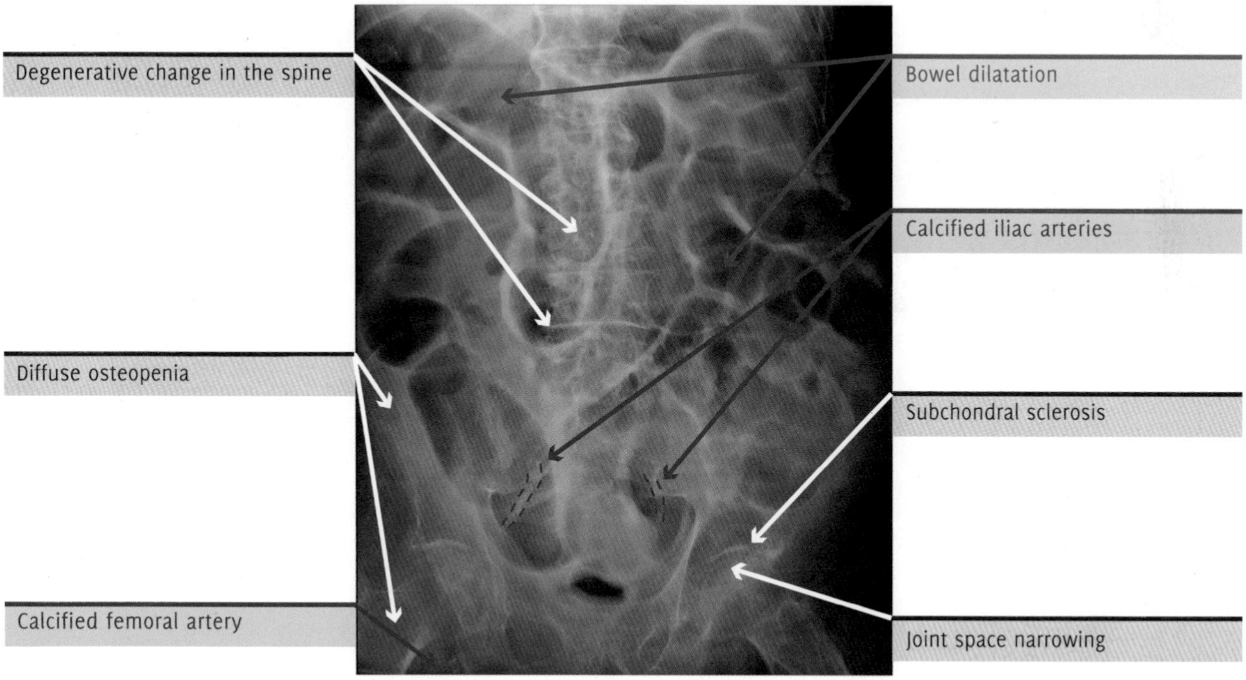

Degenerative change in the spine
Bowel dilatation
Calcified iliac arteries
Diffuse osteopenia
Subchondral sclerosis
Calcified femoral artery
Joint space narrowing

SUMMARY

This X-ray demonstrates multiple loops of dilated small and large bowel seen centrally and peripherally within the abdomen, in keeping with bowel obstruction. This is an open-loop obstruction. No cause for this is visible on the X-ray. The moderate to severe degenerative spinal changes, bilateral moderate hip joint degenerative changes and diffuse osteopenia are incidental findings.

INVESTIGATIONS AND MANAGEMENT

The patient should be resuscitated using an ABCDE approach.

Adequate analgesia and hydration should be provided.

The patient should be kept NBM and an NG tube inserted on free drainage to relieve the pressure in the small bowel. IV fluids should be commenced.

Urgent bloods should be taken, including FBC, U&Es, CRP, bone profile, LFTs, coagulation, blood gas, and group and save.

The general surgical team should be contacted urgently and a CT scan of the abdomen/pelvis with IV contrast should be considered for better visualization of the anatomy and further assessment.

Case

51

A 75-year-old female presents to ED with worsening bone pain and abdominal pain, having not opened her bowels for 5 days. Her past medical history is significant for renal cell carcinoma (awaiting surgery) and she is a nonsmoker. On examination, she has oxygen saturations of 95% in room air and a temperature of 37.1°C. Her HR is 88 bpm, RR is 19 and blood pressure is 130/75 mmHg. The abdomen is soft and nontender with normal bowel sounds. Urine dipstick is unremarkable.

An abdominal X-ray is requested to assess for possible bowel obstruction.

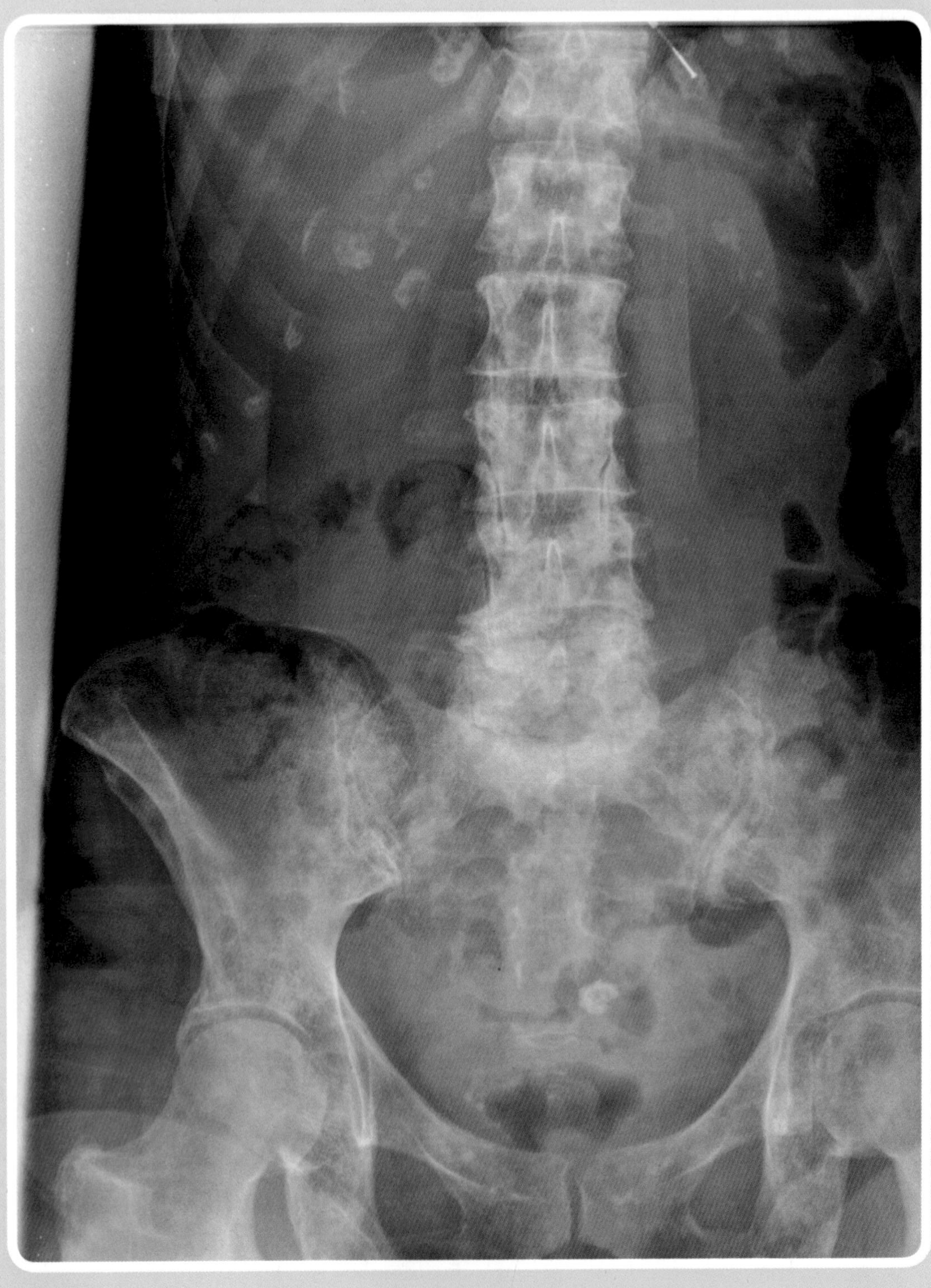

TECHNICAL INFORMATION

Patient ID: Anonymous.
Projection: AP supine.
Rotation: Adequate.
Penetration: Adequate – the spinous processes are visible.
Coverage: Inadequate – the lateral aspect of the left ilium and inferior pubic rami have not been included.

BOWEL GAS PATTERN

There is mild volume of faecal residue predominantly in the ascending colon.

BOWEL WALL

There is no evidence of mural thickening or intramural gas within the large or small bowel.

PNEUMOPERITONEUM

There is no evidence of free intraabdominal gas.

SOLID ORGANS

The solid organ contours are within normal limits with no solid organ calcification.

VASCULAR

No abnormal vascular calcification.

BONES

There are multiple mixed lytic/sclerotic bone lesions throughout the axial skeleton, including in the spine and the pelvis bilaterally.

There are moderate degenerative changes in the distal lumbar spine.

There is bilateral costochondral calcification.

SOFT TISSUES

The psoas muscle outline is visible bilaterally.

The extraabdominal soft tissues are unremarkable.

OTHER

There is a cardiac pacing lead projecting to the left of the T12 vertebral body likely within the right ventricle.

There is an area of calcification projecting within the pelvis likely to represent mesenteric lymph node calcification.

There are no vascular lines, drains or surgical clips.

REVIEW AREAS

Gallstones/renal calculi: No radiopaque calculi.
Lung bases: Not fully included.
Spine: Mixed lytic/sclerotic spinal lesions with moderate degenerative changes in the distal lumbar spine.
Femoral heads: Multiple lytic bone lesions.

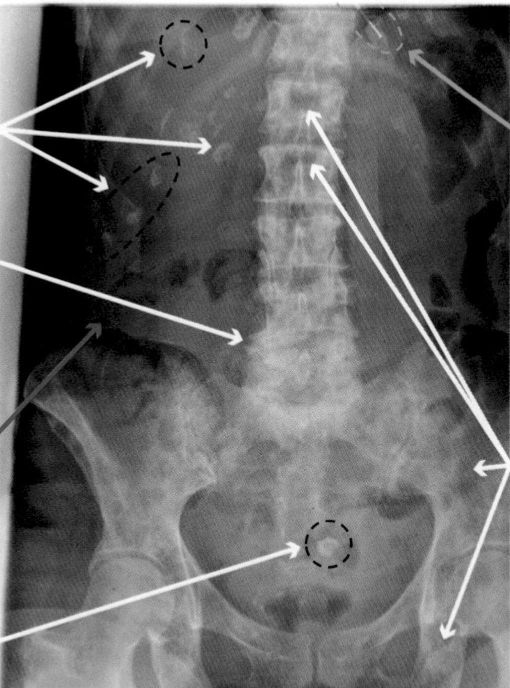

SUMMARY

This X-ray demonstrates multiple mixed lytic/sclerotic bone lesions throughout the degenerative axial skeleton likely to represent metastases secondary to the renal cell carcinoma. There is no evidence of bowel obstruction or pneumoperitoneum. Incidental note is made of the cardiac pacing wire.

INVESTIGATIONS AND MANAGEMENT

The patient should be resuscitated using an ABCDE approach.

Adequate analgesia and hydration should be provided.

Urgent bloods should be taken, including FBC, U&Es, CRP, LFTs, bone profile, blood gas and tumour markers.

If no recent imaging has been performed, a staging CT scan of the chest, abdomen and pelvis with IV contrast should be considered to assess the known renal cell carcinoma and for disease progression.

The patient should be referred to oncology for further management, which may include biopsy and MDT discussion. Treatment, which may include surgery, radiotherapy, chemotherapy or palliative treatment, will depend on the outcome of the MDT investigations and the patients' wishes.

Case

52

A 25-year-old female presents to ED with diarrhoea. Her past medical history is significant for Crohn's disease and she is a nonsmoker. On examination, she has oxygen saturations of 98% in room air and a temperature of 37.4°C. Her HR is 82 bpm, RR is 14 and blood pressure is 110/60 mmHg. The abdomen is soft and there is generalized tenderness with normal bowel sounds. Urine dipstick is unremarkable and a pregnancy test is negative.

An abdominal X-ray is requested to assess for possible colitis.

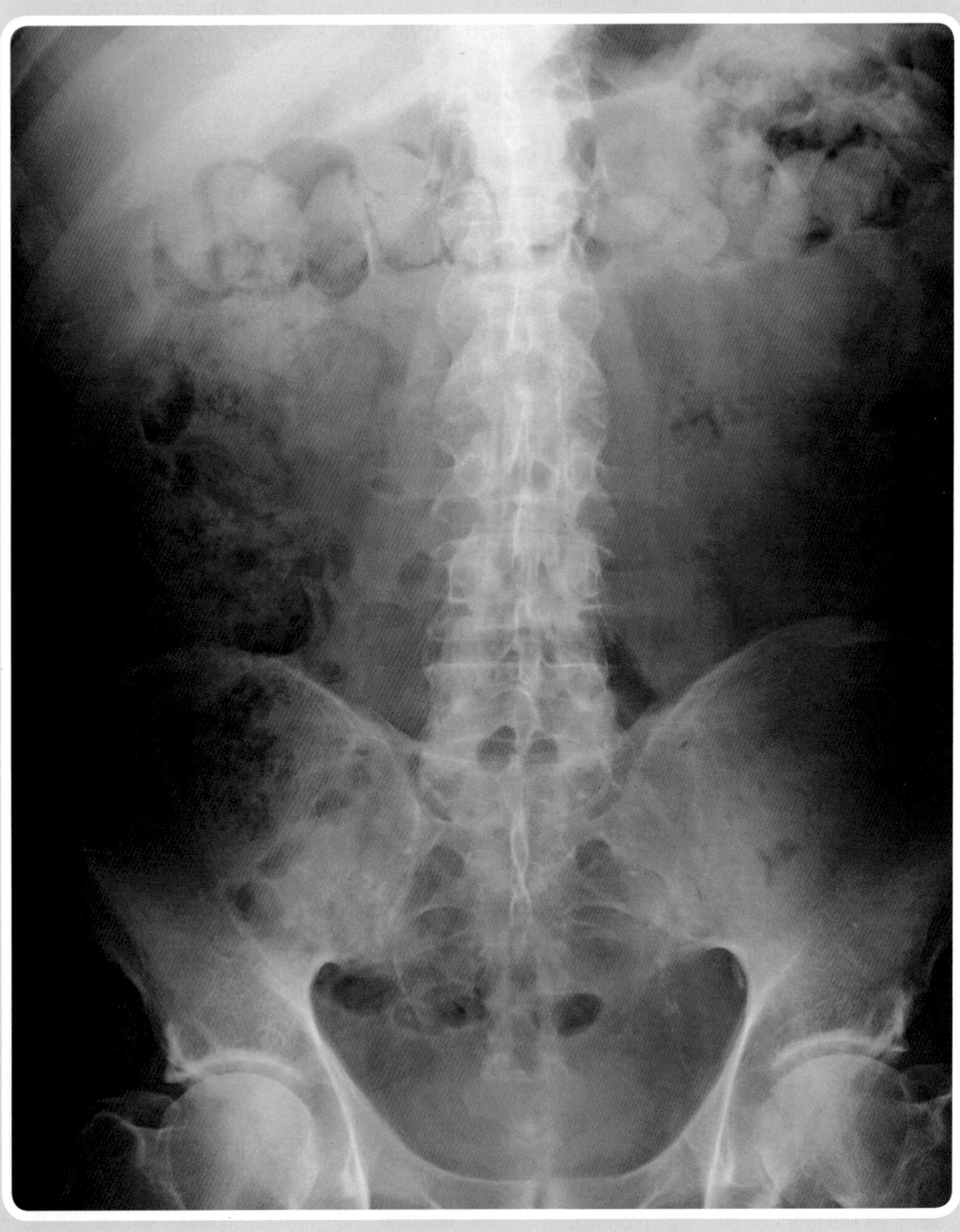

TECHNICAL INFORMATION

Patient ID: Anonymous.
Projection: AP supine.
Rotation: Adequate.
Penetration: Adequate – the spinous processes are visible.
Coverage: Inadequate – the pubic symphysis and inferior pubic rami have not been fully included.

BOWEL GAS PATTERN

The bowel gas pattern is normal.

There is a moderate volume of faecal residue present throughout the ascending colon and hard faeces within the transverse colon.

BOWEL WALL

There is no evidence of mural thickening or intramural gas within the large or small bowel.

PNEUMOPERITONEUM

There is no evidence of free intraabdominal gas.

SOLID ORGANS

The solid organ contours are within normal limits with no solid organ calcification.

VASCULAR

No abnormal vascular calcification.

BONES

There is fusion of the sacroiliac joints bilaterally.

There are no abnormalities of the imaged thoracic and lumbar spine.

SOFT TISSUES

The psoas muscle outline is visible bilaterally.

The extraabdominal soft tissues are unremarkable.

OTHER

There are no radiopaque foreign bodies.

There are no vascular lines, drains or surgical clips.

REVIEW AREAS

Gallstones/renal calculi: No radiopaque calculi.
Lung bases: Not fully included.
Spine: Normal.
Femoral heads: Normal.

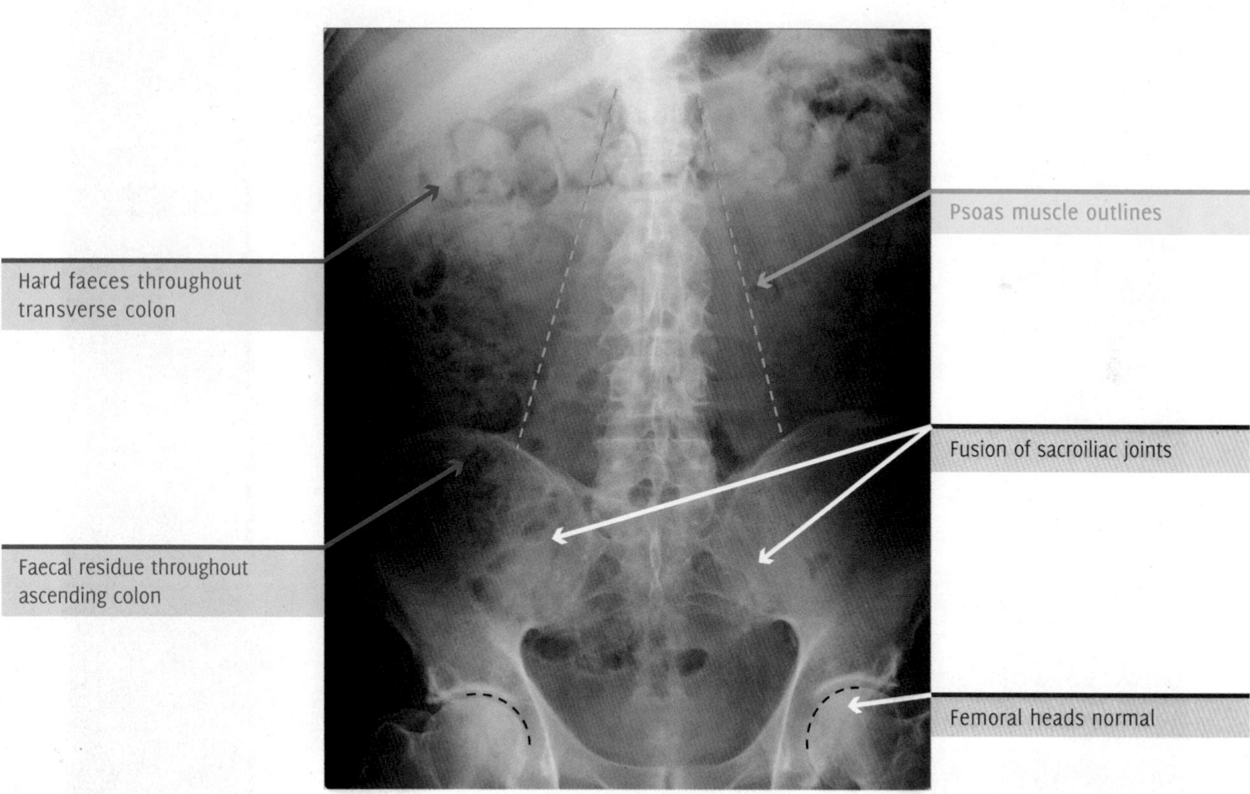

SUMMARY

This X-ray demonstrates a moderate volume of faecal residue in the ascending colon with hard faeces in the transverse colon, however no evidence of mural oedema or active colitis. Findings may suggest overflow diarrhoea given the clinical history. The bilateral fusion of the sacroiliac joints is an incidental finding and likely related to enteropathic arthritis.

INVESTIGATIONS AND MANAGEMENT

The patient should be resuscitated using an ABCDE approach.

Adequate analgesia and hydration should be provided.

Treatment should aim to disimpact the patient's bowel with either oral laxatives or an enema, and then advice should be given regarding lifestyle adjustments, including adequate fluid intake, sufficient dietary fibre and exercise.

Case

53

A 42-year-old male presents to ED with abdominal distension, night sweats, lymphadenopathy and weight loss. He is currently undergoing investigations for this. He is a nonsmoker. On examination, he has oxygen saturations of 99% in room air and a temperature of 36.2°C. His HR is 80 bpm, RR is 19 and blood pressure is 120/72 mmHg. His abdomen is soft and grossly distended and there is no tenderness. Massive hepatosplenomegaly is detected. Bowel sounds are normal. Urine dipstick is unremarkable.

An abdominal X-ray is requested to assess for possible bowel obstruction.

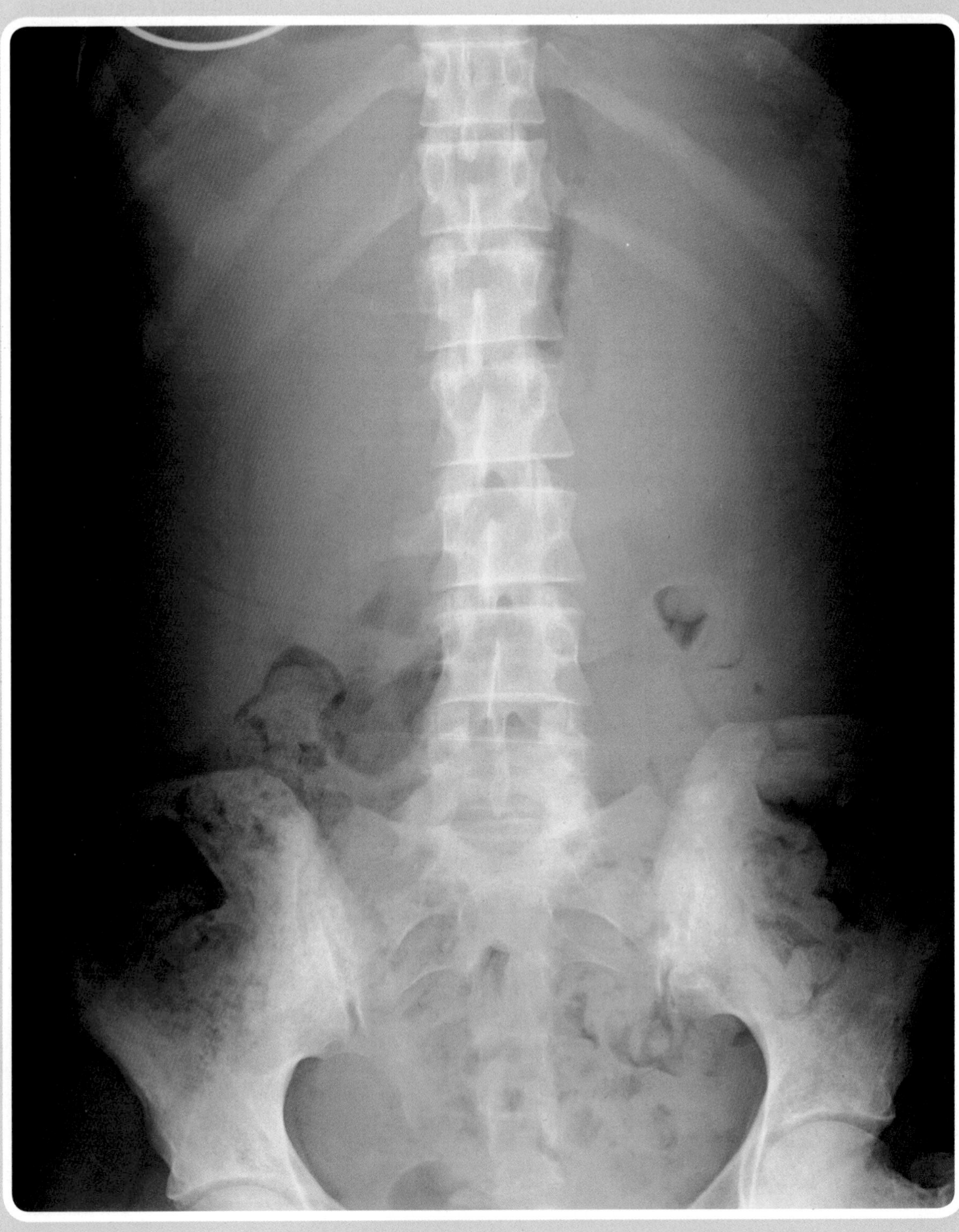

TECHNICAL INFORMATION

Patient ID: Anonymous.
Projection: AP supine.
Rotation: Adequate.
Penetration: Adequate – the spinous processes are visible.
Coverage: Inadequate – the pubic symphysis, inferior pubic rami and hip joints have not been fully included.

BOWEL GAS PATTERN

The bowel is displaced inferiorly into the lower abdomen and pelvis by a homogeneous opacification in the upper abdomen.

There is faecal residue present throughout the large bowel.

BOWEL WALL

There is no evidence of mural thickening or intramural gas within the large or small bowel.

PNEUMOPERITONEUM

There is no evidence of free intraabdominal gas.

SOLID ORGANS

There is a large homogeneous opacification projecting across the upper abdomen bilaterally, in keeping with massive hepatosplenomegaly.

VASCULAR

No abnormal vascular calcification.

BONES

There are no abnormalities of the imaged thoracic and lumbar spine.

SOFT TISSUES

The psoas muscle outline is visible bilaterally.

The extraabdominal soft tissues are unremarkable.

OTHER

There is a radiopaque line projected over the region of the right upper quadrant, likely representing an external line.

There are no vascular lines, drains or surgical clips.

REVIEW AREAS

Gallstones/renal calculi: No radiopaque calculi.
Lung bases: Not fully included.
Spine: Normal.
Femoral heads: Not visible.

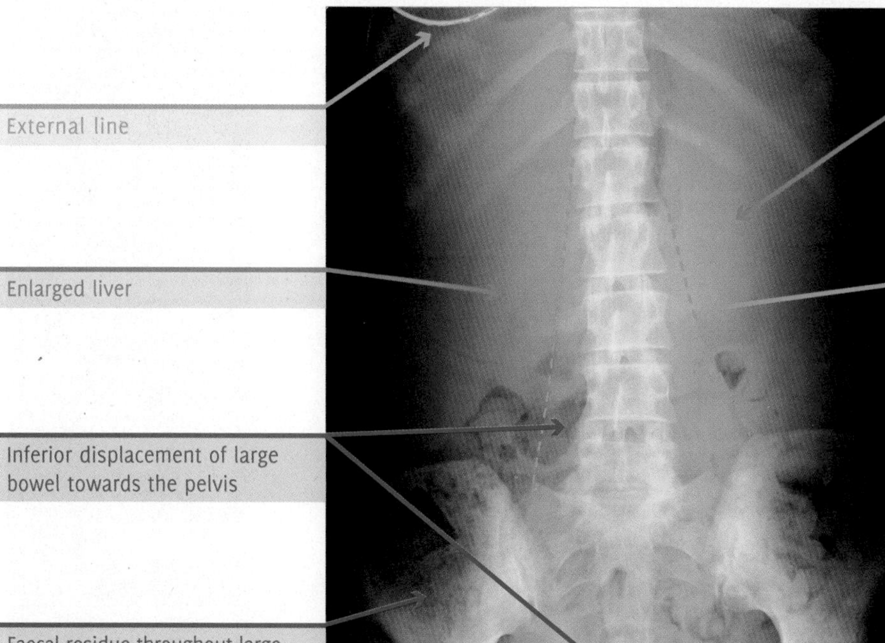

SUMMARY

This X-ray demonstrates a large homogeneous opacification in the upper abdomen causing inferior displacement of the bowel into the lower abdomen and pelvis, in keeping with massive hepatosplenomegaly.

INVESTIGATIONS AND MANAGEMENT

The patient should be resuscitated using an ABCDE approach.

Adequate analgesia and hydration should be provided.

Urgent bloods should be taken, including FBC, U&Es, CRP, ESR, LFTs, bone profile, LDH, hepatitis screening, CMV and EBV screening, clotting, tumour markers, blood gas and blood film.

An USS of the abdomen should be considered in the first instance to image the liver and spleen more clearly and to assess for any associated portal hypertension.

A CT scan of the chest, abdomen and pelvis with IV contrast should be considered for further evaluation and to assess for nodal enlargement elsewhere.

Depending on the test results, a referral to haematology and/or oncology services should be considered for further management, which may include biopsy and MDT discussion. Treatment, which may include surgery, radiotherapy, chemotherapy or palliative treatment, will depend on the outcome of the MDT, investigations and the patient's wishes.

Case

54

A 12-day-old baby boy born at 34 weeks gestation presents to ED with abdominal distension and vomiting. He has not opened his bowels for over 24 hours. He has no significant past medical history. On examination, he has oxygen saturations of 97% in room air and a temperature of 37.0°C. His HR is 220 bpm and RR is 62. The abdomen is soft and a hernia is noted in the left groin. Urine dipstick is unremarkable.

An abdominal X-ray is requested to assess for possible bowel obstruction.

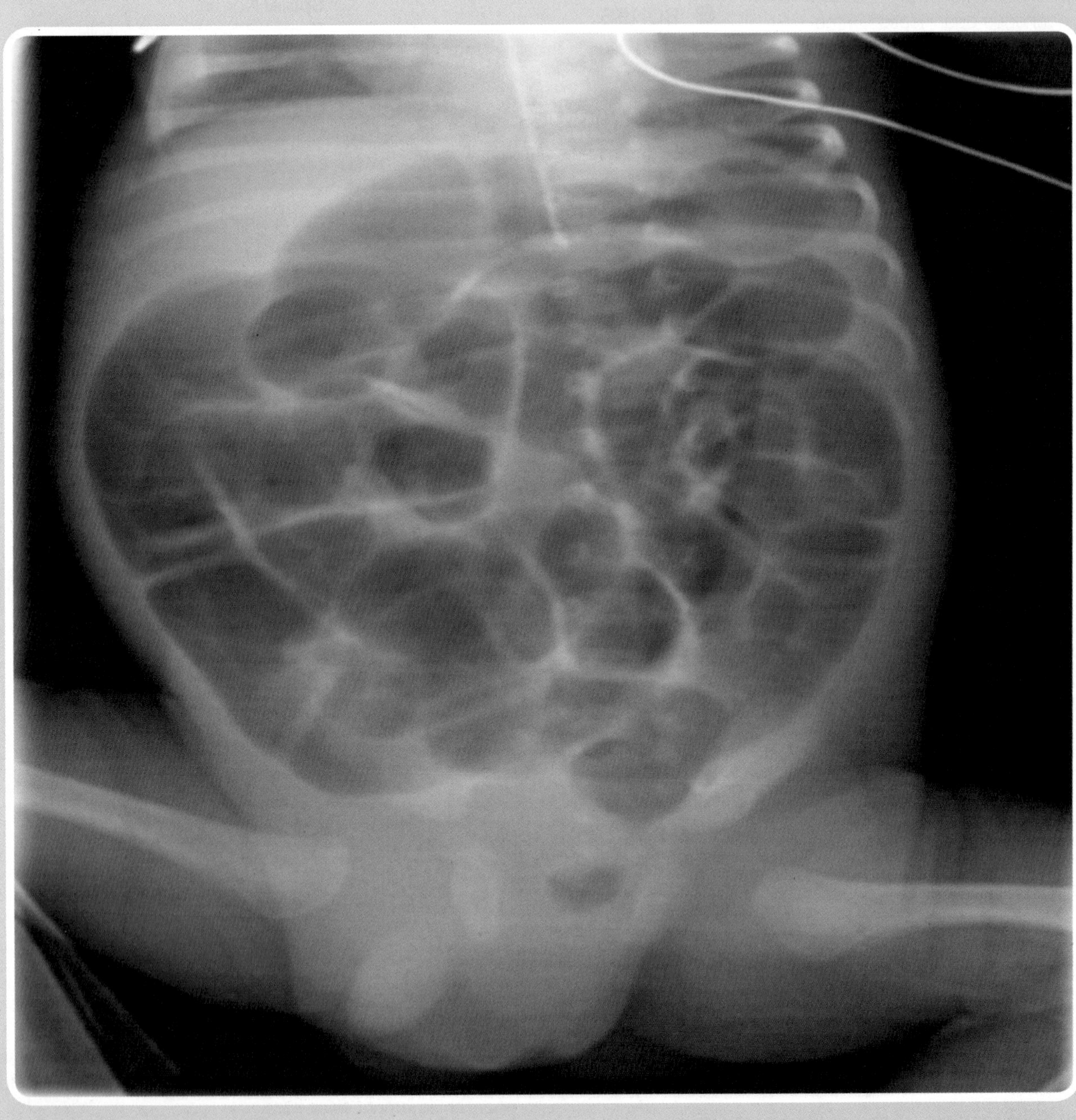

TECHNICAL INFORMATION

Patient ID: Anonymous.
Projection: AP supine – frog leg lateral view.
Rotation: Asymmetrical appearances of the pelvis with deviation of the spine to the left due to patient rotation to the right.
Penetration: Adequate – the spine is visible.
Coverage: Adequate – the anterior ribs are visible superiorly and the inferior pubic rami are visible.

BOWEL GAS PATTERN

There are multiple loops of dilated bowel seen centrally in the abdomen.

There is an air-filled loop of bowel seen within the pelvis in the inguinal region, most likely to represent an incarcerated inguinal hernia.

BOWEL WALL

There is no evidence of mural thickening or intramural gas within the large or small bowel.

PNEUMOPERITONEUM

There is no evidence of free intraabdominal gas.

SOLID ORGANS

The solid organ contours are within normal limits with no solid organ calcification.

VASCULAR

No abnormal vascular calcification.

BONES

The spine appears to be deviated to the left which is due to the rotation of the patient to the right.

There is cartilage present between the pelvic bones and femurs as they have not yet fused, which is a normal finding in a child of this age.

SOFT TISSUES

The psoas muscle outline is not visible bilaterally, which is nonspecific, particularly in a child of this age.

The extraabdominal soft tissues are unremarkable.

OTHER

There is an NG tube in situ, with its tip seen in the left upper quadrant.

There are radiopaque lines projected over the upper abdomen and chest on the left which likely represent external lines.

There are no vascular lines, drains or surgical clips.

REVIEW AREAS

Gallstones/renal calculi: No radiopaque calculi.
Lung bases: Normal.
Spine: Deviated to the left due to the rotation of the patient to the right.
Femoral heads: Normal – growth plates present.

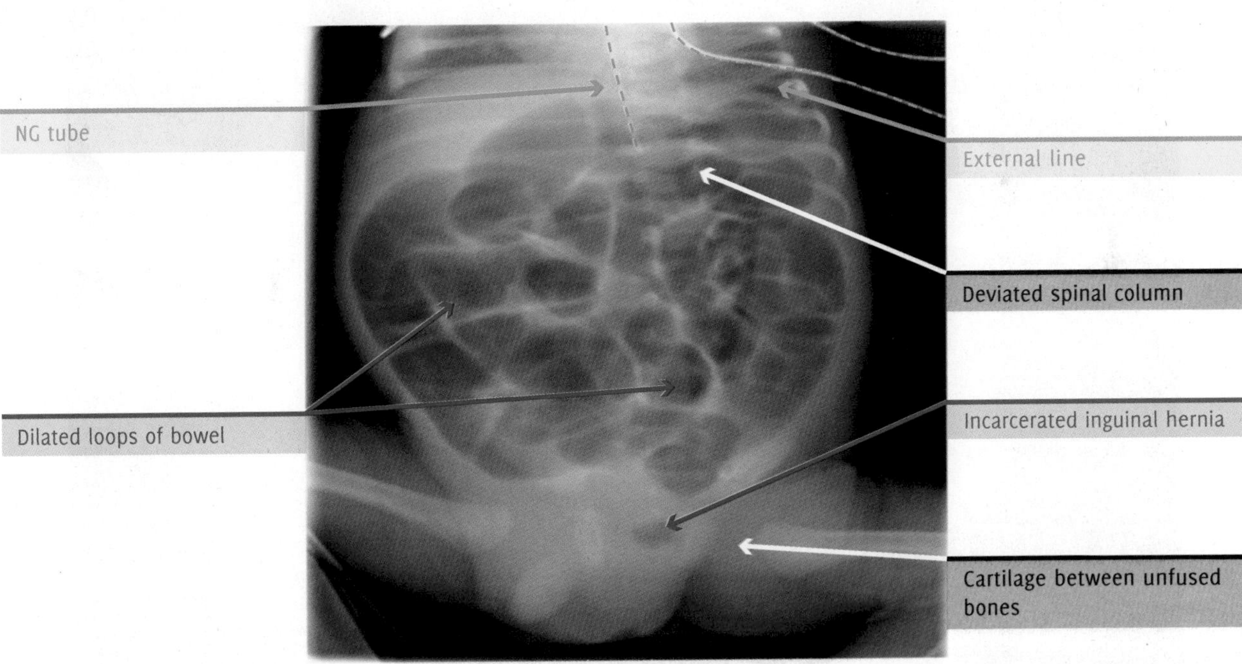

SUMMARY

This X-ray demonstrates multiple loops of dilated bowel seen centrally within the abdomen and an air-filled loop of bowel within the left inguinal region. This is likely to represent bowel obstruction secondary to an incarcerated left inguinal hernia. There is an NG tube in situ but it may be worth advancing to ensure it is in the body of the stomach.

INVESTIGATIONS AND MANAGEMENT

The baby should be resuscitated using an ABCDE approach.

Adequate analgesia and hydration should be provided.

The baby should be started on broad-spectrum antibiotics, made NBM and commenced on IV fluids.

Urgent bloods should be taken, including FBC, U&Es, blood culture, blood gas, coagulation, group and save, and CRP.

The baby should be referred urgently to the neonatal surgeons for hernia assessment and repair.

Case

55

A 48-year-old male presents to ED with generalized abdominal pain and abdominal distension. He is unable to pass flatus or open his bowels. He has no significant past medical history and is a smoker. On examination he has oxygen saturations of 94% in air and a temperature of 35.9°C. His HR is 104 bpm, RR is 26 and blood pressure is 140/90 mmHg. The abdomen is peritonitic and there are tinkling bowel sounds. Urine dipstick is unremarkable.

An abdominal X-ray is requested to assess for possible bowel obstruction.

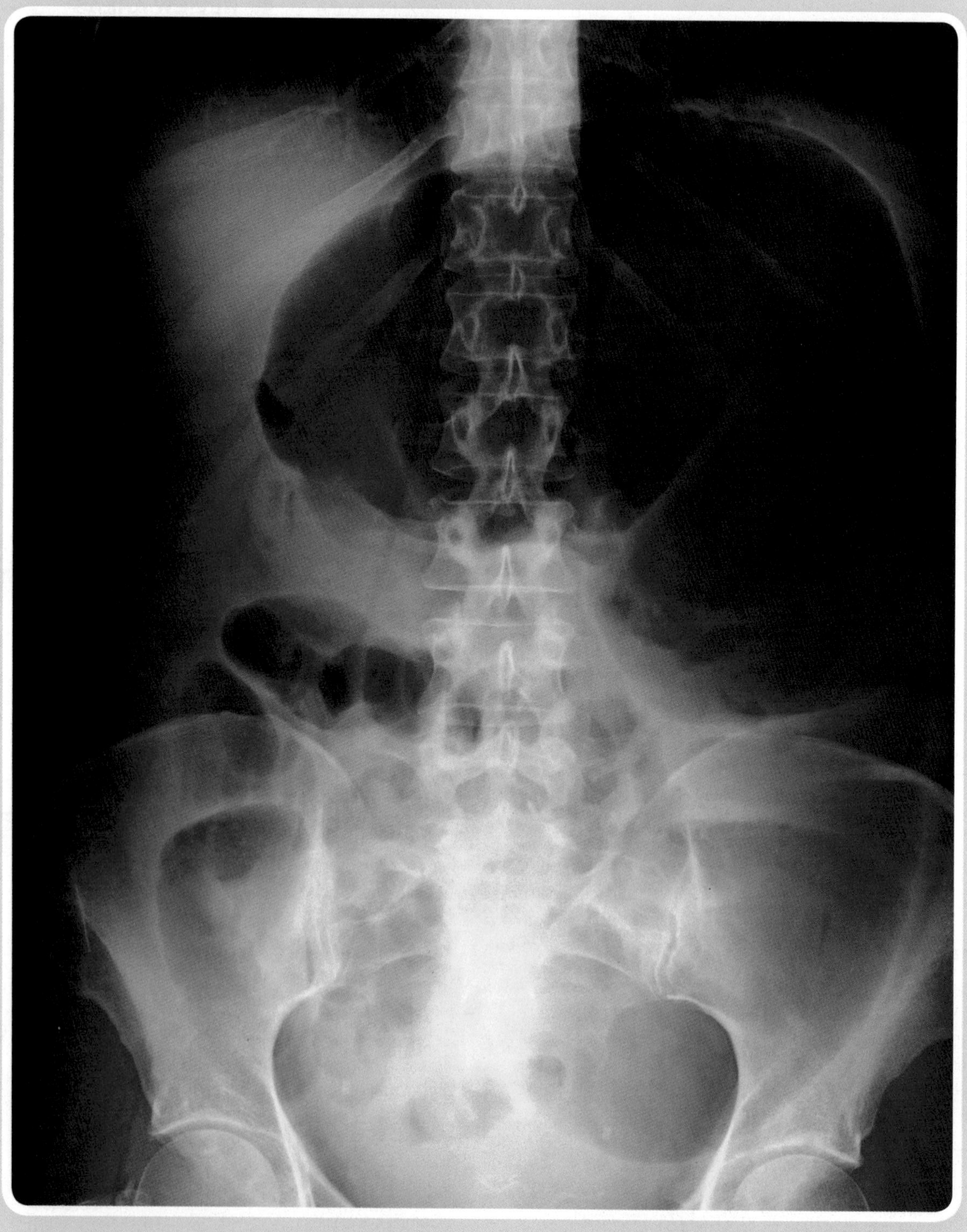

TECHNICAL INFORMATION

Patient ID: Anonymous.
Projection: AP supine.
Rotation: Adequate.
Penetration: Adequate – the spinous processes are visible.
Coverage: Inadequate – the pubic symphysis, inferior pubic rami and hip joints have not been included.

BOWEL GAS PATTERN

The caecum is very distended and in an abnormal position. There are no dilated small bowel loops.

BOWEL WALL

There is no evidence of mural thickening or intramural gas within the large or small bowel.

PNEUMOPERITONEUM

There is no evidence of free intraabdominal gas.

SOLID ORGANS

The solid organ contours are within normal limits with no solid organ calcification.

VASCULAR

No abnormal vascular calcification.

BONES

There are no abnormalities of the imaged thoracic and lumbar spine, or within the pelvis.

SOFT TISSUES

The psoas muscle outline is not visible on the left side, which is nonspecific.

The extraabdominal soft tissues are unremarkable.

OTHER

There are no radiopaque foreign bodies.

There are no vascular lines, drains or surgical clips.

REVIEW AREAS

Gallstones/renal calculi: No radiopaque calculi.
Lung bases: Not fully included.
Spine: Normal.
Femoral heads: Normal.

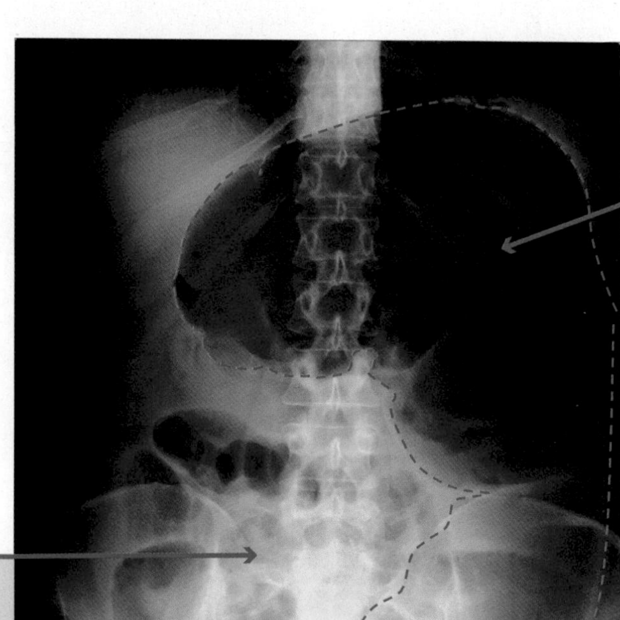

SUMMARY

This X-ray demonstrates a large gas-filled loop of large bowel in keeping with caecal volvulus.

INVESTIGATIONS AND MANAGEMENT

The patient should be resuscitated using an ABCDE approach.

Adequate analgesia and hydration should be provided.

The patient should be kept NBM and an NG tube inserted on free drainage. IV fluids should be commenced.

Urgent bloods should be taken, including FBC, U&Es, CRP, LFTs, coagulation, blood gas, and group and save.

The general surgical team should be contacted urgently. Management will be with either endoscopic decompression or surgical intervention via detorsion and caecotomy.

Case

56

An 18-year-old female presents to ED with severe lower abdominal pain. She has no significant past medical history and is a nonsmoker. On examination, she has oxygen saturations of 97% in air and a temperature of 37.2°C. Her HR is 80 bpm, RR is 18 and blood pressure is 120/85 mmHg. The abdomen is rigid and there is generalized tenderness, particularly in the left iliac fossa, with normal bowel sounds. Urine dipstick is unremarkable and a pregnancy test is negative.

An abdominal X-ray is requested to assess for possible bowel obstruction.

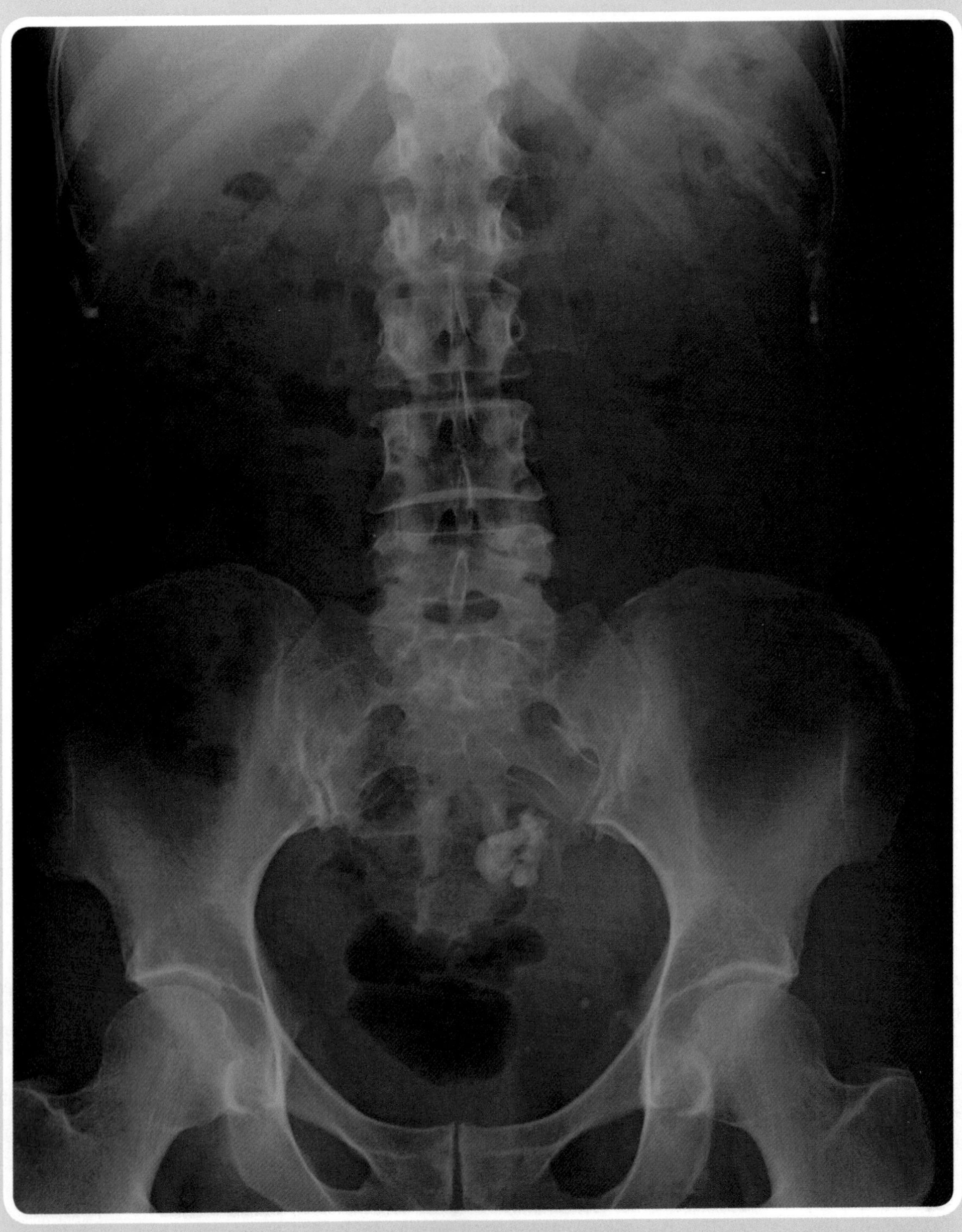

TECHNICAL INFORMATION

Patient ID: Anonymous.
Projection: AP supine.
Rotation: Adequate.
Penetration: Adequate – the spinous processes are visible.
Coverage: Adequate – the anterior ribs are visible superiorly and the inferior pubic rami are visible.

BOWEL GAS PATTERN

The bowel gas pattern is normal.

BOWEL WALL

There is no evidence of mural thickening or intramural gas within the large or small bowel.

PNEUMOPERITONEUM

There is no evidence of free intraabdominal gas.

SOLID ORGANS

The solid organ contours are within normal limits with no solid organ calcification.

VASCULAR

No abnormal vascular calcification.

BONES

There are no abnormalities of the imaged thoracic and lumbar spine, or within the pelvis.

SOFT TISSUES

The psoas muscle outline is visible bilaterally.

The extraabdominal soft tissues are unremarkable.

OTHER

There is a rounded radiopaque density projected over the region of the left hemipelvis, which demonstrates tooth-like calcifications and may represent an ovarian dermoid cyst.

There are several rounded radiopaque densities projected over the lower pelvis that most likely represent phleboliths.

There are no vascular lines, drains or surgical clips.

REVIEW AREAS

Gallstones/renal calculi: No radiopaque calculi.
Lung bases: Not fully included.
Spine: Normal.
Femoral heads: Normal.

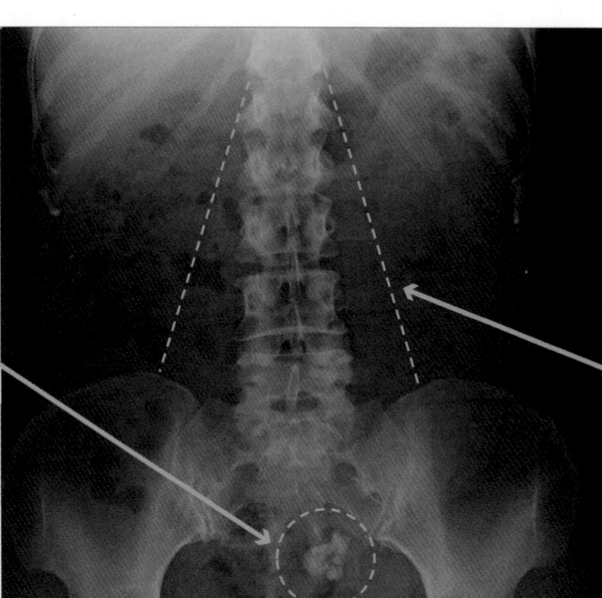

SUMMARY

This X-ray demonstrates a circular radiopaque density projected over the region of the left hemipelvis with tooth-like calcification, which may represent a potentially torted ovarian dermoid cyst (teratoma) or a fibroid. There is no evidence of bowel obstruction.

INVESTIGATIONS AND MANAGEMENT

The patient should be resuscitated using an ABCDE approach.

Adequate analgesia and hydration should be provided.

Urgent bloods should be taken, including FBC, U&Es, CRP, bone profile, LFTs, tumour markers, coagulation, blood gas, and group and save.

An ultrasound scan of the pelvis should be considered to better assess the pelvic lesion and the patient should be referred urgently to gynaecology. Whilst the most likely diagnosis is an ovarian dermoid cyst (teratoma), other differential diagnoses should be considered depending on the blood test results and clinical findings.

An MRI scan of the pelvis may be required depending on the ultrasound results to further assess the pelvic lesion.

Case

57

A 79-year-old female presents to ED with severe central abdominal pain, nausea, vomiting and diarrhoea. Her past medical history is significant for hypertension, atrial fibrillation and osteoporosis. She is a nonsmoker. On examination, she has oxygen saturations of 94% on 4 L of oxygen and a temperature of 39.0°C. Her HR is 100 bpm, RR is 22 and blood pressure is 96/52 mmHg. The abdomen is rigid and there is generalized tenderness with normal bowel sounds. Rectal examination reveals liquid faeces with a small amount of fresh blood. Urine dipstick is unremarkable.

An abdominal X-ray is requested to assess for possible colitis.

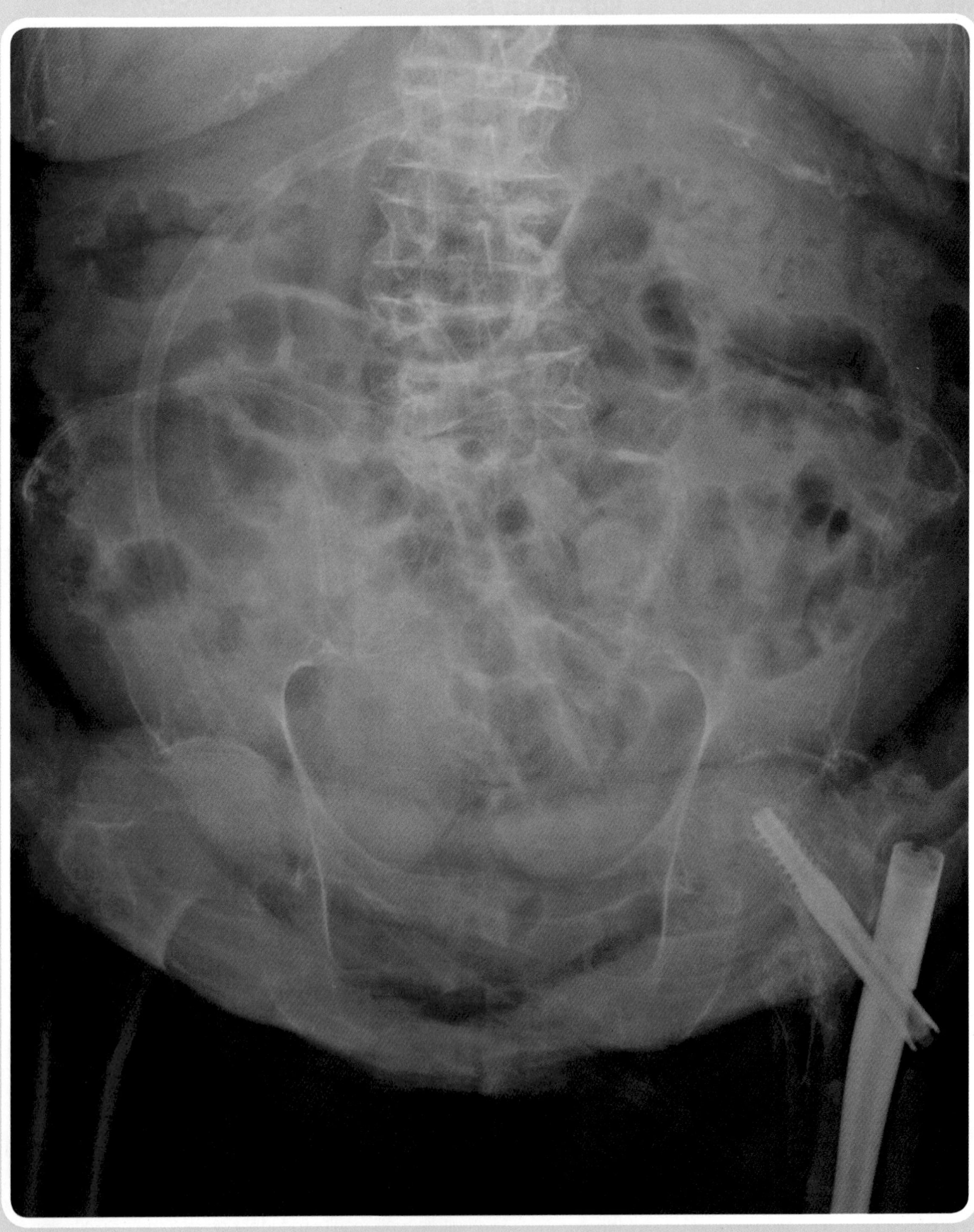

TECHNICAL INFORMATION

Patient ID: Anonymous.
Projection: AP supine.
Rotation: Adequate.
Penetration: Adequate – the spinous processes are visible.
Coverage: Inadequate – the upper abdomen and diaphragm have not been included.

BOWEL GAS PATTERN

Bowel gas pattern is normal.

BOWEL WALL

There is no evidence of mural thickening or intramural gas within the large or small bowel.

PNEUMOPERITONEUM

There is no evidence of free intraabdominal gas.

SOLID ORGANS

The solid organ contours are within normal limits with no solid organ calcification.

VASCULAR

No abnormal vascular calcification.

BONES

There is diffuse osteopenia of the skeleton, particularly of the vertebrae.

There are significant degenerative changes throughout the spine and in the sacroiliac and hip joints.

There are vertebral body compression (likely insufficiency) fractures at L3, L4 and L5.

There is an old left subtrochanteric femoral fracture, which has been repaired by internal fixation using a proximal femoral nail. Bony remodelling and heterotopic ossification is seen adjacent to this.

SOFT TISSUES

The psoas muscle outline is not visible bilaterally, which is nonspecific.

The extraabdominal soft tissues are unremarkable.

OTHER

There is a left-sided proximal femoral nail in situ but there are no other radiopaque foreign bodies.

There is an external line projected over the right side of the abdomen and the pelvis, which most likely represents oxygen tubing. The patient's hands are visible across the pelvis.

There are no vascular lines, drains or surgical clips.

REVIEW AREAS

Gallstones/renal calculi: No radiopaque calculi.
Lung bases: Not visible.
Spine: Vertebral body compression fractures at L3, L4 and L5.
Femoral heads: Old left subtrochanteric fracture with left-sided proximal femoral nail in situ.

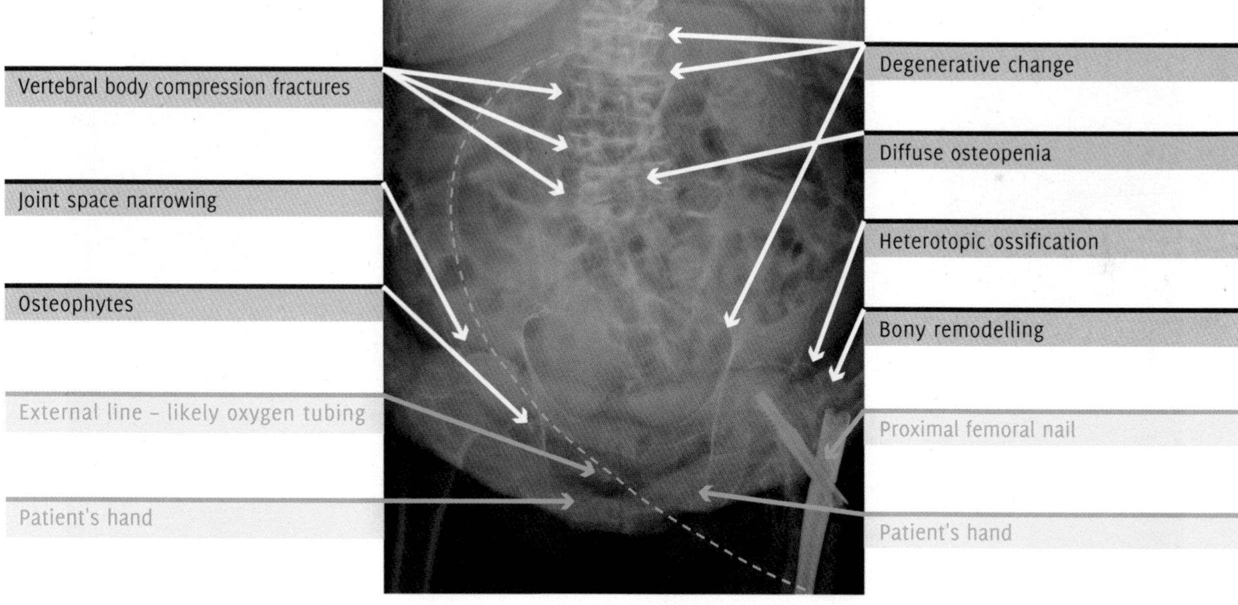

SUMMARY

This X-ray demonstrates a normal bowel appearance with no evidence of colitis, intramural gas or pneumoperitoneum. It also demonstrates age-indeterminate vertebral body compression (insufficiency) fractures at L3, L4 and L5, on a background of diffuse osteopenia and significant degenerative changes throughout the spine, sacroiliac and hip joints. The left-sided proximal femoral nail is an incidental finding in keeping with a previous subtrochanteric femur fracture with associated bony remodelling and heterotopic ossification.

INVESTIGATIONS AND MANAGEMENT

The patient should be resuscitated using an ABCDE approach.

Adequate analgesia and hydration should be provided.

Urgent bloods should be taken, including FBC, U&Es, LFTs, amylase, CRP, blood gas, coagulation, blood gas, and group and save. Broad-spectrum antibiotics should be prescribed.

There are no clear findings on the abdominal X-ray to explain the patient's clinical presentation.

A CT scan of the abdomen and pelvis with IV contrast should be considered for further assessment and the patient should be referred to general surgery.

Chronic management of vertebral crush fractures may involve lifestyle modification, physiotherapy and pain medication, but further history/examination should be sought, and previous images reviewed.

Case

58

A 42-year-old male presents to ED following a collapse and abdominal pain at home. She is diagnosed with septic shock secondary to pneumonia. He has no significant past medical history and is a nonsmoker. On examination, he has oxygen saturations of 80% in room air and a temperature of 38.4°C. His HR is 95 bpm, RR is 30 and blood pressure is 90/50 mmHg. The abdomen is firm and there is some tenderness centrally with normal bowel sounds. Urine dipstick is unremarkable. He is intubated and vascular access is established as part of his ABCDE resuscitation.

An abdominal X-ray is requested to assess the position of his femoral line and assess for possible bowel obstruction.

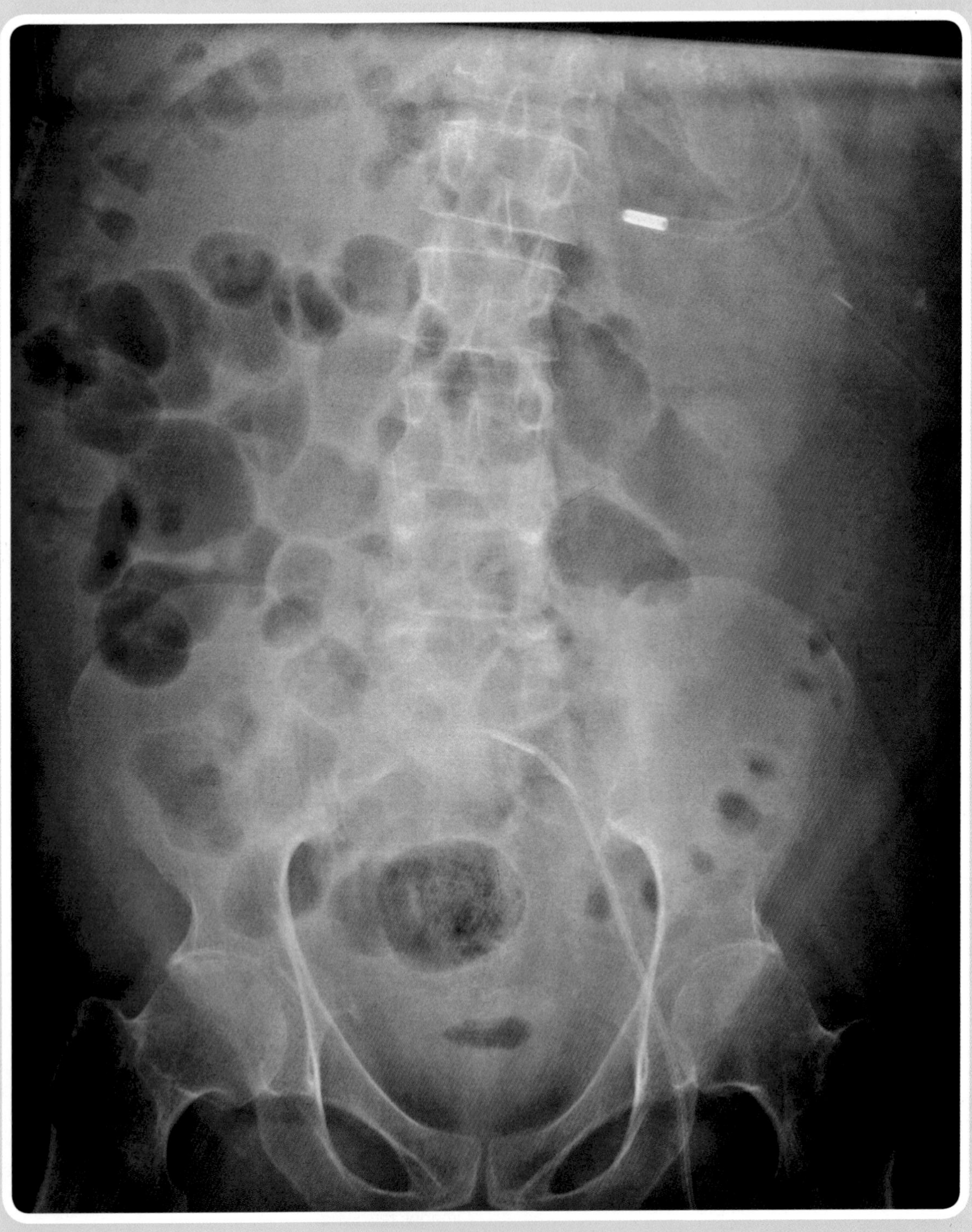

TECHNICAL INFORMATION

Patient ID: Anonymous.
Projection: AP supine.
Rotation: Adequate.
Penetration: Adequate – the spinous processes are visible.
Coverage: Adequate – the anterior ribs are visible superiorly and the inferior pubic rami are visible.

BOWEL GAS PATTERN

The bowel gas pattern is normal.

BOWEL WALL

There is no evidence of mural thickening or intramural gas within the large or small bowel.

PNEUMOPERITONEUM

There is no evidence of free intraabdominal gas.

SOLID ORGANS

The solid organ contours are within normal limits with no solid organ calcification.

VASCULAR

There is a left-sided femoral venous catheter with its tip projecting over the inferior endplate of L5, likely at the site of the inferior vena cava bifurcation.

The abdominal aorta appears normal.

BONES

There are no abnormalities of the imaged thoracic and lumbar spine, or within the pelvis.

SOFT TISSUES

The psoas muscle outline is visible bilaterally.

The extraabdominal soft tissues are unremarkable.

OTHER

There is an NG tube in situ, with its tip seen in the left upper quadrant within the stomach.

There are no drains or surgical clips.

REVIEW AREAS

Gallstones/renal calculi: No radiopaque calculi.
Lung bases: Not fully included.
Spine: Normal.
Femoral heads: Normal.

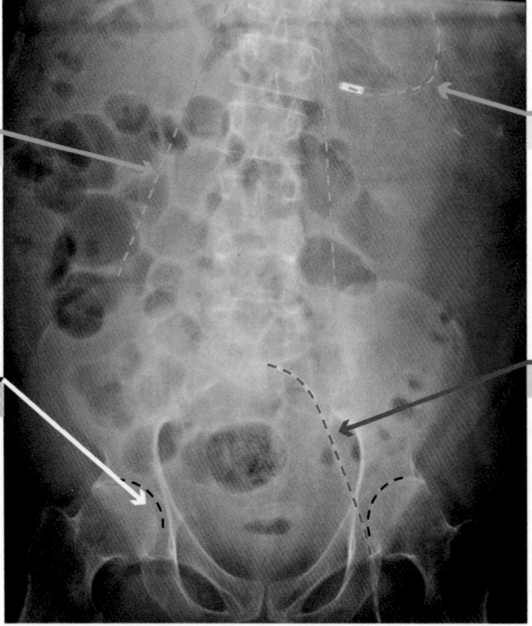

SUMMARY

This X-ray demonstrates an NG tube in situ, with its tip situated within the gastric fundus. It also demonstrates a left-sided femoral venous catheter with its tip projecting over the proximal left common iliac vein. There is no evidence of any other significant abnormality.

INVESTIGATIONS AND MANAGEMENT

The patient should be resuscitated using an ABCDE approach.

Adequate analgesia and hydration should be provided.

Urgent bloods should be taken, including FBC, U&Es, CRP, bone profile, LFTs, coagulation, blood culture, blood gas, and group and save.

The Sepsis 6 pathway should be started immediately, including administration of oxygen, IV broad-spectrum antibiotics and consideration of a fluid bolus as well as measurement of lactate and urinary output and blood cultures.

The patient should be made NBM and started on IV fluids.

There are no clear findings on the abdominal X-ray to explain the patient's abdominal pain. A CT scan of the abdomen/pelvis with IV contrast may be considered for further evaluation of the abdomen and the general surgical team should be involved.

Intensive care should be informed about the patient as their input may be required.

Case

59

A 1-day-old baby boy is currently admitted to NICU after a premature birth at 34 weeks. On examination, he has oxygen saturations of 99%, is intubated with 40% oxygen and has a temperature of 36.5°C. His HR is 190 bpm and RR is 40. The abdomen is soft and bowel sounds are normal.

An abdominal X-ray is requested to assess the position of the ET tube and umbilical lines that have just been inserted.

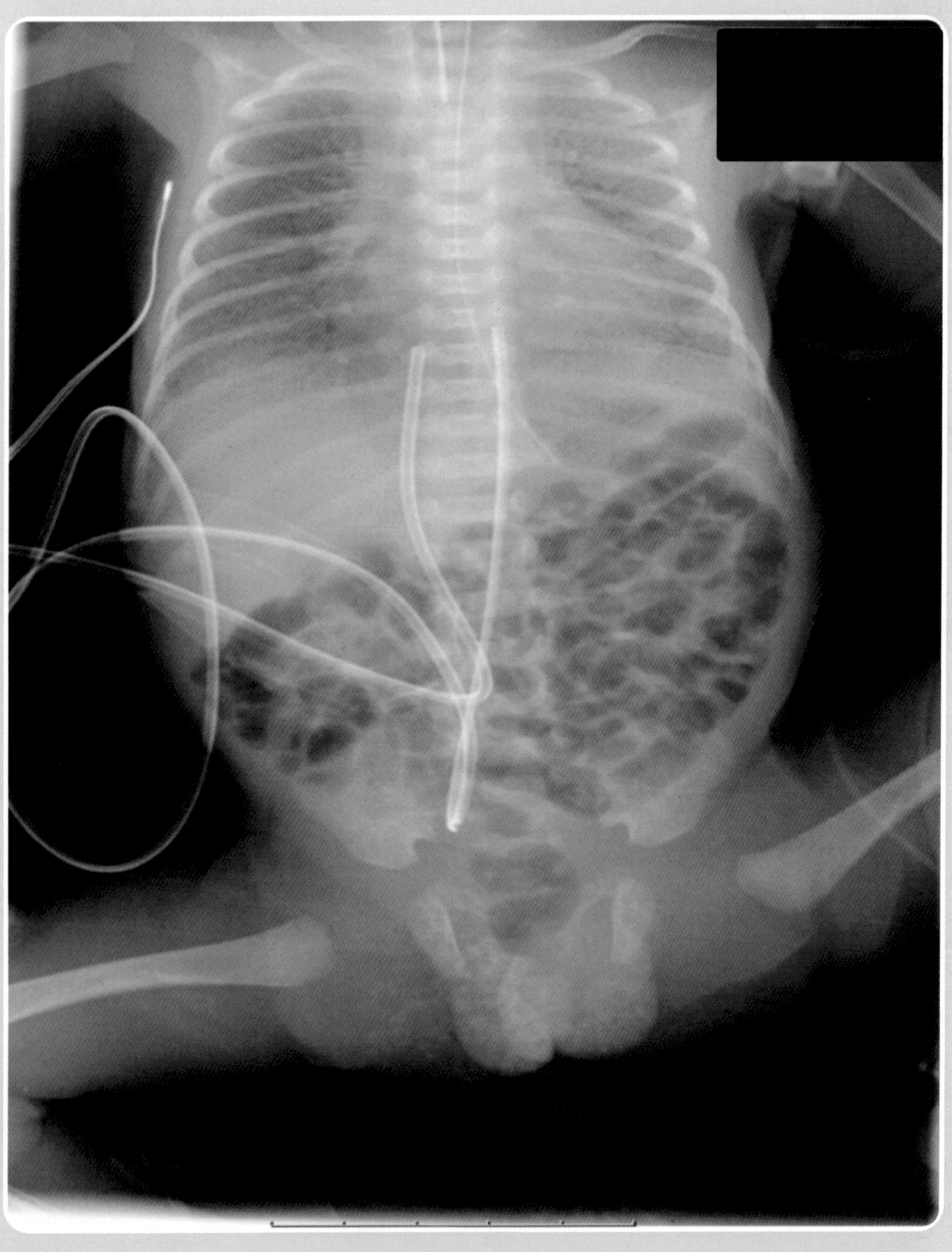

TECHNICAL INFORMATION

Patient ID: Anonymous.
Projection: AP supine.
Rotation: Adequate.
Penetration: Adequate – the spine is visible.
Coverage: Adequate – the anterior ribs are visible superiorly and the inferior pubic rami are visible.

BOWEL GAS PATTERN

The bowel gas pattern is normal. There is faeces projecting over the pelvis and external to the patient with a nappy.

BOWEL WALL

There is no evidence of mural thickening or intramural gas within the large or small bowel.

PNEUMOPERITONEUM

There is no evidence of free intraabdominal gas.

SOLID ORGANS

The solid organ contours are within normal limits with no solid organ calcification.

There is bilateral ground glass shadowing in the lung fields.

VASCULAR

No abnormal vascular calcification.

There is an umbilical artery catheter. Its tip is seen appropriately sited at the level of T9.

There is an umbilical venous catheter with its tip seen appropriately sited projecting over the diaphragm at the level of T9/10 in the inferior vena cava.

BONES

There are no abnormalities of the imaged thoracic and lumbar spine, or within the pelvis.

There is cartilage present between the pelvic bones and femurs as they have not yet fused, which is a normal finding in a child of this age.

There is cartilage seen between vertebrae which is a normal finding in a child of this age.

SOFT TISSUES

The psoas muscle outline is not visible bilaterally, which is nonspecific, particularly in a child of this age.

The extraabdominal soft tissues are unremarkable.

OTHER

There is an NG tube in situ, with its tip seen in the left upper quadrant of the abdomen, within the stomach.

There is an ET tube in situ, with its tip seen in the midline between the medial border of the clavicles and above the carina in a satisfactory position.

There is an electrode and lead external to the patient, in keeping with a skin temperature probe.

There are no drains or surgical clips.

REVIEW AREAS

Gallstones/renal calculi: No radiopaque calculi.
Lung bases: Bilateral ground glass shadowing.
Spine: Normal – cartilage between vertebrae.
Femoral heads: Normal – growth plates present.

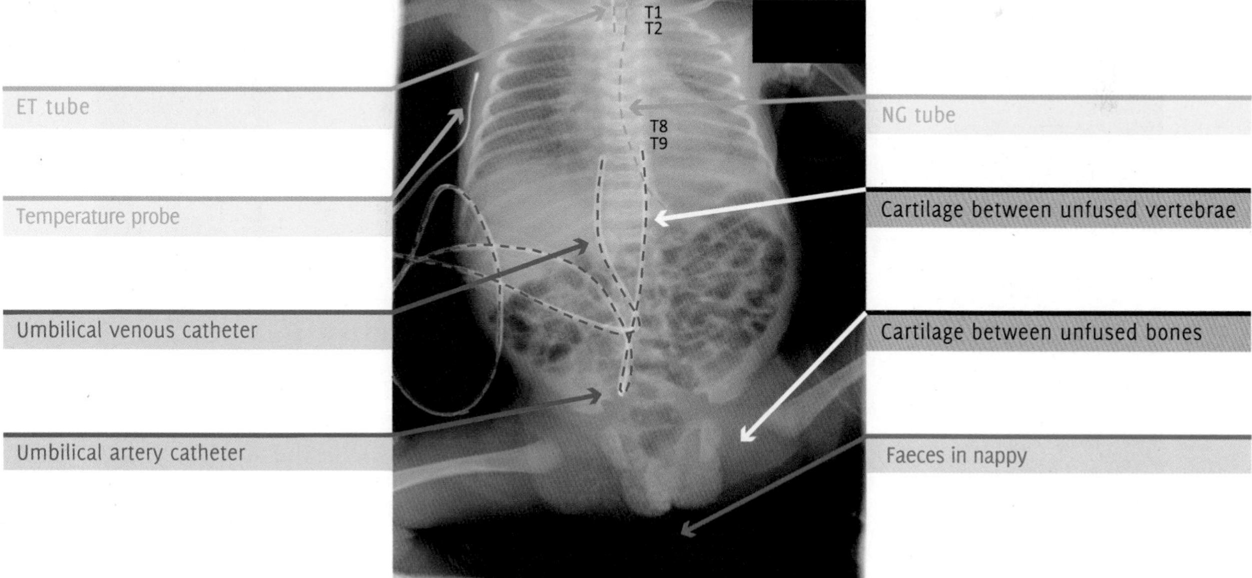

SUMMARY

This X-ray demonstrates an NG tube, ET tube, skin temperature probe, umbilical artery catheter and umbilical venous catheter, all appropriately sited. There is bilateral ground glass shadowing in the lung fields, in keeping with respiratory distress syndrome.

INVESTIGATIONS AND MANAGEMENT

The ET tube and vascular lines are in satisfactory positions.

If not already done, surfactant should be given. The baby should be started on broad-spectrum antibiotics and kept NBM on IV fluids.

Case

60

A 39-year-old female presents to ED with abdominal distension and increasing frequency of diarrhoea and passing mucus. Her past medical history is significant for ulcerative colitis and she is a smoker. On examination, she has oxygen saturations of 99% in room air and a temperature of 38.1°C. Her HR is 88 bpm, RR is 19 and blood pressure is 125/65 mmHg. The abdomen is soft and there is generalized tenderness with normal bowel sounds. Urine dipstick is unremarkable and a pregnancy test is negative.

An abdominal X-ray is requested to assess for active colitis.

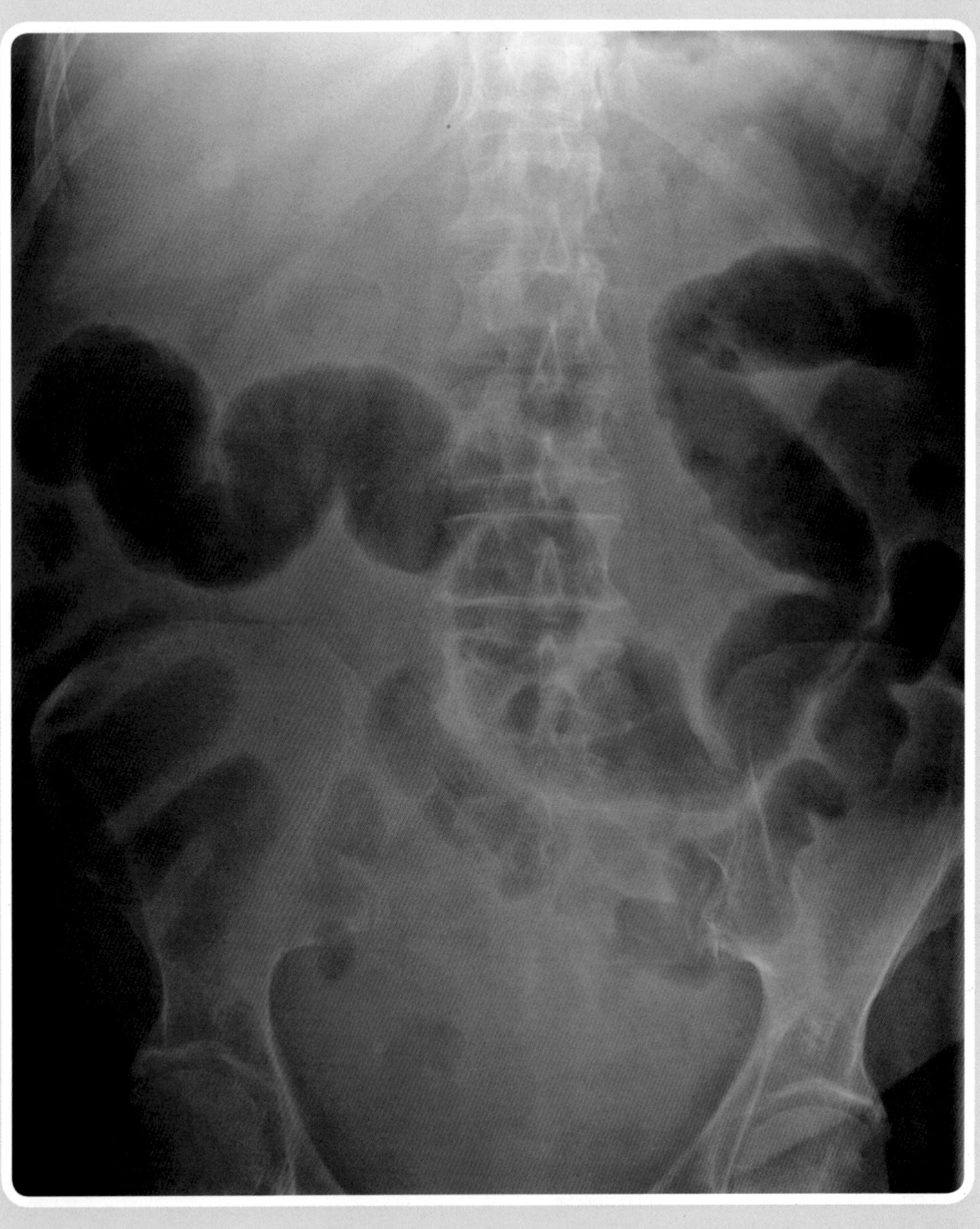

TECHNICAL INFORMATION

Patient ID: Anonymous.
Projection: AP supine.
Rotation: Adequate.
Penetration: Adequate – the spinous processes are visible.
Coverage: Inadequate – the pubic symphysis and inferior pubic rami have not been included.

BOWEL GAS PATTERN

There is dilatation of the large bowel, in particular, the ascending and transverse colon.

BOWEL WALL

There is mural thickening of the entire transverse colon in the right and left upper quadrants, and of the sigmoid colon, with loss of the normal colonic haustral folds, in keeping with mural oedema. This is termed 'lead pipe colon'.

There is no evidence of intramural gas within the large or small bowel.

PNEUMOPERITONEUM

There is no evidence of free intraabdominal gas.

SOLID ORGANS

The solid organ contours are within normal limits with no solid organ calcification.

VASCULAR

No abnormal vascular calcification.

BONES

There are no abnormalities of the imaged thoracic and lumbar spine, or within the pelvis.

SOFT TISSUES

The psoas muscle outline is visible bilaterally.

The extraabdominal soft tissues are unremarkable.

OTHER

There are no radiopaque foreign bodies.

There are no vascular lines, drains or surgical clips.

REVIEW AREAS

Gallstones/renal calculi: No radiopaque calculi.
Lung bases: Not fully included.
Spine: Normal.
Femoral heads: Normal.

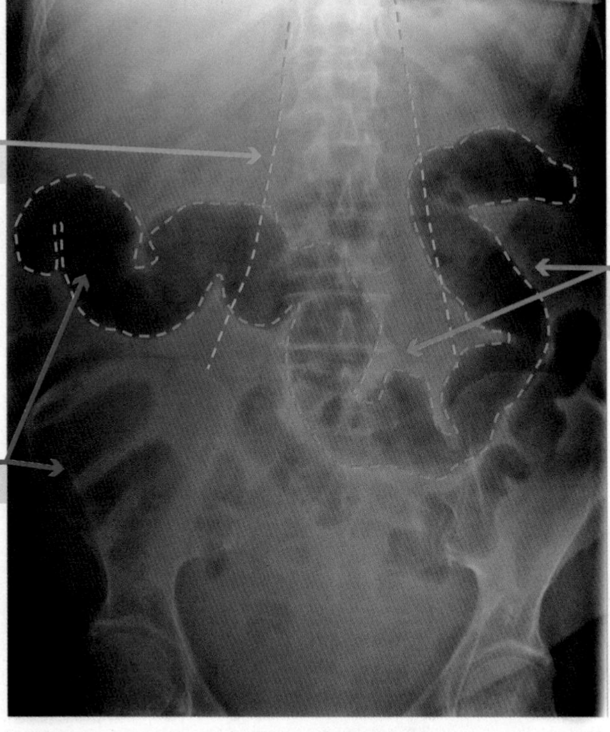

SUMMARY

This X-ray demonstrates mural oedema of the transverse and sigmoid colon with loss of the normal colonic haustral folds. There is also dilatation of the ascending and transverse colon. Given the clinical history, findings are in keeping with an acute exacerbation of ulcerative colitis.

INVESTIGATIONS AND MANAGEMENT

The patient should be resuscitated using an ABCDE approach.

Adequate analgesia and hydration should be provided.

Urgent bloods should be taken, including FBC, U&Es, LFTs, ESR, CRP, iron studies, folate, blood gas, and group and save. A stool sample should be sent.

Urgent referral to the gastroenterology team should be considered.

A CT scan of the abdomen/pelvis with IV contrast should be considered for better visualization of the anatomy and to assess the extent of the disease.

Treatment will depend on the results of further investigations, as well as the clinical state of the patient.

Case

61

A 70-year-old male presents to ED with a 2-day history of nausea, vomiting and not passing flatus or opening his bowels. He has no significant past medical history and is a nonsmoker. On examination, he has oxygen saturations of 98% in room air and a temperature of 36.5°C. His HR is 95 bpm, RR is 26 and blood pressure is 135/75 mmHg. The abdomen is rigid and there is generalized tenderness with tinkling bowel sounds. Urine dipstick is unremarkable.

An abdominal X-ray is requested to assess for possible bowel obstruction.

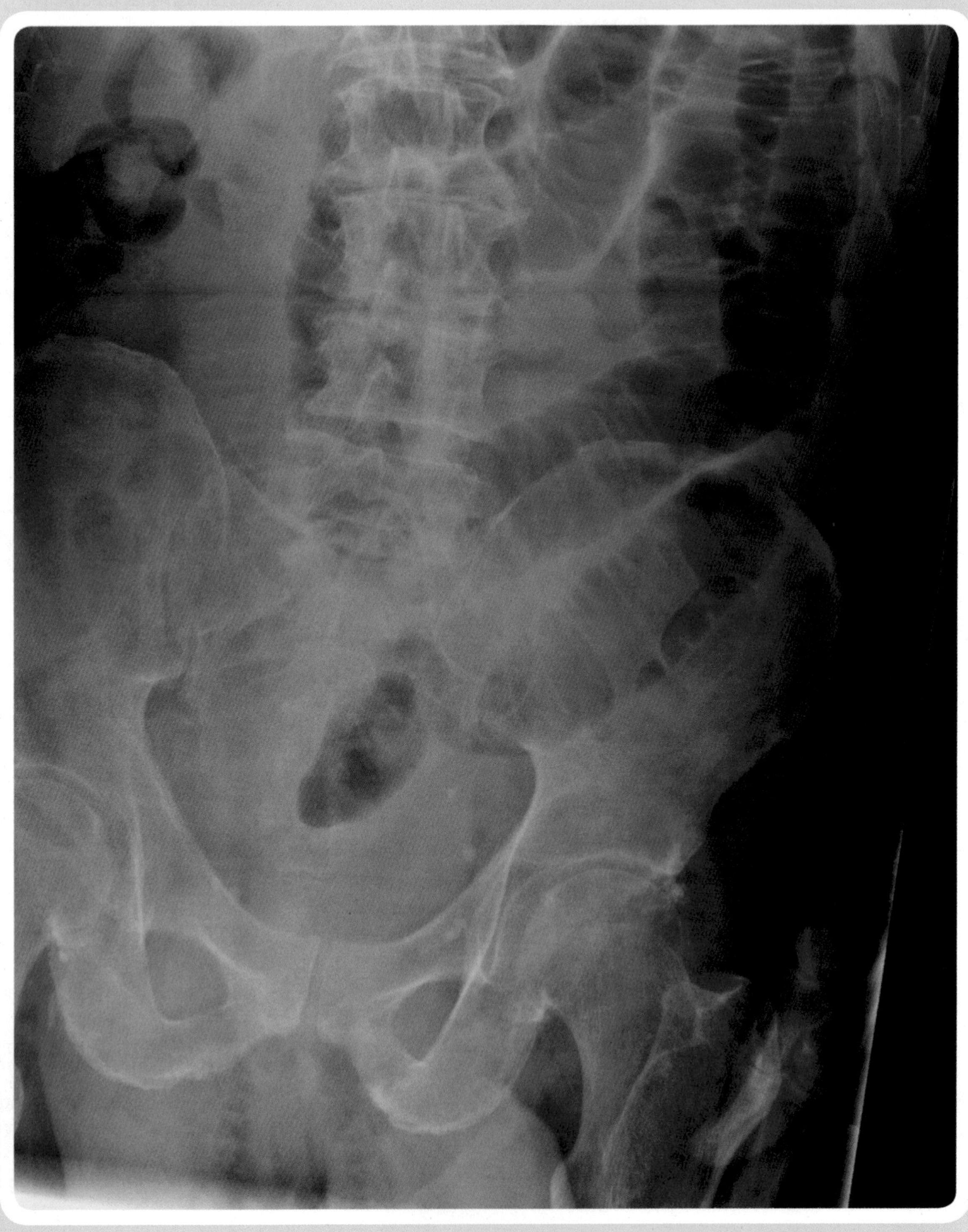

TECHNICAL INFORMATION

Patient ID: Anonymous.
Projection: AP supine.
Rotation: Adequate.
Penetration: Adequate – the spinous processes are visible.
Coverage: Inadequate – the anterior ribs, right hip joint and right ilium have not been fully included.

BOWEL GAS PATTERN

There are multiple loops of dilated bowel seen centrally within the abdomen, which demonstrate valvulae conniventes in keeping with small bowel obstruction.

There is abnormal bowel gas projecting over the groin below the inguinal ligament towards the scrotum, suggestive of an incarcerated indirect inguinal hernia.

BOWEL WALL

There is no evidence of mural thickening or intramural gas within the large or small bowel.

PNEUMOPERITONEUM

There is no evidence of free intraabdominal gas.

SOLID ORGANS

The solid organ contours are within normal limits with no solid organ calcification.

VASCULAR

There is calcification of the iliac arteries bilaterally.

BONES

There is moderate degenerative change in the spine with osteophyte formation and mild degenerative change in the hip joints with osteophyte formation and subchondral sclerosis.

SOFT TISSUES

The psoas muscle outline is not visible.

The extraabdominal soft tissues are unremarkable.

OTHER

There are multiple rounded radiopaque densities projected over the region of the pelvis, most likely phleboliths.

A hand has been exposed in the lower left-hand side of the radiograph.

There are no vascular lines, drains or surgical clips.

REVIEW AREAS

Gallstones/renal calculi: No radiopaque calculi.
Lung bases: Not included.
Spine: Moderate degenerative change.
Femoral heads: Mild degenerative change.

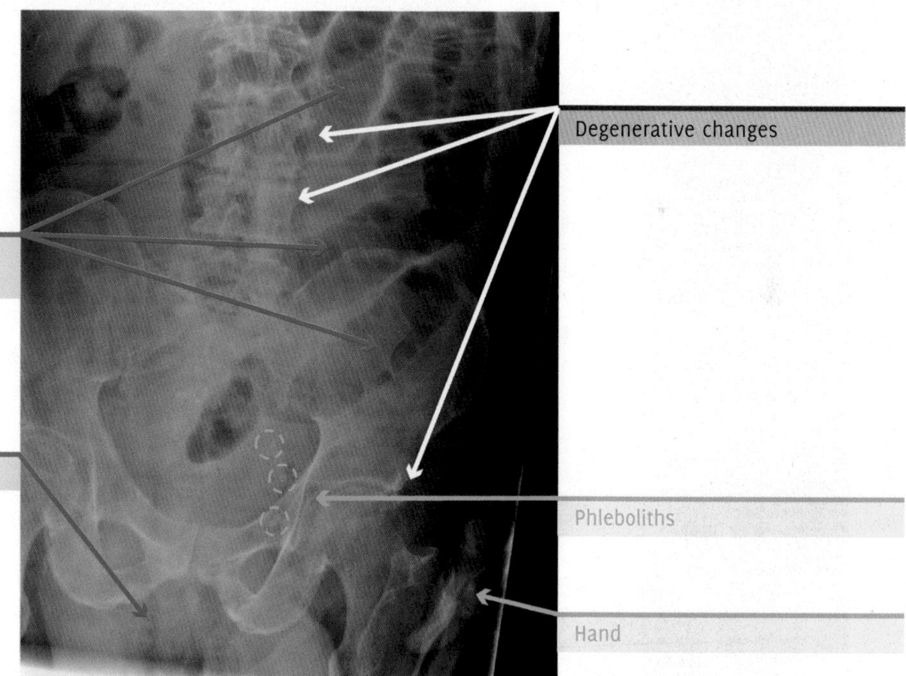

SUMMARY

This X-ray demonstrates multiple loops of dilated bowel seen centrally within the abdomen demonstrating valvulae conniventes, in keeping with small bowel obstruction. There is bowel gas seen projecting over the groin towards the scrotum, which most likely represents an incarcerated indirect inguinal hernia. The moderate degenerative changes in the spine, mild left hip degenerative changes and pelvic phleboliths are incidental findings.

INVESTIGATIONS AND MANAGEMENT

The patient should be resuscitated using an ABCDE approach.

Adequate analgesia and hydration should be provided.

The patient should be kept NBM and an NG tube inserted on free drainage to relieve the pressure in the small bowel. IV fluids should be commenced.

Urgent bloods should be taken, including FBC, U&Es, CRP, LFTs, coagulation, blood gas, and group and save.

The general surgical team should be contacted urgently for consideration of hernia repair.

Case 62

A 50-year-old male presents to ED with abdominal distension and generalized abdominal pain. He has not passed flatus or opened his bowels for 24 hours. He has chronic constipation and is a smoker. On examination, he has oxygen saturations of 99% in room air and a temperature of 36.5°C. His HR is 101 bpm, RR is 24 and blood pressure is 135/80 mmHg. The abdomen is rigid and there is generalized tenderness with tinkling bowel sounds. Urine dipstick is unremarkable.

An abdominal X-ray is requested to assess for possible bowel obstruction.

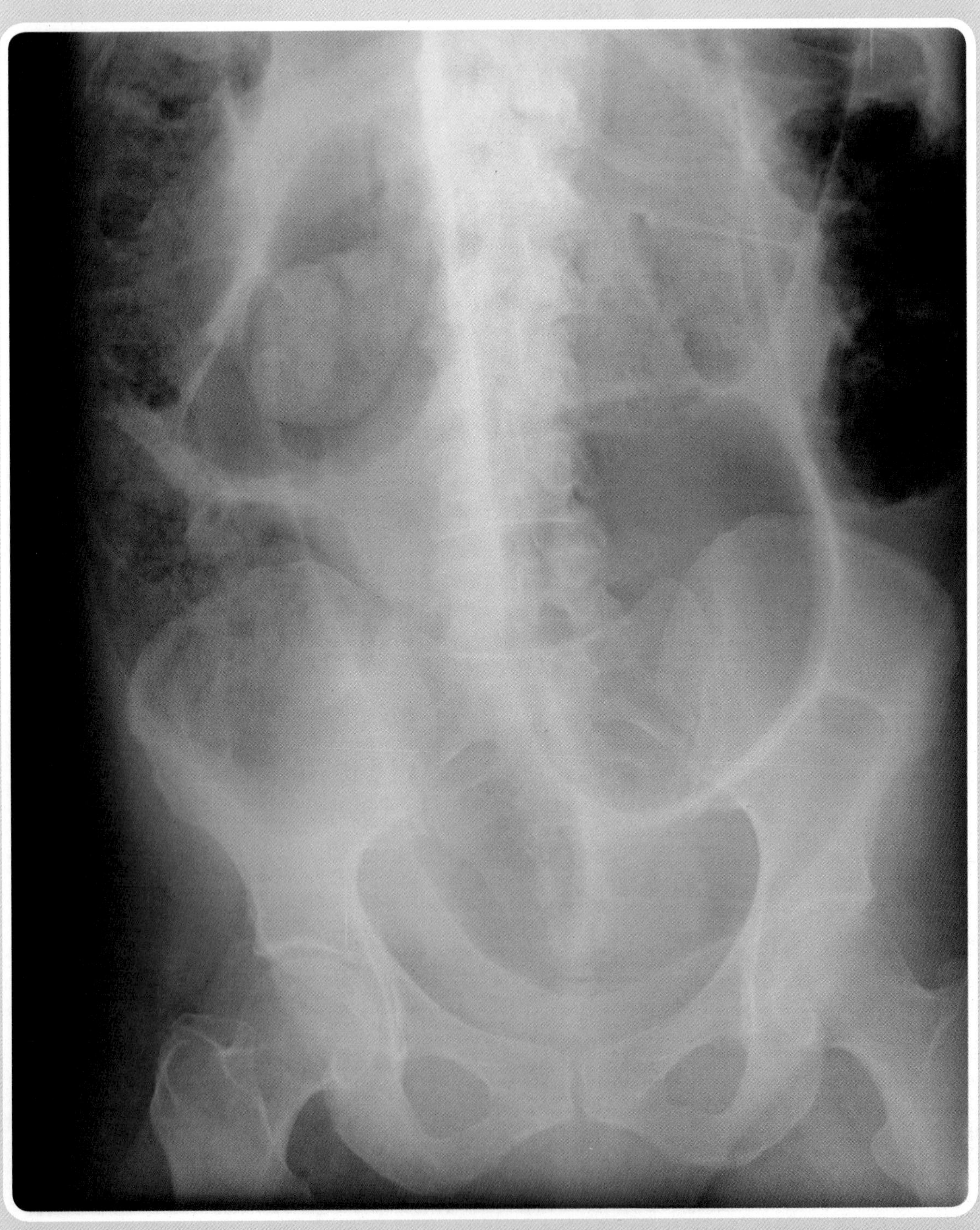

TECHNICAL INFORMATION

Patient ID: Anonymous.
Projection: AP supine.
Rotation: Adequate.
Penetration: Adequate – the spinous processes are visible.
Coverage: Adequate – the anterior ribs are visible superiorly and the inferior pubic rami are visible.

BOWEL GAS PATTERN

There is a large gas-filled loop of large bowel in the centre of the abdomen, with loss of the normal haustral markings, extending from the pelvis to the upper abdomen.

There are multiple loops of dilated bowel seen within the abdomen demonstrating haustra, in keeping with large bowel dilatation.

Bowel gas is not seen in the rectum.

There is a moderate volume of faecal residue present within the ascending colon.

BOWEL WALL

There is no evidence of mural thickening or intramural gas within the large or small bowel.

PNEUMOPERITONEUM

There is no evidence of free intraabdominal gas.

SOLID ORGANS

The solid organ contours are within normal limits with no solid organ calcification.

VASCULAR

No abnormal vascular calcification.

BONES

There is mild degenerative change in the spine.

There is mild osteoarthritic change seen within both hip joints, including subchondral sclerosis and narrowing of the joint spaces.

SOFT TISSUES

The psoas muscle outline is not visible bilaterally, which is nonspecific.

The extraabdominal soft tissues are unremarkable.

OTHER

There are no radiopaque foreign bodies.

There are no vascular lines, drains or surgical clips.

REVIEW AREAS

Gallstones/renal calculi: No radiopaque calculi.
Lung bases: Normal.
Spine: Mild degenerative change.
Femoral heads: Moderate degenerative change.

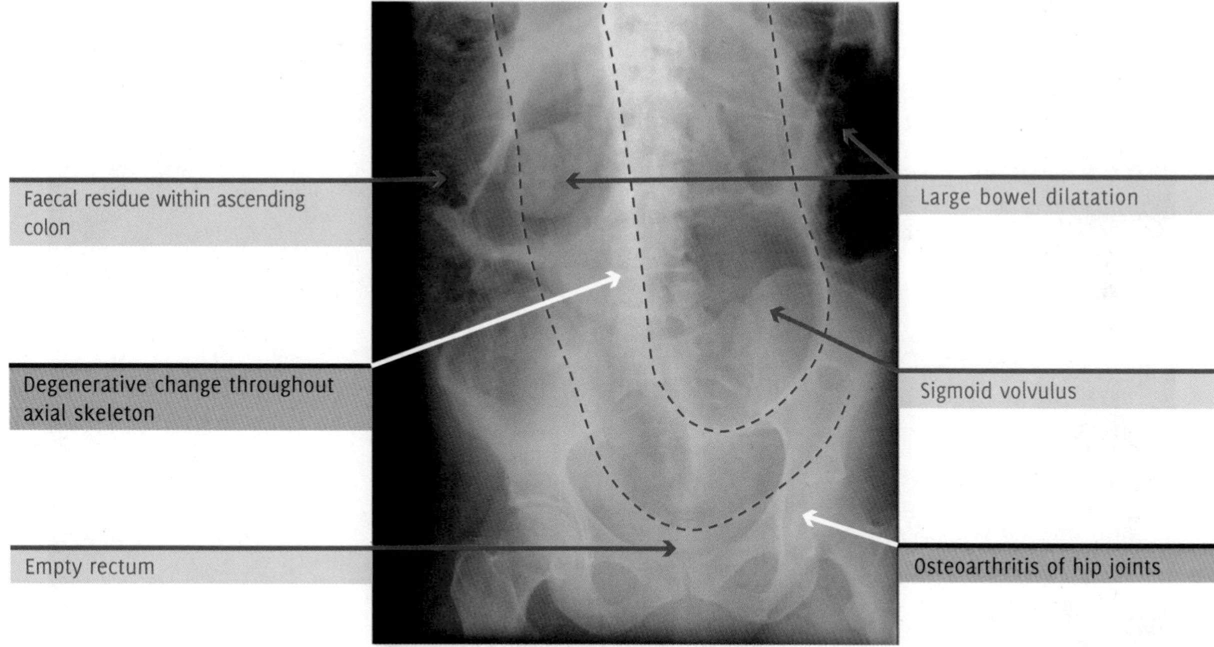

SUMMARY

This X-ray demonstrates a large gas-filled loop of large bowel, with loss of normal haustral markings. There is dilatation of the large bowel proximal to this, and an absence of bowel gas seen within the rectum distally. Findings are in keeping with sigmoid volvulus. The mild degenerative changes in the spine and hip joints are incidental findings.

INVESTIGATIONS AND MANAGEMENT

The patient should be resuscitated using an ABCDE approach.

Adequate analgesia and hydration should be provided.

Urgent bloods should be taken, including FBC, U&Es, CRP, blood gas, coagulation, and group and save.

The general surgical team should be contacted urgently.

Urgent decompression with sigmoidoscopy is required to relieve the obstruction, with a flatus tube left in situ.

Elective sigmoidectomy with primary anastomosis may then be undertaken to prevent reoccurrence.

Arthritic changes in the first instance should be managed with lifestyle changes and analgesia, depending on symptoms.

Case

63

A 55-year-old female presents to ED with a 4-day history of generalized abdominal pain. She has not opened her bowels in that time and feels nauseated but has not vomited. Her past medical history is significant for chronic back pain, for which she takes regular co-codamol and ibuprofen. She has no other significant past medical history and is a smoker. On examination, she has oxygen saturations of 95% in room air and a temperature of 36.5°C. Her HR is 77 bpm, RR is 18 and blood pressure is 118/64 mmHg. The abdomen is mildly distended with voluntary guarding and there is tenderness in the left iliac fossa with sluggish bowel sounds. Urine dipstick is unremarkable.

An abdominal X-ray is requested to assess for possible bowel obstruction.

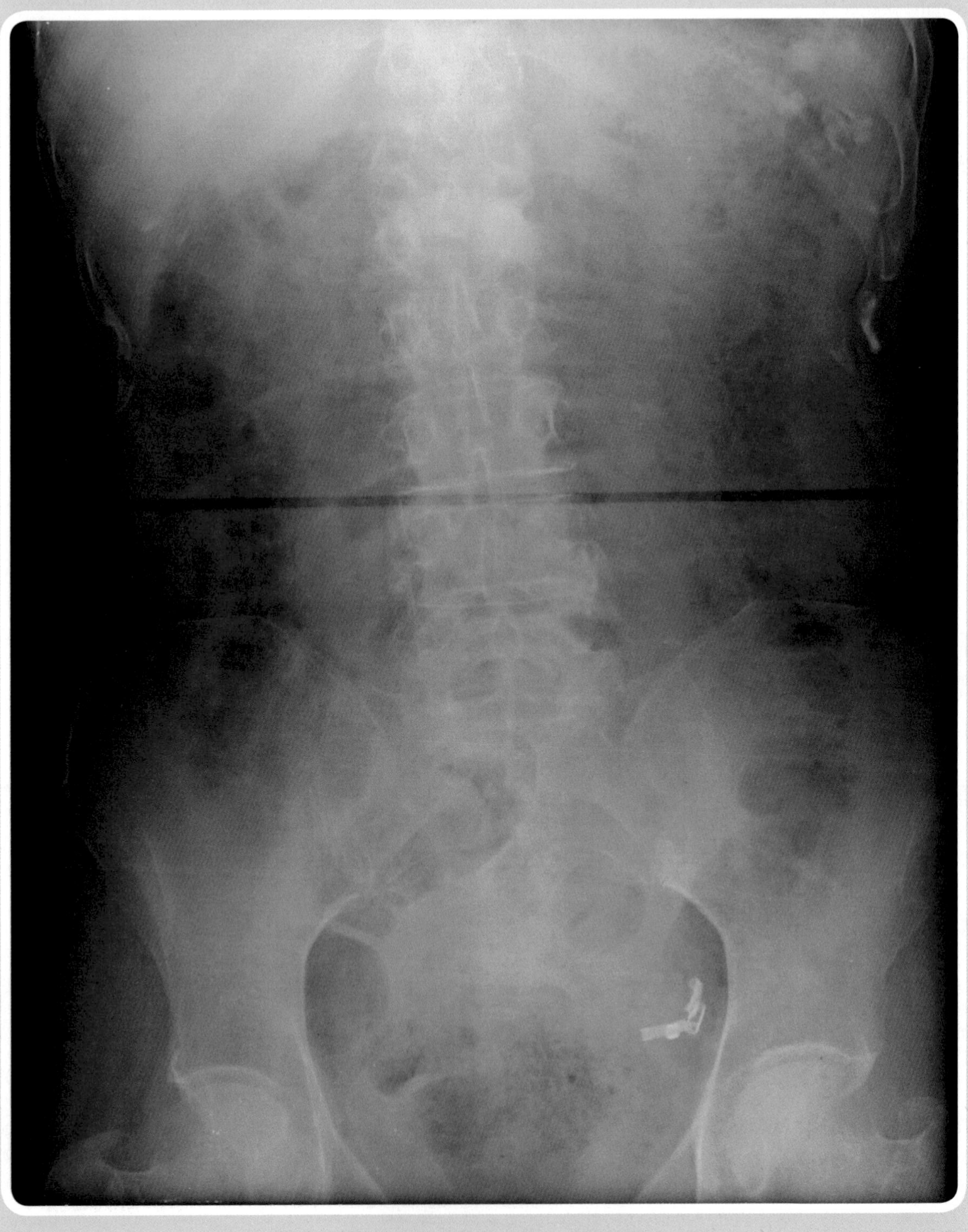

TECHNICAL INFORMATION

Patient ID: Anonymous.
Projection: AP supine.
Rotation: Adequate.
Penetration: Adequate – the spinous processes are visible.
Coverage: Inadequate – the pubic symphysis and inferior pubic rami have not been fully included.

BOWEL GAS PATTERN

There is a paucity of bowel gas but no bowel dilatation is visible.

There is a moderate amount of faecal material present throughout the large bowel, extending from caecum to rectum.

BOWEL WALL

There is no evidence of mural thickening or intramural gas within the large or small bowel.

PNEUMOPERITONEUM

There is no evidence of free intraabdominal gas.

SOLID ORGANS

The solid organ contours are within normal limits with no solid organ calcification.

VASCULAR

No abnormal vascular calcification.

BONES

There is degenerative change visible in the imaged thoracic and lumbar spine.

No fractures or destructive bone lesions are visible in the imaged skeleton.

SOFT TISSUES

The psoas muscle outline is visible bilaterally.

The extraabdominal soft tissues are unremarkable.

OTHER

There are two sterilization clips projecting over the left pelvis, indicating that one may have become loose.

There are no vascular lines or drains.

REVIEW AREAS

Gallstones/renal calculi: No radiopaque calculi.
Lung bases: Not fully included.
Spine: Degenerative change.
Femoral heads: Normal.

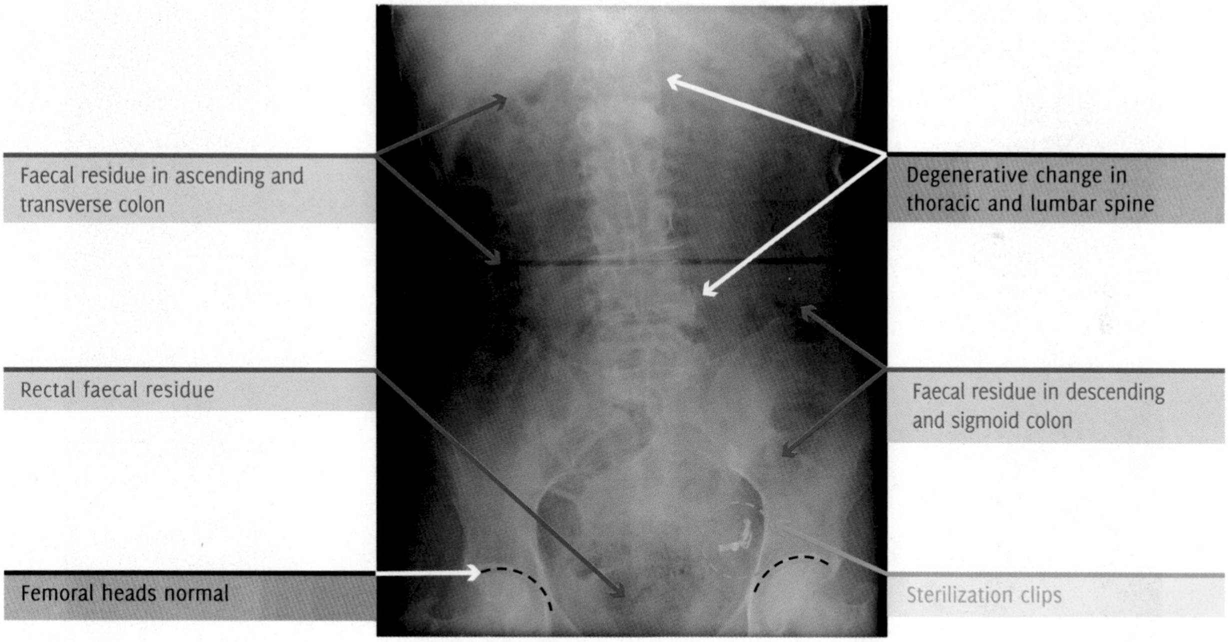

Faecal residue in ascending and transverse colon
Degenerative change in thoracic and lumbar spine
Rectal faecal residue
Faecal residue in descending and sigmoid colon
Femoral heads normal
Sterilization clips

SUMMARY

This X-ray demonstrates a moderate volume of faecal residue throughout the large bowel. There are two sterilization clips projecting over the left pelvis, indicating that one may have become loose. There is no evidence of bowel obstruction or pneumoperitoneum. There are moderate degenerative changes in the spine.

INVESTIGATIONS AND MANAGEMENT

If the patient is otherwise well, no further investigation or imaging is required.

If the patient is clinically constipated, current medications should be reviewed and laxatives considered. Advice should be given regarding lifestyle adjustments, including adequate fluid intake, sufficient dietary fibre and exercise if clinically appropriate.

In a premenopausal woman, the loose sterilization clip would be of clinical importance as the patient may not be protected from conception and additional contraception may be required.

Case

64

A 25-year-old female presents to ED with right-sided abdominal pain. Her past medical history is significant for congenital hydrocephalus, for which she has a VP shunt, and she is a nonsmoker. On examination, she has oxygen saturations of 98% in room air and a temperature of 36.5°C. Her HR is 88 bpm, RR is 23 and blood pressure is 130/82 mmHg. The abdomen is soft and there is widespread tenderness over the right side of the abdomen with normal bowel sounds. Urine dipstick is unremarkable and a pregnancy test is negative.

An abdominal X-ray is requested to assess for a possible bowel obstruction.

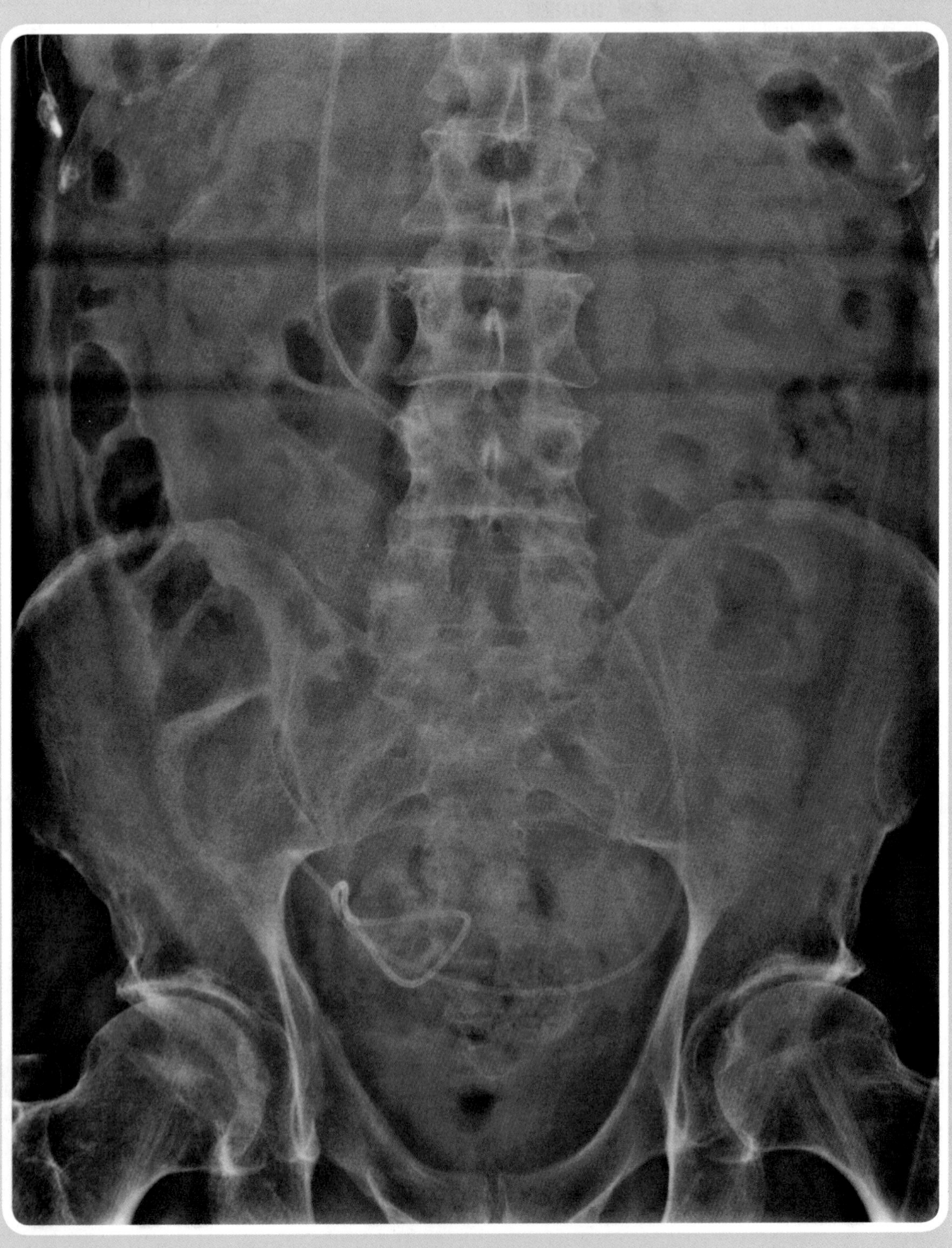

TECHNICAL INFORMATION

Patient ID: Anonymous.
Projection: AP supine.
Rotation: Adequate.
Penetration: Adequate – the spinous processes are visible.
Coverage: Inadequate – the pubic symphysis and inferior pubic rami have not been included.

BOWEL GAS PATTERN

The bowel gas pattern is normal.

BOWEL WALL

There is no evidence of mural thickening or intramural gas within the large or small bowel.

PNEUMOPERITONEUM

There is no evidence of free intraabdominal gas.

SOLID ORGANS

The solid organ contours are within normal limits with no solid organ calcification.

VASCULAR

No abnormal vascular calcification.

BONES

There are no abnormalities of the imaged thoracic and lumbar spine, or within the pelvis.

SOFT TISSUES

The psoas muscle outline is visible bilaterally.

The extraabdominal soft tissues are unremarkable.

OTHER

There is a radiopaque line projecting over the right upper quadrant, crossing the midline and with its tip terminating within the pelvis in keeping with the known VP shunt, which appears intact.

There are no vascular lines, drains or surgical clips.

REVIEW AREAS

Gallstones/renal calculi: No radiopaque calculi.
Lung bases: Not fully included.
Spine: Normal.
Femoral heads: Normal.

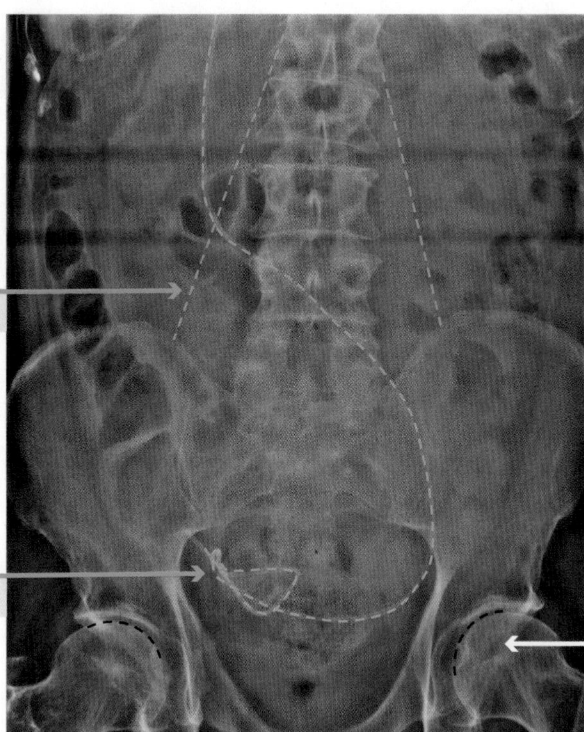

SUMMARY

This X-ray demonstrates a VP shunt with its tip projecting within the pelvis, which appears intact. There is no evidence of pneumoperitoneum.

INVESTIGATIONS AND MANAGEMENT

The patient should be resuscitated using an ABCDE approach.

Adequate analgesia and hydration should be provided.

Urgent bloods should be taken, including FBC, U&Es, LFTs, amylase, bone profile, blood culture, blood gas and CRP.

There are no clear findings on the abdominal X-ray to explain the patient's clinical presentation.

An ultrasound scan of the abdomen should be considered in the first instance to exclude gallstones, renal calculi and abdominal/pelvic collections, which may account for the patient's symptoms. The patient is also at risk of a VP shunt infection, so this should be considered as a differential.

Case

65

A 3-year-old male presents to ED with worsening abdominal distension, nausea and vomiting. He has not opened his bowels for the past 24 hours. He has no significant past medical history. On examination, he has oxygen saturations of 97% in room air and a temperature of 37.4°C. His HR is 135 bpm and RR is 36. The abdomen is rigid and there is generalized tenderness with tinkling bowel sounds. Urine dipstick is unremarkable.

An abdominal X-ray is requested to assess for possible bowel obstruction.

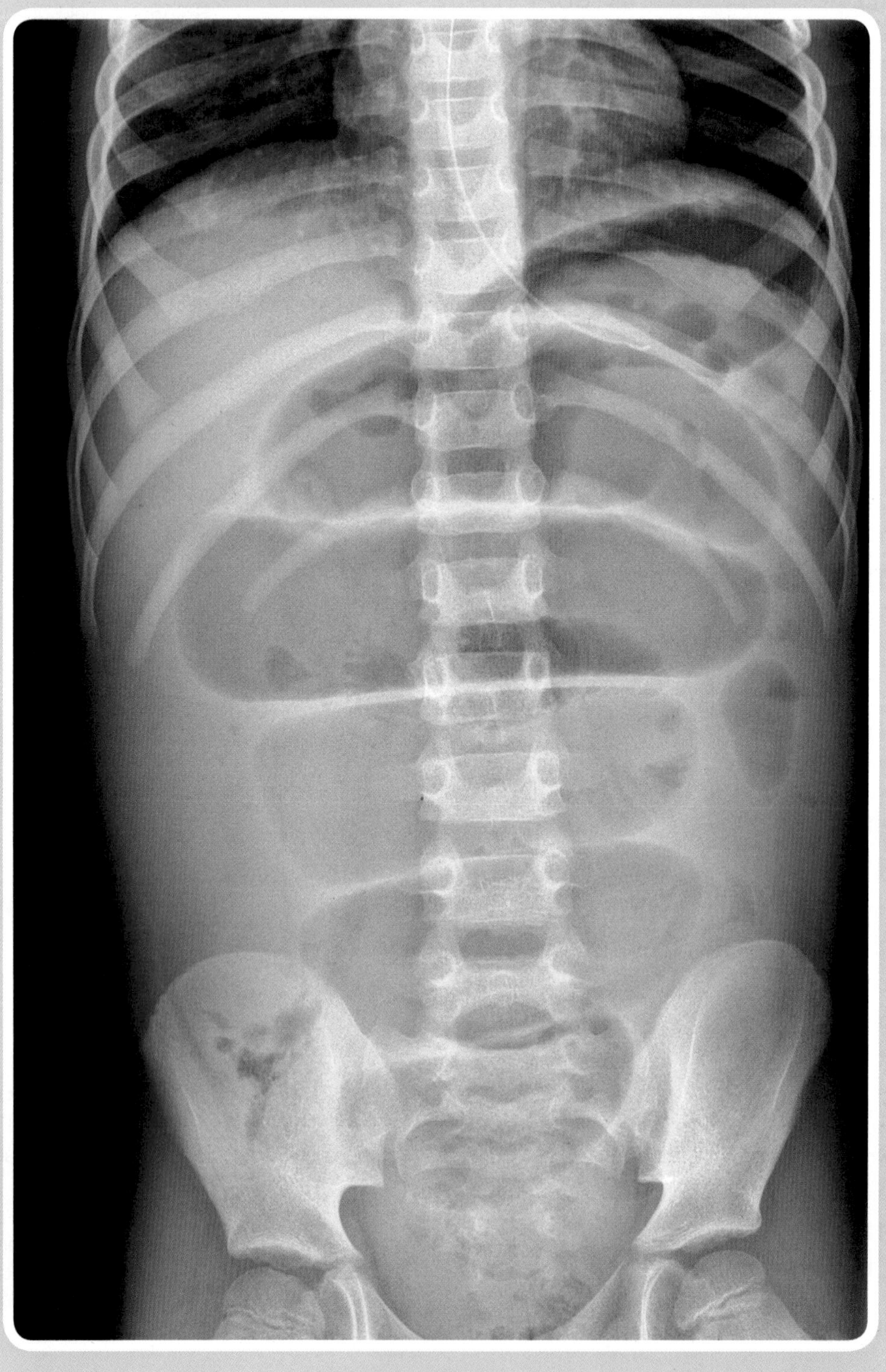

TECHNICAL INFORMATION

Patient ID: Anonymous.
Projection: AP supine.
Rotation: Adequate.
Penetration: Adequate – the spinous processes are visible.
Coverage: Inadequate – the pubic symphysis and inferior pubic rami have not been included.

BOWEL GAS PATTERN

There are multiple loops of dilated bowel seen centrally in the abdomen. Valvulae conniventes are not seen and there is probable mural thickening in keeping with mural oedema. There is a small amount of bowel gas projecting in the right lower quadrant at the caecum and within the lower pelvis in the rectum.

BOWEL WALL

There is mural thickening of the dilated small bowel loops. There is no evidence of intramural gas within the large or small bowel.

PNEUMOPERITONEUM

There is no evidence of free intraabdominal gas.

SOLID ORGANS

The solid organ contours are within normal limits with no solid organ calcification.

VASCULAR

No abnormal vascular calcification.

BONES

There are no abnormalities of the imaged thoracic and lumbar spine, or within the pelvis.

There are growth plates at the femoral head and acetabulum as the ossification centres have not yet fused, which is a normal finding in a child of this age.

SOFT TISSUES

The psoas muscle outline is not visible bilaterally, which is nonspecific, particularly in a child of this age.

The extraabdominal soft tissues are unremarkable.

OTHER

There is an NG tube in situ with its tip projecting in the left upper quadrant, in the fundus of the stomach.

There are no vascular lines, drains or surgical clips.

REVIEW AREAS

Gallstones/renal calculi: No radiopaque calculi.
Lung bases: Not fully included.
Spine: Normal.
Femoral heads: Normal – growth plates present.

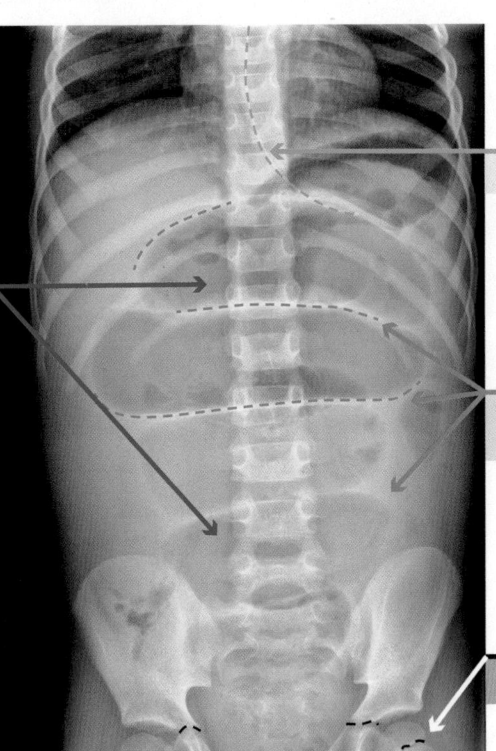

SUMMARY

This X-ray demonstrates multiple loops of dilated bowel seen centrally within the abdomen, with loss of the normal pattern of valvulae conniventes, and mural oedema, in keeping with small bowel obstruction, with no cause visible on X-ray. There is an NG tube in situ with its tip in the fundus of the stomach.

INVESTIGATIONS AND MANAGEMENT

The patient should be resuscitated using an ABCDE approach.

Adequate analgesia and hydration should be provided.

The patient should be kept NBM, have their NG tube put on free drainage and be commenced on IV fluids.

Urgent bloods should be taken, including FBC, U&Es, CRP, LFTs, coagulation, blood gas, and group and save.

The paediatric surgical team should be contacted urgently and further radiological imaging of the abdomen and pelvis should be considered for better visualization of the anatomy and further assessment.

Case

66

A 59-year-old male presents to his doctor with worsening abdominal distension and is transferred to ED by ambulance. He has no significant past medical history and is a nonsmoker. On examination, he has oxygen saturations of 92% on 4 L of oxygen and a temperature of 36.7°C. His HR is 88 bpm, RR is 22 and blood pressure is 130/78 mmHg. The abdomen is peritonitic and there are tinkling bowel sounds. Urine dipstick is unremarkable.

An abdominal X-ray is requested to assess for possible bowel obstruction.

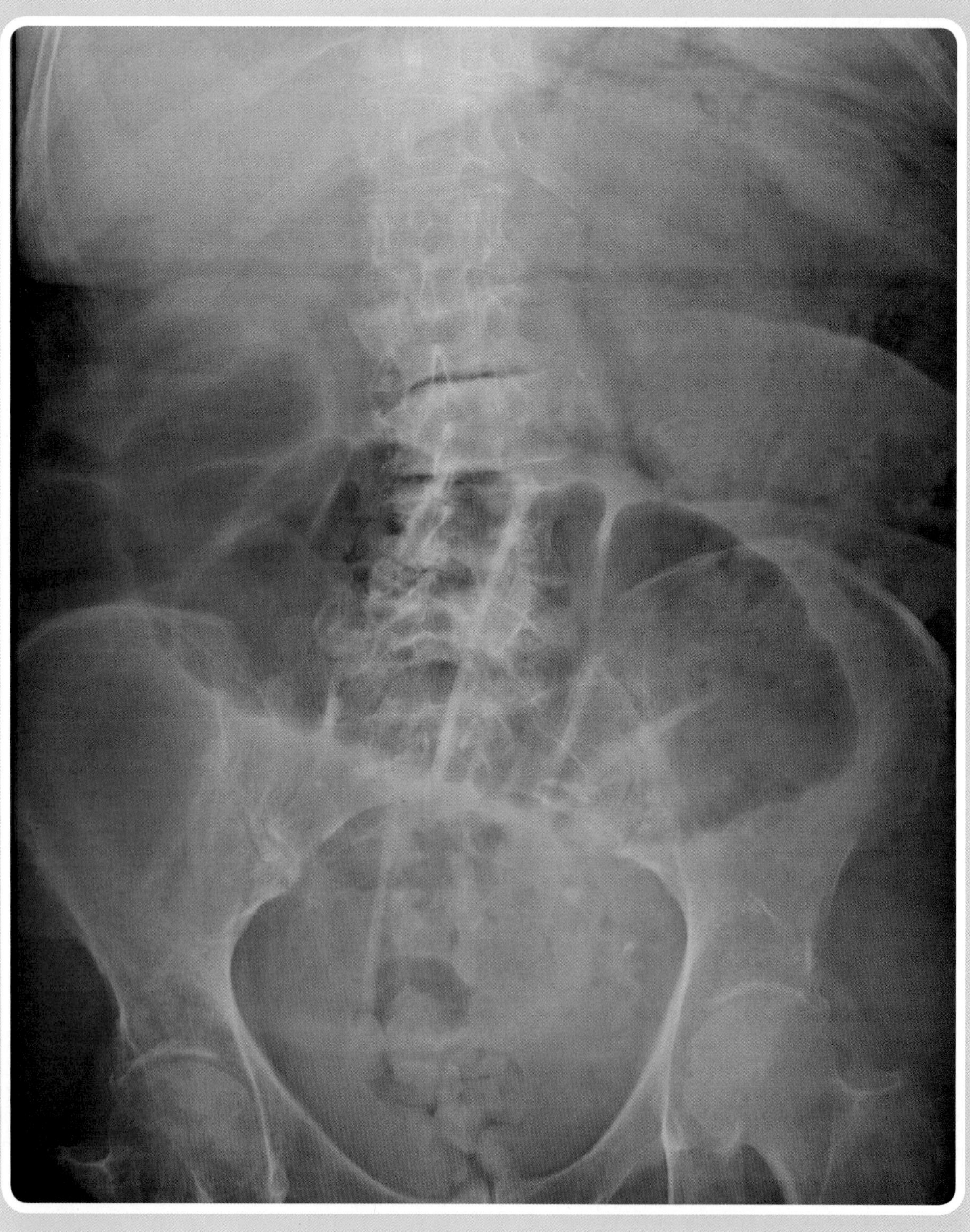

TECHNICAL INFORMATION

Patient ID: Anonymous.
Projection: AP supine.
Rotation: Adequate.
Penetration: Adequate – the spinous processes are visible.
Coverage: Inadequate – the anterior ribs, pubic symphysis and inferior pubic rami have not been fully included.

BOWEL GAS PATTERN

There is a loop of dilated bowel seen centrally within the abdomen demonstrating haustra, suggestive of large bowel obstruction.

BOWEL WALL

There is no evidence of mural thickening or intramural gas within the large or small bowel.

PNEUMOPERITONEUM

There is no evidence of free intraabdominal gas.

SOLID ORGANS

The solid organ contours are within normal limits with no solid organ calcification.

VASCULAR

No abnormal vascular calcification.

BONES

There is severe degenerative change seen throughout the lower lumbar spine.

There is loss of height of the L5 vertebral body, in keeping with a compression fracture.

The L4 vertebral body demonstrates right-sided loss of height with a wedge-shaped appearance suggestive of a probable compression fracture.

There is moderate lumbar scoliosis seen convex to the left, centred on the L4 vertebral body, secondary to degenerative change.

SOFT TISSUES

The psoas muscle outline is not visible bilaterally, which is nonspecific.

The extraabdominal soft tissues are unremarkable.

OTHER

There are no radiopaque foreign bodies.

There are no vascular lines, drains or surgical clips.

REVIEW AREAS

Gallstones/renal calculi: No radiopaque calculi.
Lung bases: Not fully included.
Spine: Degenerative change in lumbar spine with loss of height of L5 vertebral body and scoliosis.
Femoral heads: Normal.

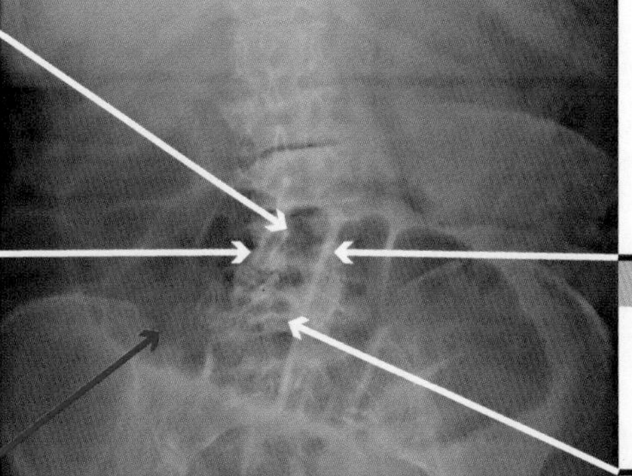

SUMMARY

This X-ray demonstrates a loop of dilated bowel seen centrally within the abdomen demonstrating haustra, suggestive of large bowel obstruction. There is severe degenerative disease of the lower lumbar spine, with degenerative scoliosis convex to the left centred on the L4 vertebral body and a compression fracture of the L5 vertebral body. There is a further probable L4 compression fracture. Malignancy with secondary bony metastases should be suspected.

INVESTIGATIONS AND MANAGEMENT

The patient should be resuscitated using an ABCDE approach.

Adequate analgesia and hydration should be provided.

The patient should be kept NBM and an NG tube inserted. IV fluids should be commenced.

Urgent bloods should be taken, including FBC, U&Es, CRP, LFTs, coagulation, blood gas, and group and save.

The general surgical team should be contacted urgently and a CT scan of the abdomen/pelvis with IV contrast should be considered for better visualization of the anatomy and further assessment.

Arthritic changes in the first instance should be managed with lifestyle changes and analgesia, but depending on symptoms, orthopaedic referral may be considered.

Chronic management of vertebral compression fractures may involve lifestyle modification, physiotherapy and pain medication, but further history/examination should be sought, and previous images reviewed.

Case

67

A 67-year-old male presents to ED with generalized abdominal pain and distension. He has not passed flatus or opened his bowels for over 24 hours. He has no significant past medical history and is a nonsmoker. On examination, he has oxygen saturations of 94% in room air and a temperature of 37.2°C. His HR is 90 bpm, RR is 28 and blood pressure is 120/68 mmHg. The abdomen is soft with central tenderness and associated lumbar back pain. Bowel sounds are normal and urine dipstick is unremarkable.

An abdominal X-ray is requested to assess for possible bowel obstruction.

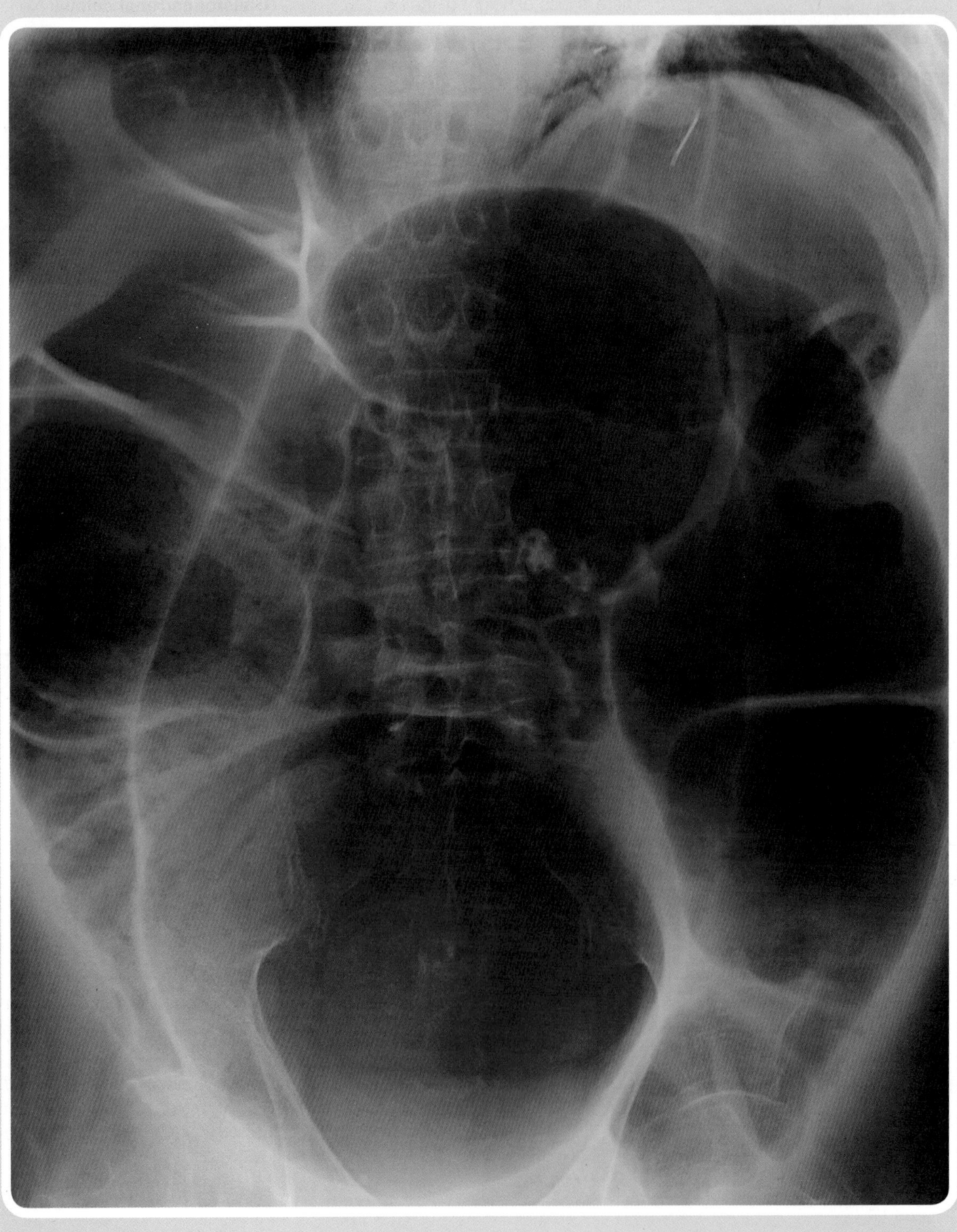

TECHNICAL INFORMATION

Patient ID: Anonymous.
Projection: AP supine.
Rotation: Adequate.
Penetration: Adequate – the spinous processes are visible.
Coverage: Inadequate – the anterior ribs, pubic symphysis and inferior pubic rami have not been included.

BOWEL GAS PATTERN

There is a large gas-filled loop of bowel centrally in the abdomen demonstrating haustra, arising from the pelvis, with its tip pointing towards the upper abdomen, in keeping with sigmoid volvulus. There are further loops of dilated bowel seen peripherally in the abdomen, demonstrating haustra, in keeping with large bowel dilatation.

BOWEL WALL

There is no evidence of mural thickening or intramural gas within the large or small bowel.

PNEUMOPERITONEUM

There is no evidence of free intraabdominal gas.

SOLID ORGANS

The solid organ contours are within normal limits with no solid organ calcification.

VASCULAR

No abnormal vascular calcification.

BONES

There is mild to moderate degenerative change seen throughout the lower lumbar spine.

There is mild osteoarthritic change seen within both hip joints with joint space narrowing and subchondral sclerosis.

There is diffuse osteopenia of the bones.

SOFT TISSUES

The psoas muscle outline is not visible bilaterally, which is nonspecific.

The extraabdominal soft tissues are unremarkable.

OTHER

There is a radiopacity projecting in the epigastrium, which likely represents film artefact.

There are no radiopaque foreign bodies.

There are no vascular lines, drains or surgical clips.

REVIEW AREAS

Gallstones/renal calculi: No radiopaque calculi.
Lung bases: Not fully included.
Spine: Degenerative change in lower lumbar spine.
Femoral heads: Mild osteoarthritic change.

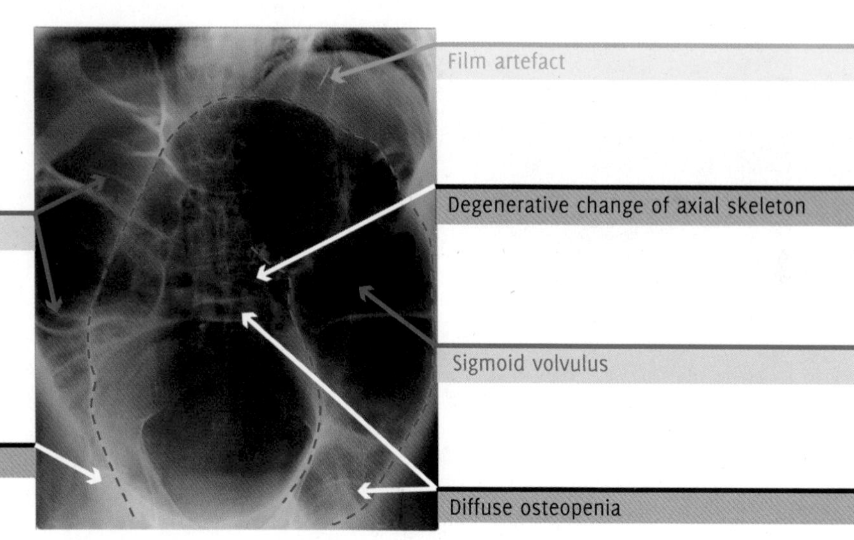

SUMMARY

This X-ray demonstrates a large gas-filled loop of bowel centrally within the abdomen displaying haustra, in keeping with sigmoid volvulus. There are further dilated large bowel loops seen peripherally in keeping with large bowel obstruction secondary to the volvulus. The mild to moderate lower lumbar spine degenerative changes, mild osteoarthritic hip changes and diffuse osteopenia are incidental findings.

INVESTIGATIONS AND MANAGEMENT

The patient should be resuscitated using an ABCDE approach.

Adequate analgesia and hydration should be provided.

The patient should be kept NBM and an NG tube inserted on free drainage. IV fluids should be commenced.

Urgent bloods should be taken, including FBC, U&Es, bone profile, CRP, LFTs, coagulation, blood gas, and group and save.

The general surgical team should be contacted urgently.

Urgent decompression with sigmoidoscopy is required to relieve the obstruction, with a flatus tube left in situ. Elective sigmoidectomy with primary anastomosis may then be undertaken to prevent reoccurrence.

Case

68

A 50-year-old female is currently admitted to the urology ward with longstanding dysuria and the inability to pass urine over the last 12 hours. She has no other significant past medical history and is a nonsmoker. On examination, she has oxygen saturations of 95% in room air and a temperature of 37.0°C. Her HR is 84 bpm, RR is 14 and blood pressure is 118/80 mmHg. The abdomen is soft and there is tenderness in both flanks with normal bowel sounds. Urine dipstick shows blood ++.

An abdominal X-ray is requested to assess for possible renal calculi.

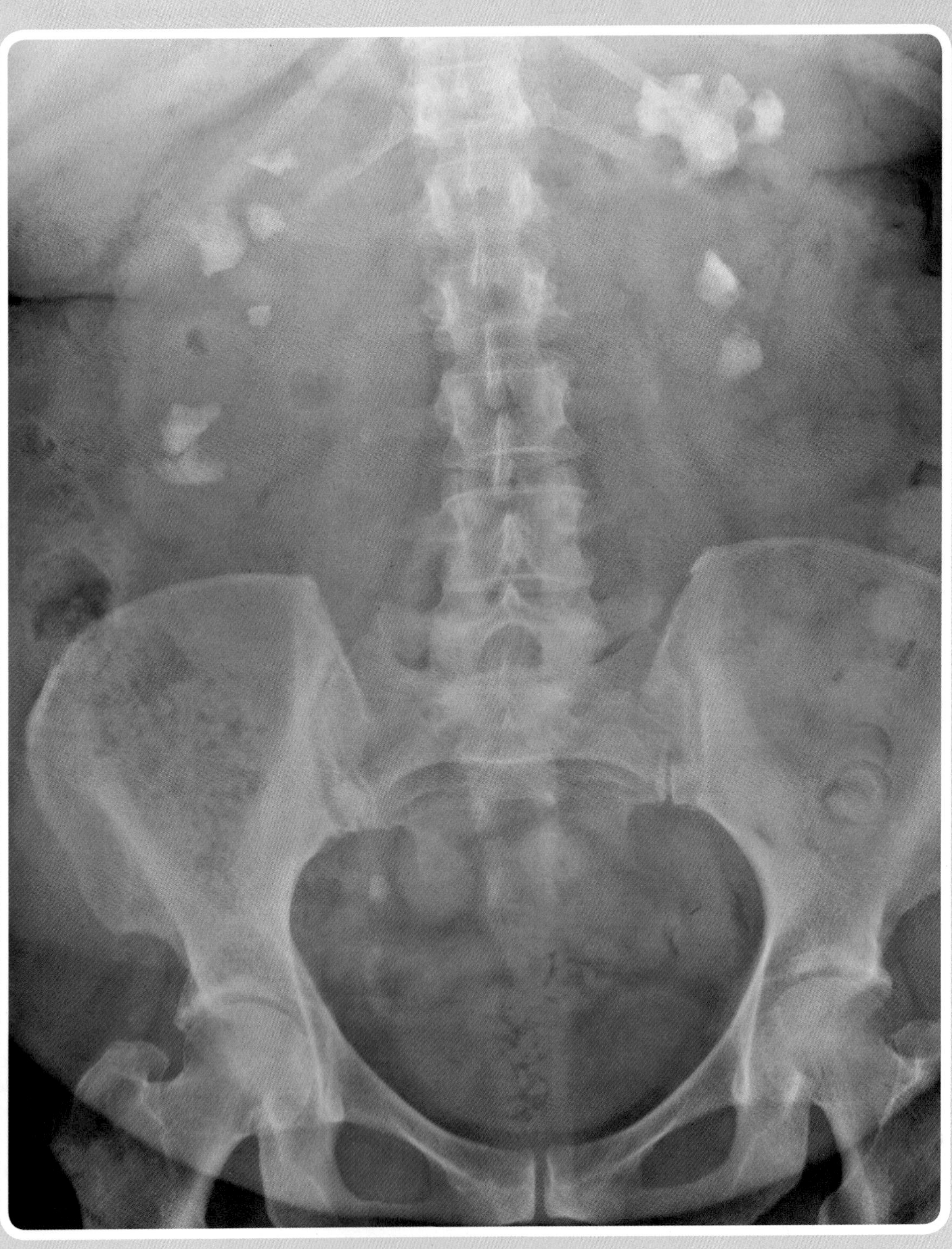

TECHNICAL INFORMATION

Patient ID: Anonymous.
Projection: AP supine.
Rotation: Adequate.
Penetration: Adequate – the spinous processes are visible.
Coverage: Adequate – the anterior ribs are visible superiorly and the inferior pubic rami are visible.

BOWEL GAS PATTERN

There is a paucity of bowel gas but no bowel dilatation is visible.

There is a small to moderate volume of faecal residue present throughout the large bowel.

BOWEL WALL

There is no evidence of mural thickening or intramural gas within the large or small bowel.

PNEUMOPERITONEUM

There is no evidence of free intraabdominal gas.

SOLID ORGANS

There are multiple large irregular radiopaque densities projected over the regions of both kidneys. The largest density is projecting over the left upper pole conforming to the shape of the renal calyces in keeping with a staghorn calculus.

VASCULAR

No abnormal vascular calcification.

BONES

There are no abnormalities of the imaged thoracic and lumbar spine, or within the pelvis.

SOFT TISSUES

The psoas muscle outline is visible bilaterally.

The extraabdominal soft tissues are unremarkable.

OTHER

There are no radiopaque foreign bodies.

There are no vascular lines, drains or surgical clips.

REVIEW AREAS

Gallstones/renal calculi: Likely staghorn calculus in the upper pole of the left kidney with multiple bilateral smaller calculi or renal tissue calcifications in the region of both kidneys.
Lung bases: Not fully included.
Spine: Normal.
Femoral heads: Normal.

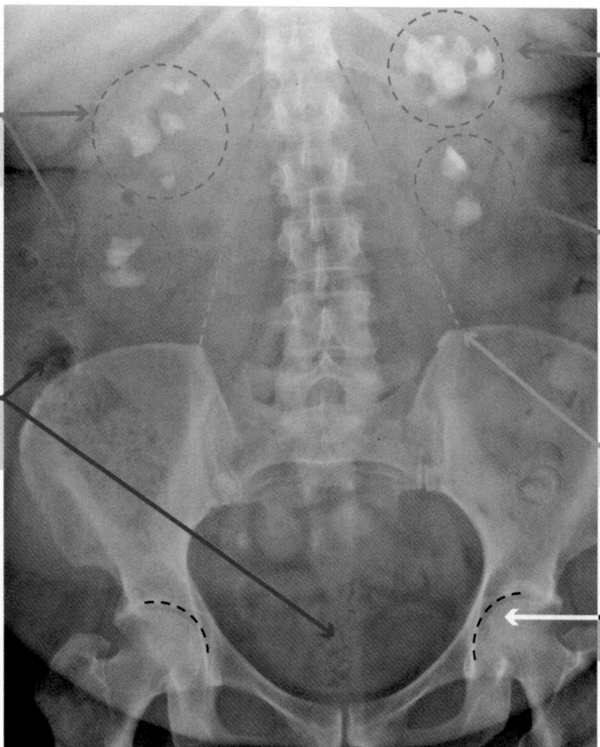

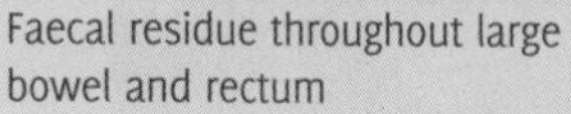

SUMMARY

This X-ray demonstrates multiple radiopaque densities projected over the regions of both kidneys, in keeping with medullary nephrocalcinosis with an associated staghorn calculus in the left upper pole.

INVESTIGATIONS AND MANAGEMENT

Adequate analgesia and hydration should be provided.

Urgent bloods should be taken, including FBC, U&Es, CRP, LFTs, blood gas and bone profile.

The patient should be assessed for acute kidney injury, and if present, an ultrasound of the urinary tract in the first instance would be beneficial in assessing for hydronephrosis. A CT scan of the kidneys, ureters and bladder may be useful for better visualization of the anatomy.

The patient should be discussed with the urology team for further assessment of the medullary nephrocalcinosis.

Case

69

A 20-year-old male presents to ED with generalized abdominal pain. He has no significant past medical history and is a nonsmoker. On examination, he has oxygen saturations of 99% in room air and a temperature of 38.0°C. His HR is 106 bpm, RR is 22 and blood pressure is 120/65 mmHg. The abdomen is rigid and there is generalized tenderness. Urine dipstick is unremarkable.

An abdominal X-ray is requested to assess for possible bowel obstruction.

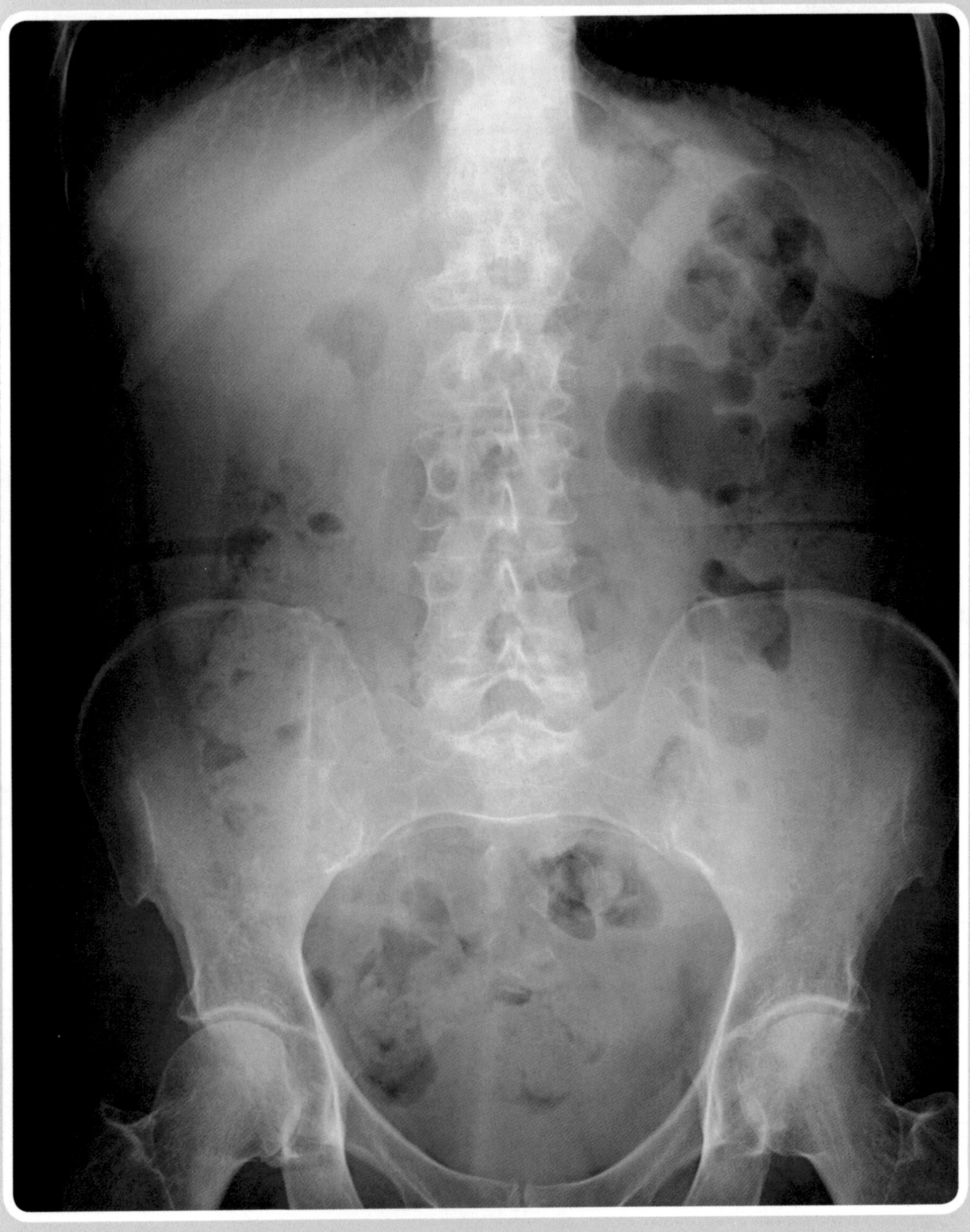

TECHNICAL INFORMATION

Patient ID: Anonymous.
Projection: AP supine.
Rotation: Adequate.
Penetration: Adequate – the spinous processes are visible.
Coverage: Inadequate – the pubic symphysis and inferior pubic rami have not been fully included.

BOWEL GAS PATTERN

The bowel gas pattern is normal.

There is a mild to moderate volume of faecal residue throughout the colon and rectum.

BOWEL WALL

There is no evidence of mural thickening or intramural gas within the large or small bowel. There is mild faecal loading throughout the large bowel and within the rectum.

PNEUMOPERITONEUM

There is no evidence of free intraabdominal gas.

SOLID ORGANS

The right lobe of the liver extends inferiorly beyond the lower margin of the right kidney, with a tongue-like appearance, in keeping with a Riedel's lobe.

VASCULAR

No abnormal vascular calcification.

BONES

There are no abnormalities of the imaged thoracic and lumbar spine, or within the pelvis.

SOFT TISSUES

The psoas muscle outline is visible bilaterally.

The extraabdominal soft tissues are unremarkable.

OTHER

There are no radiopaque foreign bodies.

There are no vascular lines, drains or surgical clips.

REVIEW AREAS

Gallstones/renal calculi: No radiopaque calculi.
Lung bases: Normal.
Spine: Normal.
Femoral heads: Normal.

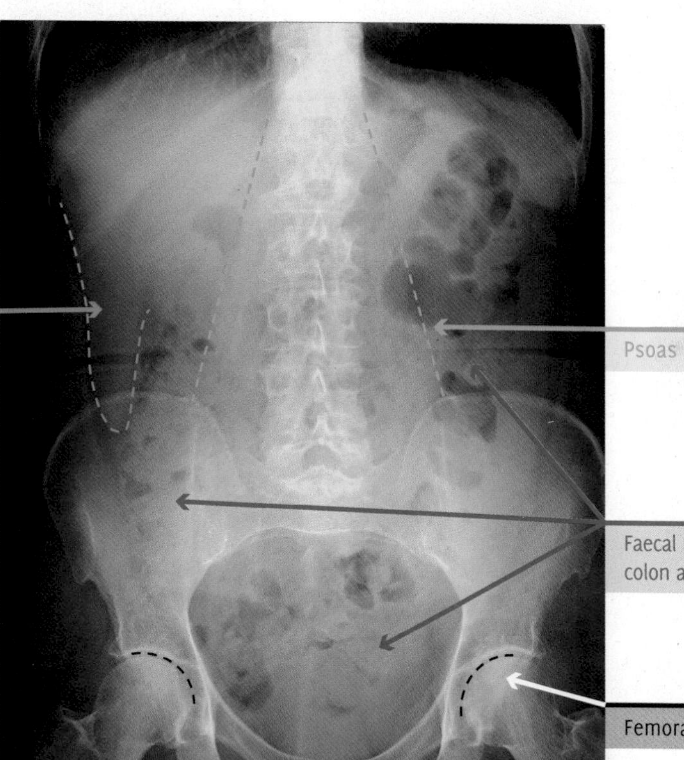

SUMMARY

This X-ray demonstrates a normal abdominal appearance with no evidence of bowel obstruction or pneumoperitoneum. There is an incidental Riedel's lobe of the liver, which is a normal anatomical variant.

INVESTIGATIONS AND MANAGEMENT

The patient should be resuscitated using an ABCDE approach.

Adequate analgesia and hydration should be provided.

Bloods should be taken, including FBC, U&Es, LFTs, amylase, bone profile, blood gas, blood cultures, group and save, and CRP.

The Sepsis 6 pathway should be started immediately, including administration of oxygen, IV broad-spectrum antibiotics and consideration of a fluid bolus as well as measurement of lactate and urinary output and blood cultures.

The patient should be made NBM and started on IV fluids.

There are no clear findings on the abdominal X-ray to explain the patient's clinical presentation. An ultrasound scan of the abdomen and pelvis should be considered in the first instance for further assessment.

Case

70

A 6-day-old baby girl is currently admitted to NICU, having had operative intervention on day 5 of life for Hirschsprung disease. On examination, she has oxygen saturations of 98% in room air and a temperature of 36.6°C. Her HR is 160 bpm and RR is 42. The abdomen is soft with normal bowel sounds.

You are asked to review her postoperative X-ray.

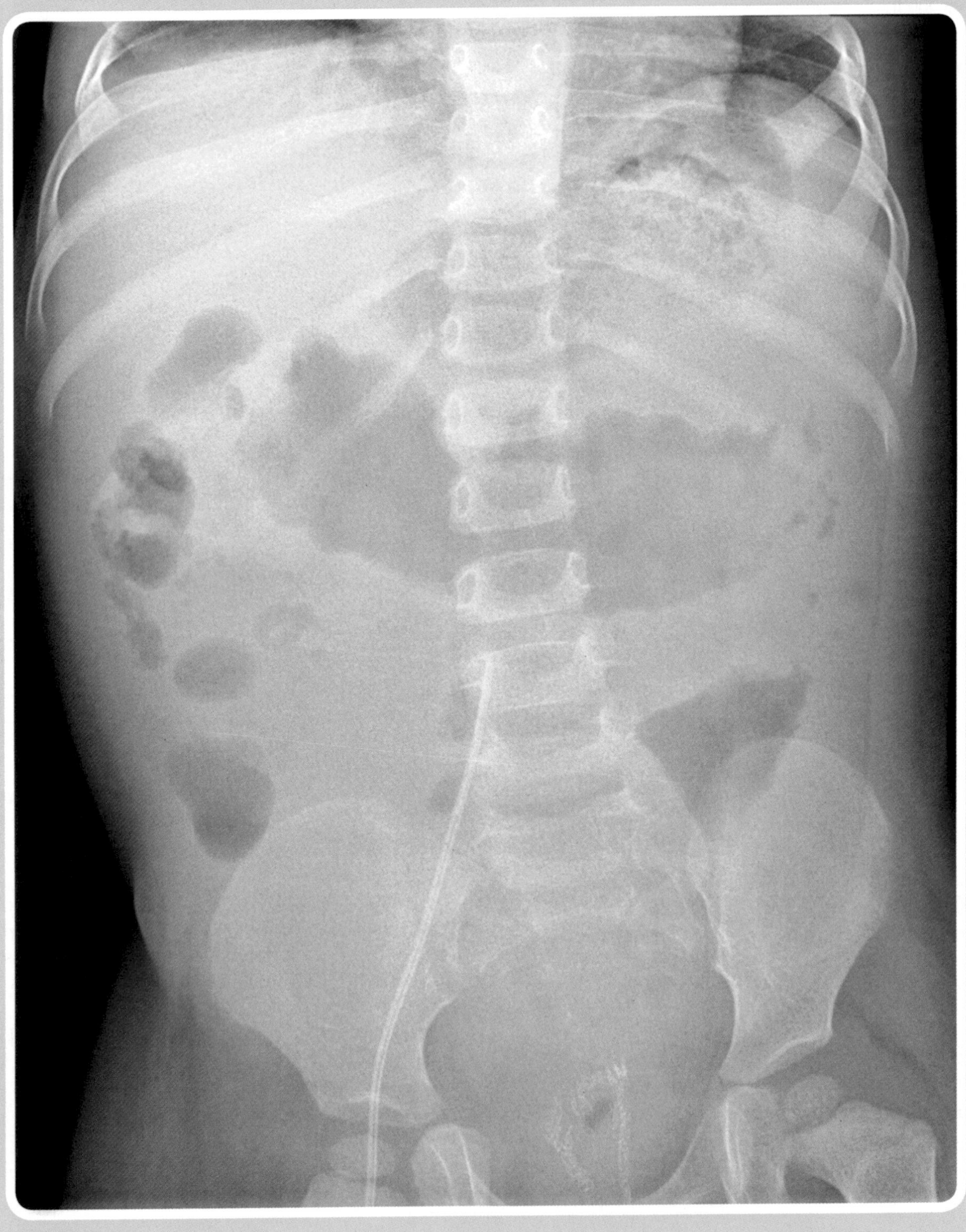

TECHNICAL INFORMATION

Patient ID: Anonymous.
Projection: AP supine.
Rotation: Asymmetrical appearances of the pelvis in keeping with mild patient rotation.
Penetration: Adequate – the spine is visible.

Coverage: Inadequate – the pubic symphysis and inferior pubic rami have not been included.

BOWEL GAS PATTERN

There is prominence of the transverse colon, which is nonspecific.

There is a paucity of bowel gas seen within the distal descending and sigmoid colon, but there is gas in the rectum.

BOWEL WALL

There is evidence of mural thickening of the transverse colon in the left and right upper quadrants of the abdomen with evidence of 'thumbprinting', in keeping with mural oedema.

There is no evidence of intramural gas within the large or small bowel.

PNEUMOPERITONEUM

There is no evidence of free intraabdominal gas.

SOLID ORGANS

The solid organ contours are within normal limits with no solid organ calcification.

VASCULAR

No abnormal vascular calcification.

BONES

There are no abnormalities of the imaged thoracic and lumbar spine, or within the pelvis.

There are growth plates at the femoral head and acetabulum as the ossification centres have not yet fused, which is a normal finding in a child of this age.

There is cartilage seen between the vertebrae, which is a normal finding in a child of this age.

SOFT TISSUES

The psoas muscle outline is not visible bilaterally, which is nonspecific, particularly in a child of this age.

The extraabdominal soft tissues are unremarkable.

OTHER

There is a radiopaque line seen projected over the region of the right hemipelvis with its tip projecting at the level of the right L4 vertebral pedicle, in keeping with a right-sided femoral venous catheter appropriately sited in the inferior vena cava.

There are radiopaque surgical sutures seen within the rectum, in keeping with previous bowel surgery.

REVIEW AREAS

Gallstones/renal calculi: No radiopaque calculi.
Lung bases: Normal.
Spine: Normal – cartilage between vertebrae.
Femoral heads: Normal – growth plates present.

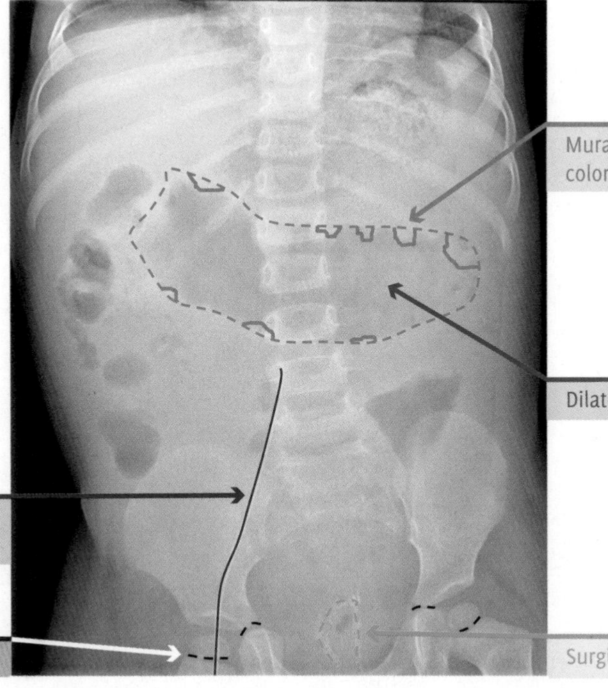

SUMMARY

This X-ray demonstrates dilatation of the transverse colon with mural thickening. Given the history of Hirschsprung disease and recent surgery, findings may represent residual colitis in the transverse colon.

INVESTIGATIONS AND MANAGEMENT

Appearances are within normal postoperative limits; however, there is possible residual colitis in the transverse colon.

Current management should continue and correlation with clinical findings and biochemical markers should guide further management.

The patient should remain NBM and on total parenteral nutrition (TPN), with careful monitoring of fluid balance, broad-spectrum antibiotics and electrolytes.

Regular surgical review is required until discharge.

Case 71

A 60-year-old male on the general surgical ward develops severe abdominal pain, vomiting and abdominal distention. His past medical history is significant for recent drainage of an abdominal abscess. On examination, he has oxygen saturations of 93% in room air and a temperature of 38.3°C. His HR is 100 bpm and RR is 25. The abdomen is rigid and there is generalized tenderness. Urine dipstick is unremarkable.

An abdominal X-ray is requested to assess for possible bowel obstruction.

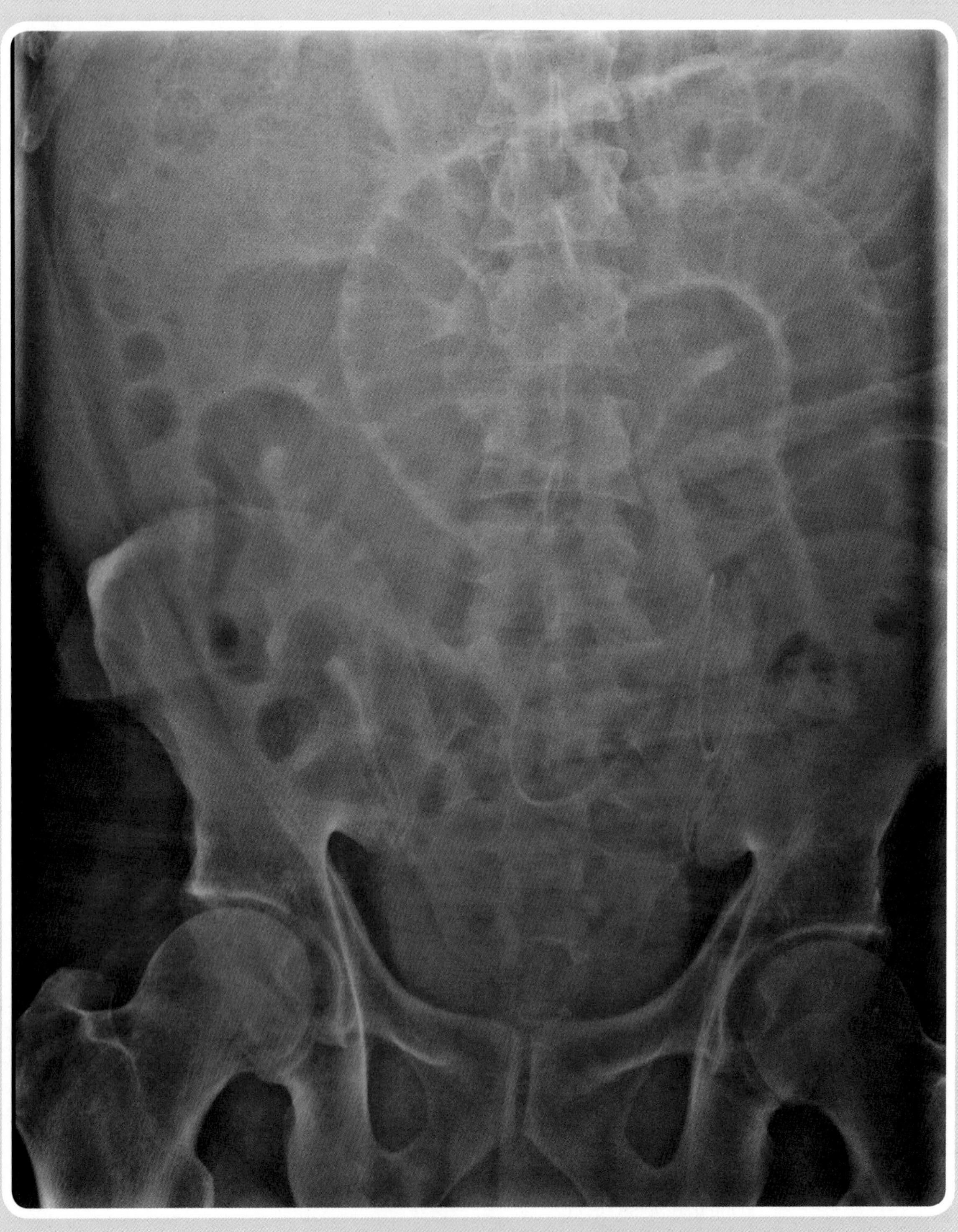

TECHNICAL INFORMATION

Patient ID: Anonymous.
Projection: AP supine.
Rotation: Adequate.
Penetration: Adequate.
Coverage: Inadequate – left and right hemidiaphragms not included.

BOWEL GAS PATTERN

There are multiple loops of prominent small bowel seen centrally in the abdomen demonstrating valvulae conniventes, in keeping with small bowel obstruction.

BOWEL WALL

There is mural thickening of the dilated small bowel loops. There is no evidence of intramural gas within the large or small bowel.

PNEUMOPERITONEUM

There is no evidence of free intraabdominal gas.

SOLID ORGANS

The solid organ contours are within normal limits with no solid organ calcification.

VASCULAR

No abnormal vascular calcification.

BONES

There are no abnormalities of the imaged thoracic and lumbar spine, or within the pelvis.

SOFT TISSUES

The psoas muscle outline is not visible bilaterally, which is nonspecific.

Extraabdominal soft tissues are unremarkable.

OTHER

There are no radiopaque foreign bodies.

There is a radiopaque line in the lower left quadrant with its tip projecting over the left sacroiliac joint, which likely represents an abdominal drain.

There are no surgical clips.

REVIEW AREAS

Gallstones/renal calculi: No radiopaque calculi.
Lung bases: Not fully included.
Spine: Normal.
Femoral heads: Normal.

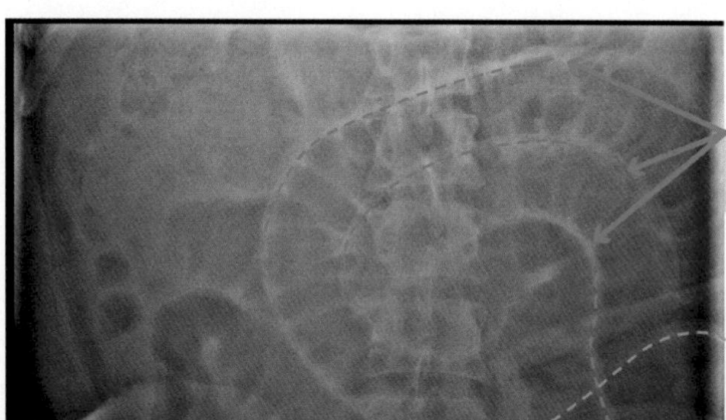

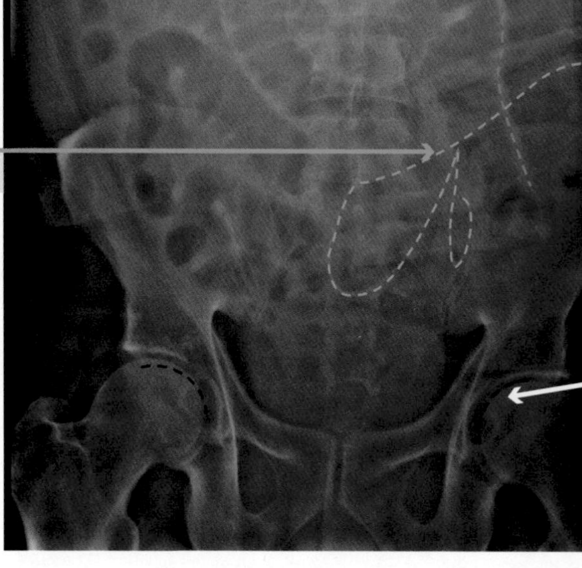

SUMMARY

This X-ray demonstrates dilatation of small bowel loops, which demonstrate mural thickening in keeping with small bowel obstruction and related inflammatory changes. No cause is visible, although ileus is most likely given the recent abdominal drainage. There is an abdominal drain in situ with its tip projecting over the left sacroiliac joint.

INVESTIGATIONS AND MANAGEMENT

The patient should be resuscitated using an ABCDE approach.

The Sepsis 6 pathway should be started immediately, including administration of oxygen, IV broad-spectrum antibiotics and consideration of a fluid bolus as well as measurement of lactate, urinary output and blood cultures.

The patient should be made NBM and started on IV fluids, and have an NG tube inserted.

Urgent bloods should be taken, including FBC, U&Es, CRP, bone profile, LFTs, coagulation, blood cultures, blood gas, and group and save.

A CT scan of the abdomen/pelvis with IV contrast should be considered for further evaluation of the abdomen and the general surgical team should be involved.

Case 72

A 60-year-old female presents to ED with abdominal pain, vomiting and severe abdominal distention. She has no significant past medical history. On examination, she has oxygen saturations of 94% in room air and a temperature of 37.4°C. Her HR is 100 bpm and RR is 25. The abdomen is soft and distended, with generalized tenderness and normal bowel sounds. Urine dipstick is unremarkable.

An abdominal X-ray is requested to assess for possible bowel obstruction.

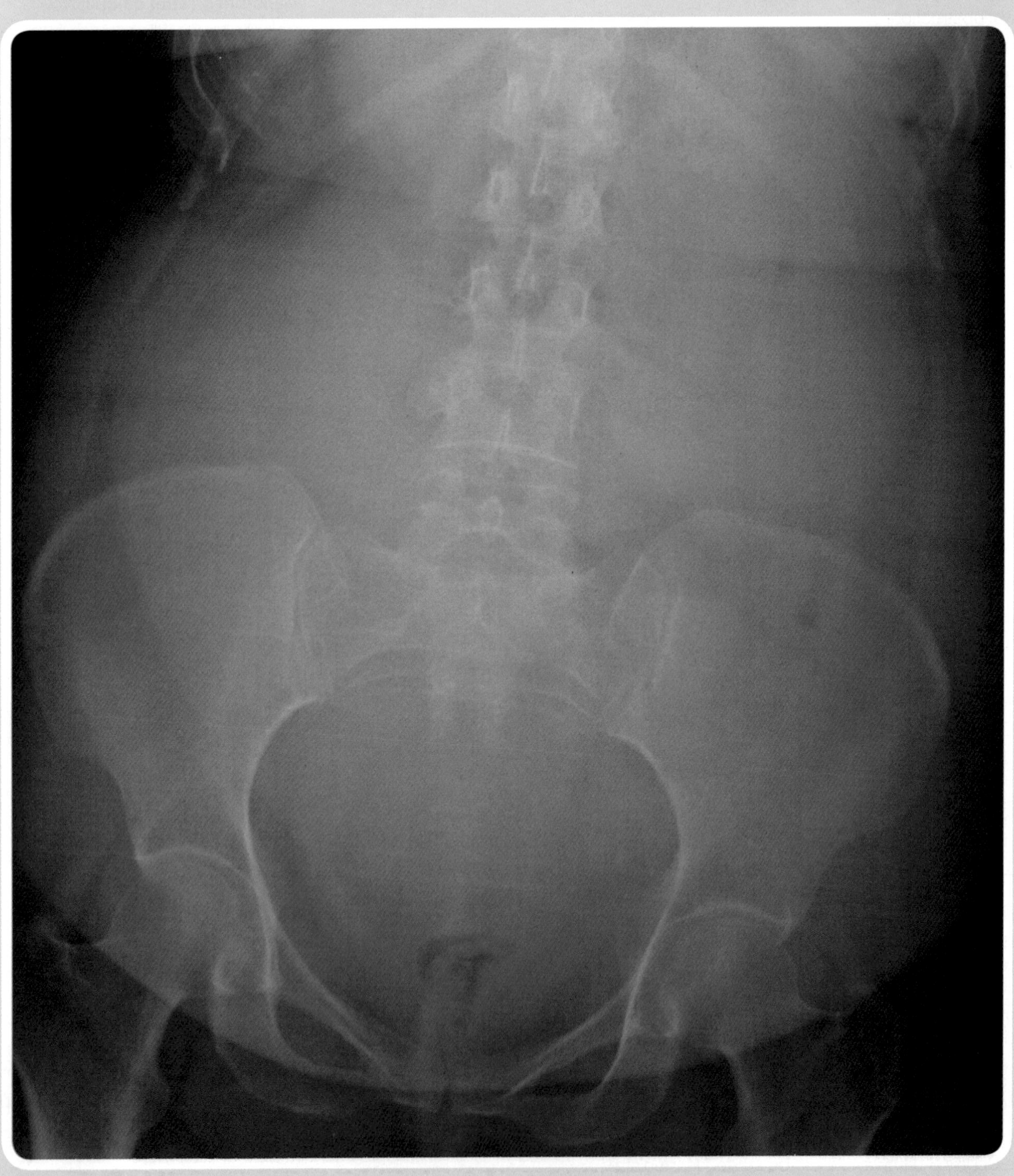

TECHNICAL INFORMATION

Patient ID: Anonymous.
Projection: AP supine.
Rotation: Adequate.
Penetration: Adequate – the spinous processes are visible.
Coverage: Inadequate – the upper abdomen is not fully included.

BOWEL GAS PATTERN

There is a generalized paucity of bowel gas. Gas is seen in the rectum.

BOWEL WALL

There is no evidence of mural thickening or intramural gas within the large or small bowel.

PNEUMOPERITONEUM

There is no evidence of free intraabdominal gas.

SOLID ORGANS

The solid organs are poorly defined due to diffusely increased density of the abdomen.

VASCULAR

No abnormal vascular calcification.

BONES

There are no abnormalities of the imaged thoracic and lumbar spine, or within the pelvis.

SOFT TISSUES

The psoas muscle outline is not visible bilaterally due to diffusely increased density of the abdomen.

Bulging of the flanks is seen.

OTHER

There are no radiopaque foreign bodies.

There are no vascular lines, drains or surgical clips.

REVIEW AREAS

Gallstones/renal calculi: No radiopaque calculi.
Lung bases: Not fully included.
Spine: Normal.
Femoral heads: Normal.

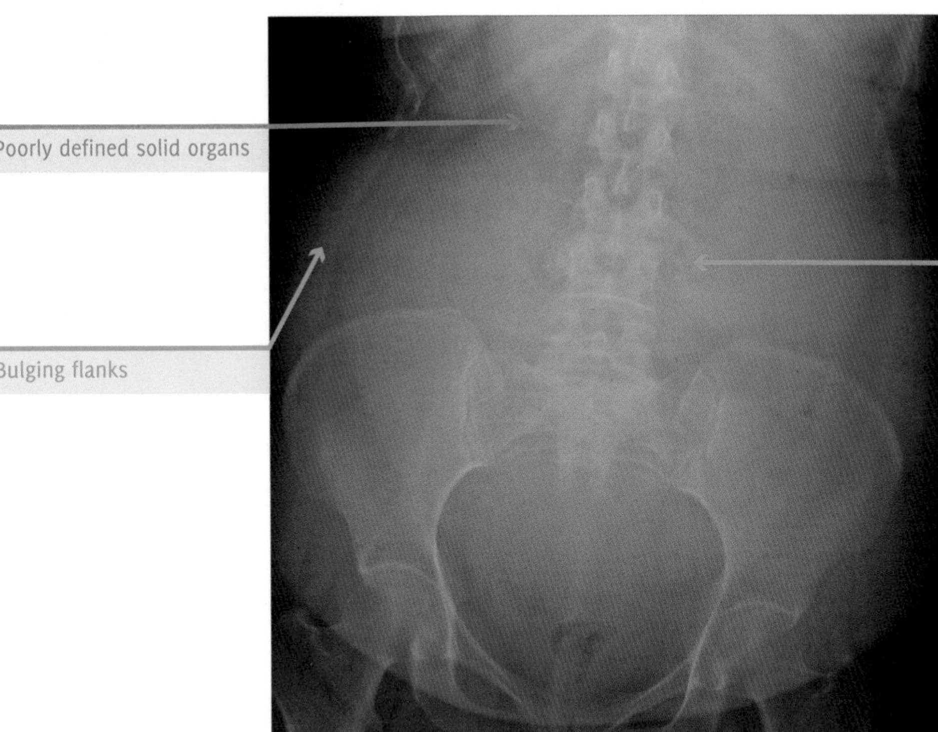

SUMMARY

This X-ray demonstrates diffuse increased density of the abdomen, with poor definition of the solid organs and other soft tissues including the psoas muscle shadow with bulging at the flanks in keeping with a large volume intraabdominal ascites. There is no evidence of pneumoperitoneum.

INVESTIGATIONS AND MANAGEMENT

The patient should be resuscitated using an ABCDE approach.

Adequate analgesia, antiemetics and hydration should be provided.

Urgent bloods should be taken, including FBC, U&Es, CRP, LFTs, TFTs, blood gas and bone profile.

A USS-guided diagnostic aspiration of the ascitic fluid should be considered to determine the cause. Therapeutic ascitic drain insertion should be considered if clinically appropriate.

Further imaging may be required depending on the underlying cause (e.g. cirrhosis, malignancy).

ADVANCED CASES

Case

73

A 75-year-old female presents to ED with worsening abdominal pain, abdominal distension, nausea and vomiting. She has no significant past medical history and is a nonsmoker. On examination, she has oxygen saturations of 94% in room air and a temperature of 37.2°C. Her HR is 98 bpm, RR is 26 and blood pressure is 100/62 mmHg. The abdomen is soft and there is generalized abdominal tenderness with tinkling bowel sounds. Urine dipstick is unremarkable.

An abdominal X-ray is requested to assess for possible bowel obstruction.

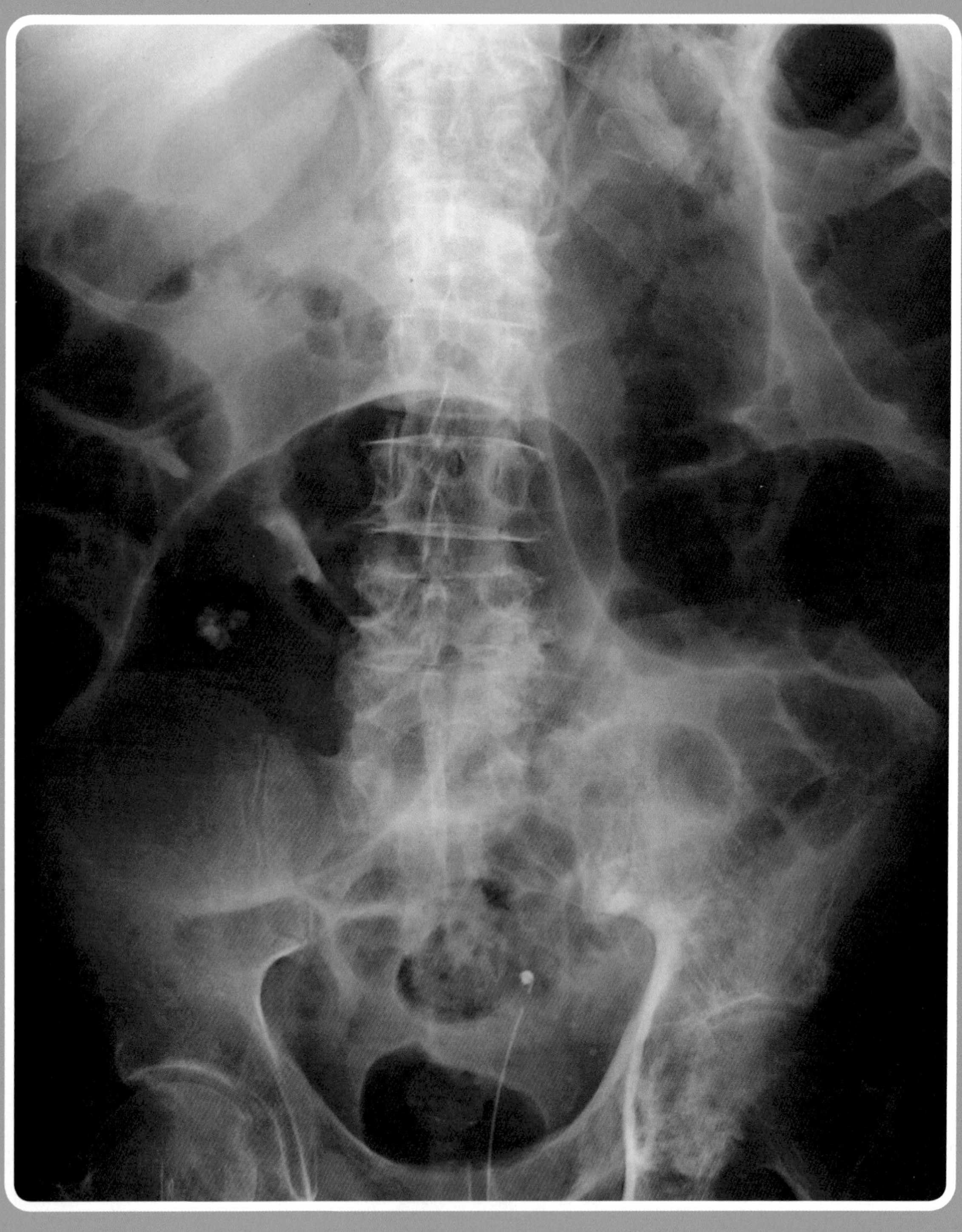

TECHNICAL INFORMATION

Patient ID: Anonymous.
Projection: AP supine.
Rotation: Adequate.
Penetration: Adequate – the spinous processes are visible.
Coverage: Inadequate – the pubic symphysis, inferior pubic rami and upper abdomen have not been fully included.

BOWEL GAS PATTERN

There are multiple loops of dilated bowel seen centrally and peripherally in the abdomen demonstrating haustra, in keeping with large bowel obstruction.

BOWEL WALL

There is no evidence of mural thickening or intramural gas within the large or small bowel.

PNEUMOPERITONEUM

There is no evidence of free intraabdominal gas.

SOLID ORGANS

The solid organ contours are within normal limits with no solid organ calcification.

VASCULAR

There is splenic artery calcification in the left upper quadrant.

BONES

There is moderate degenerative change seen in the lower lumbar spine.

There is a mixed lucent and sclerotic architecture of the left hemipelvis.

There is mild expansion of the left hemipelvis compared to the right hemipelvis and coarsening of the trabeculae with cortical thickening of the left ilioischial line.

SOFT TISSUES

The psoas muscle outline is visible bilaterally.

The extraabdominal soft tissues are unremarkable.

OTHER

There is a urinary catheter in situ within the urinary bladder.

There is an irregular radiopaque area of calcification within the right lower quadrant of the abdomen in keeping with mesenteric lymph node calcification.

There are no vascular lines, drains or surgical clips.

REVIEW AREAS

Gallstones/renal calculi: No radiopaque calculi.
Lung bases: Not fully included.
Spine: Degenerative change throughout the lower lumbar spine.
Femoral heads: Mixed lucent and sclerotic architecture.

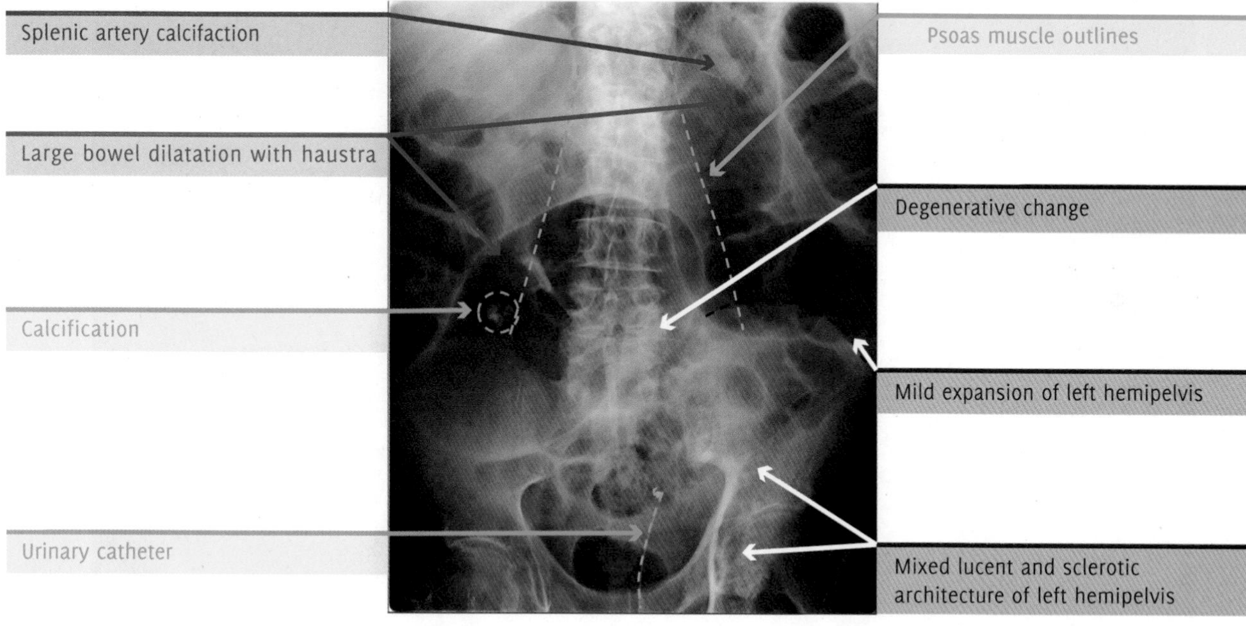

SUMMARY

This X-ray demonstrates multiple loops of dilated bowel demonstrating haustra, in keeping with large bowel obstruction. The cause for this is not demonstrated. The left hemipelvis bony expansion with coarsening of trabeculae and mixed lucent and sclerotic architecture is in keeping with Paget disease. There is a urinary catheter in situ.

INVESTIGATIONS AND MANAGEMENT

The patient should be resuscitated using an ABCDE approach.

Adequate analgesia and hydration should be provided.

The patient should be kept NBM and an NG tube inserted on free drainage. IV fluids should be commenced.

Urgent bloods should be taken, including FBC, U&Es, bone profile, CRP, LFTs, coagulation, blood gas, and group and save.

The general surgical team should be contacted urgently and a CT scan of the abdomen/pelvis with IV contrast should be considered for better visualization of the anatomy and further assessment.

Once the bowel obstruction has been resolved, the patient should be seen in rheumatology clinic for review of her Paget disease. Arthritic changes in the first instance should be management with lifestyle changes and analgesia, depending on symptoms.

Case 74

A 40-year-old female presents to ED with abdominal pain, having not passed flatus or opened her bowels for over 48 hours. Her past medical history is significant for a previous laparoscopic appendicectomy 6 years ago, and an IVC insertion for recurrent pulmonary embolisms. She is a smoker. On examination, she has oxygen saturations of 97% in room air and a temperature of 37.5°C. Her HR is 132 bpm, RR is 25 and blood pressure is 142/86 mmHg. The abdomen is rigid and there is generalized tenderness with tinkling bowel sounds. Urine dipstick is unremarkable and a pregnancy test is negative.

An abdominal X-ray is requested to assess for possible bowel obstruction.

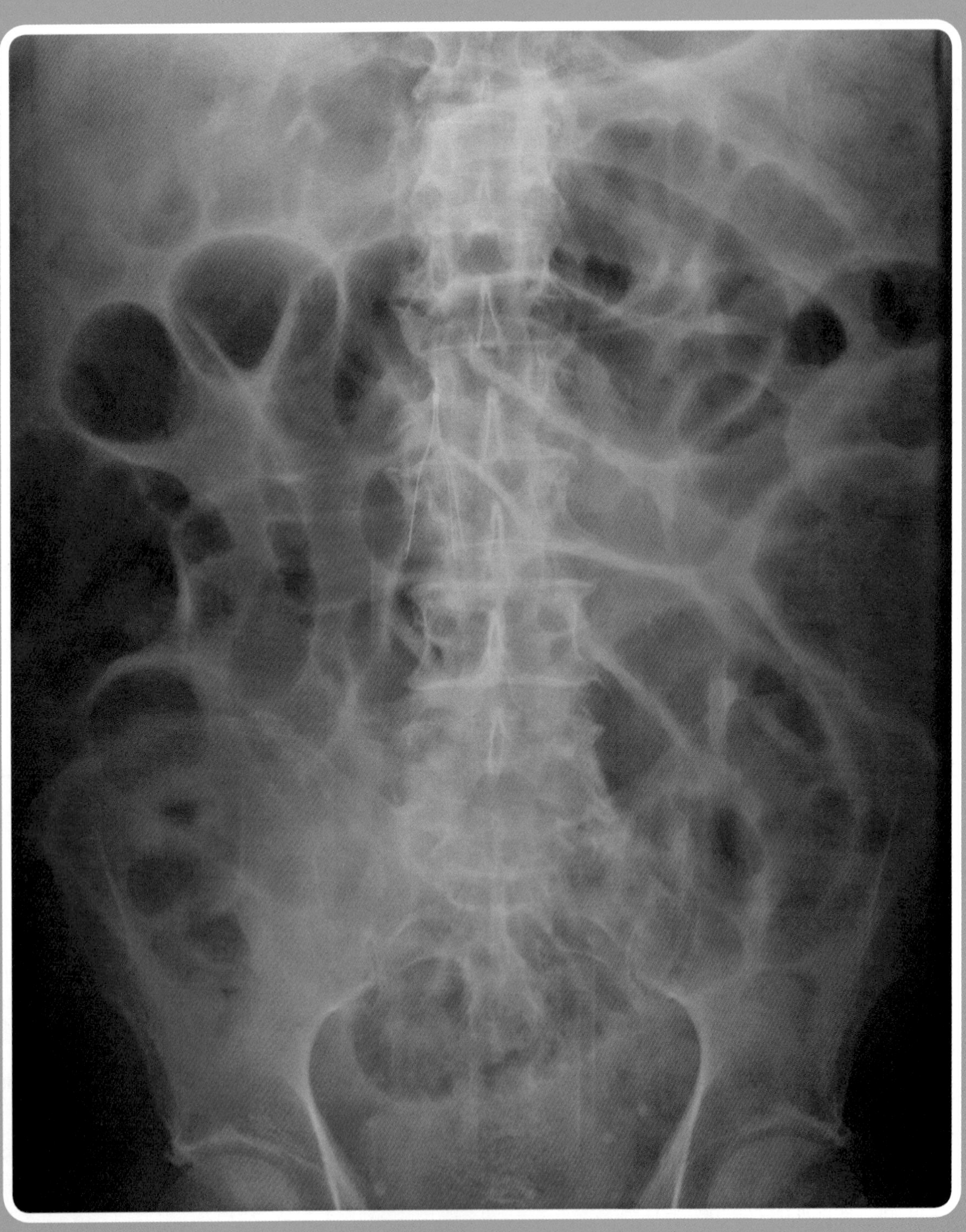

TECHNICAL INFORMATION

Patient ID: Anonymous.
Projection: AP supine.
Rotation: Adequate.
Penetration: Adequate – the spinous processes are visible.
Coverage: Inadequate – the pubic symphysis and inferior pubic rami have not been included.

BOWEL GAS PATTERN

There are multiple loops of dilated bowel seen centrally in the abdomen, which demonstrate valvulae conniventes in keeping with small bowel dilatation.

There is a small volume of faeces seen in the rectum.

BOWEL WALL

There is no evidence of mural thickening or intramural gas within the large or small bowel.

PNEUMOPERITONEUM

There is no evidence of free intraabdominal gas.

SOLID ORGANS

The solid organ contours are within normal limits with no solid organ calcification.

VASCULAR

No abnormal vascular calcification.

BONES

There is moderate degenerative change seen in the spine with osteophyte formation.

SOFT TISSUES

The psoas muscle outline is not visible bilaterally, which is nonspecific.

The extraabdominal soft tissues are unremarkable.

OTHER

There is an IVC filter projected over the right pedicles of L2 and L3, within the region of the abdominal IVC.

There are multiple rounded radiopaque densities projected over the region of the pelvis, most likely phleboliths.

There are no vascular lines, drains or surgical clips.

REVIEW AREAS

Gallstones/renal calculi: No radiopaque calculi.
Lung bases: Not fully included.
Spine: Moderate degenerative change.
Femoral heads: Normal.

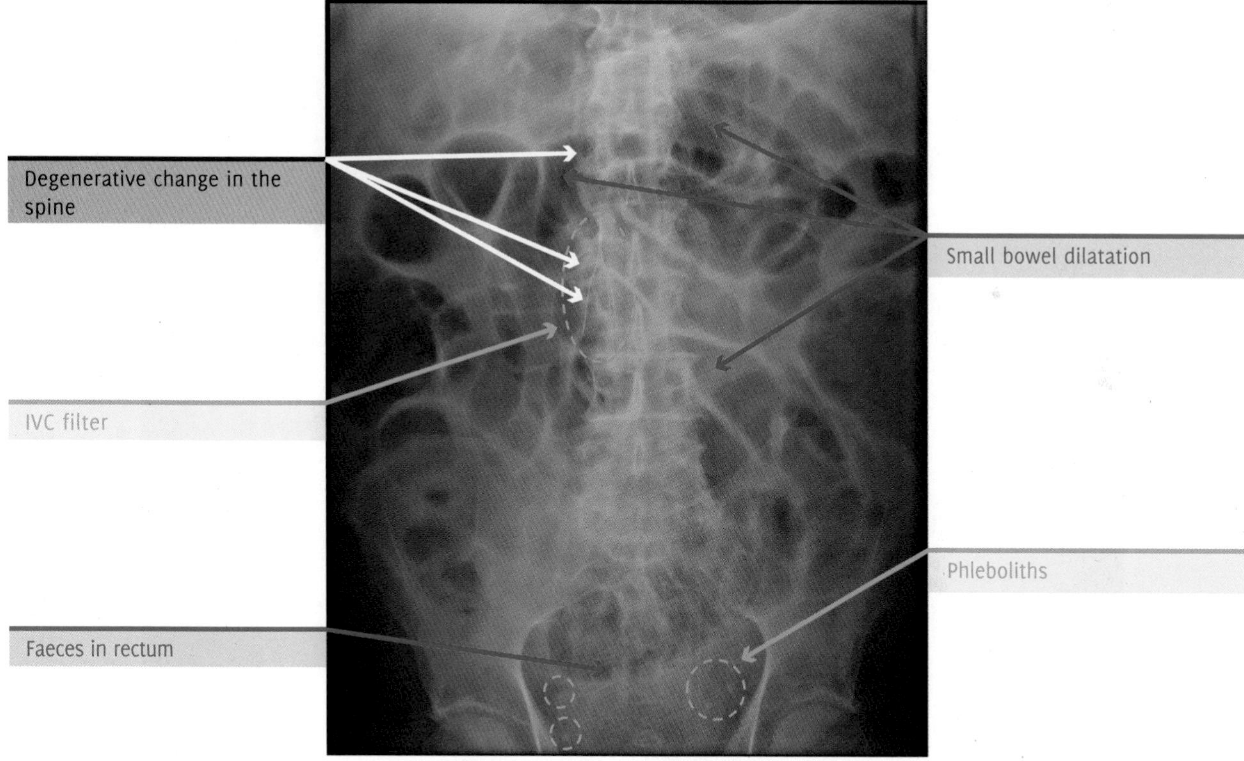

SUMMARY

This X-ray demonstrates multiple loops of dilated bowel seen centrally within the abdomen demonstrating valvulae conniventes, in keeping with small bowel obstruction. The cause for this is not demonstrated but may relate to adhesions given the previous surgery. There is an IVC filter in situ in a satisfactory position. The moderate degenerative changes in the spine and pelvic phleboliths are incidental findings.

INVESTIGATIONS AND MANAGEMENT

The patient should be resuscitated using an ABCDE approach.

Adequate analgesia and hydration should be provided.

The patient should be kept NBM and an NG tube inserted on free drainage to relieve the pressure in the small bowel. IV fluids should be commenced.

Urgent bloods should be taken, including FBC, U&Es, CRP, LFTs, coagulation, blood gas, and group and save.

The general surgical team should be contacted urgently and a CT scan of the abdomen/pelvis with IV contrast should be considered for better visualization of the anatomy and further assessment.

Case

75

A 10-year-old boy presents to the gastroenterology clinic with ongoing constipation. He has a background of chronic constipation, for which he is on laxatives, but no other significant past medical history. A colonic transit study is organized. On examination, he has oxygen saturations of 99% in room air and a temperature of 36.5°C. His HR is 88 bpm, RR is 20 and blood pressure is 110/65 mmHg. The abdomen is soft and there is no tenderness with normal bowel sounds.

An abdominal X-ray is requested for day 4 to assess the location of any remaining colonic transit markers.

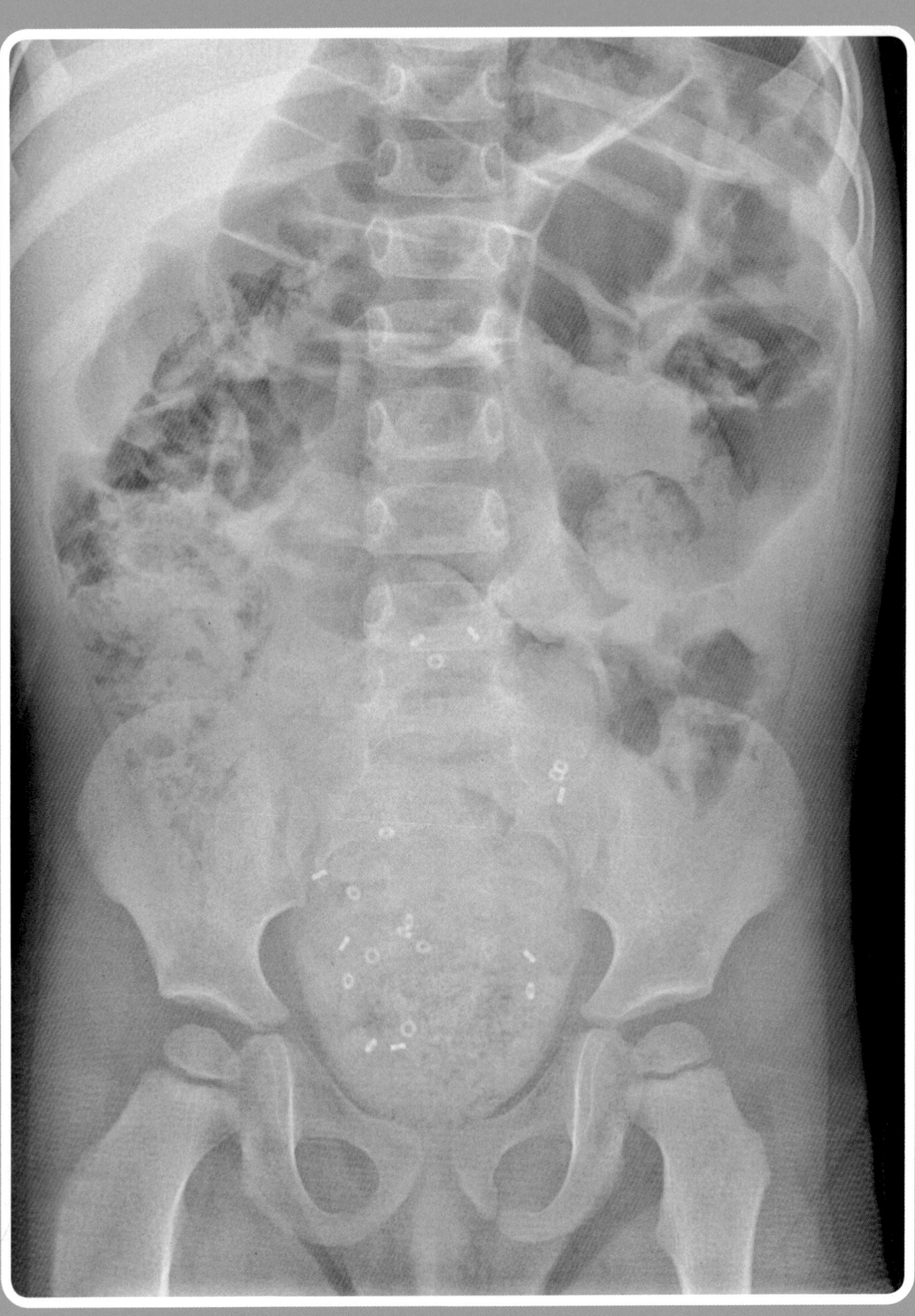

TECHNICAL INFORMATION

Patient ID: Anonymous.
Projection: AP supine.
Rotation: Adequate.
Penetration: Adequate – the spine is visible.
Coverage: Adequate – the anterior ribs are visible superiorly and the pubic rami are visible inferiorly.

BOWEL GAS PATTERN

There are loops of dilated bowel demonstrating haustra seen in the upper abdomen in keeping with large bowel dilatation, predominantly of the transverse colon.

There is a moderate volume of faecal material present throughout the large bowel from the ascending colon to the rectum. The rectum is prominent, containing a significant volume of faeces, which may be impacted.

BOWEL WALL

There is no evidence of mural thickening or intramural gas within the large or small bowel.

PNEUMOPERITONEUM

There is no evidence of free intraabdominal gas.

SOLID ORGANS

The solid organ contours are within normal limits with no solid organ calcification.

VASCULAR

No abnormal vascular calcification.

BONES

There are no abnormalities of the imaged thoracic and lumbar spine, or within the pelvis.

There are growth plates at the femoral head and acetabulum as the ossification centres have not yet fused, which is a normal finding in a child of this age.

SOFT TISSUES

The psoas muscle outline is visible bilaterally.

The extraabdominal soft tissues are unremarkable.

OTHER

There are a total of 20 rounded and linear radiopaque densities seen projected over the region of the lower abdomen and pelvis within the sigmoid colon and rectum, in keeping with the known radiopaque transit markers.

There are no vascular lines, drains or surgical clips.

REVIEW AREAS

Gallstones/renal calculi: No radiopaque calculi.
Lung bases: Not fully included.
Spine: Normal.
Femoral heads: Normal – growth plates present.

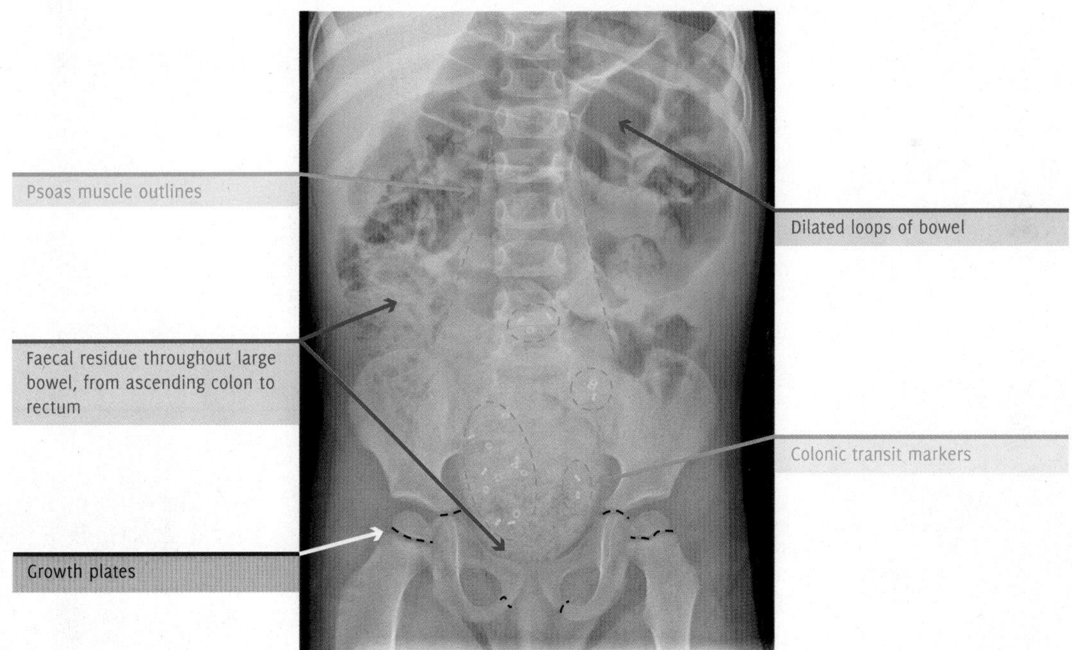

SUMMARY

This X-ray demonstrates moderate volume faecal loading throughout the colon with significant faecal impaction in the rectum, which is prominent. There are 20 ingested radiopaque transit markers projecting over the lower abdomen and pelvis, likely within the sigmoid colon and rectum.

INVESTIGATIONS AND MANAGEMENT

The colon transit study should be reviewed and interpreted by a specialist, the results of which will depend on the number of markers ingested and timings of ingestion.

Further investigations should be considered to assess the cause for the patient's ongoing constipation, and in consultation with a gastroenterologist, optimization of laxatives/enemas and lifestyle advice, including adequate fluid intake, sufficient dietary fibre and exercise, is needed.

Case

76

A 73-year-old female presents to her primary care physician with a 2-month history of generalized abdominal pain. Her past medical history is significant for chronic renal failure and she is currently on haemodialysis after a failed renal transplant. She is a nonsmoker. On examination, she has oxygen saturations of 95% in air and a temperature of 37.1°C. Her HR is 78 bpm, RR is 14 and blood pressure is 120/85 mmHg. The abdomen is soft and there is tenderness in the right iliac fossa with normal bowel sounds. Urine dipstick is unremarkable.

An abdominal X-ray is requested to assess for possible bowel obstruction.

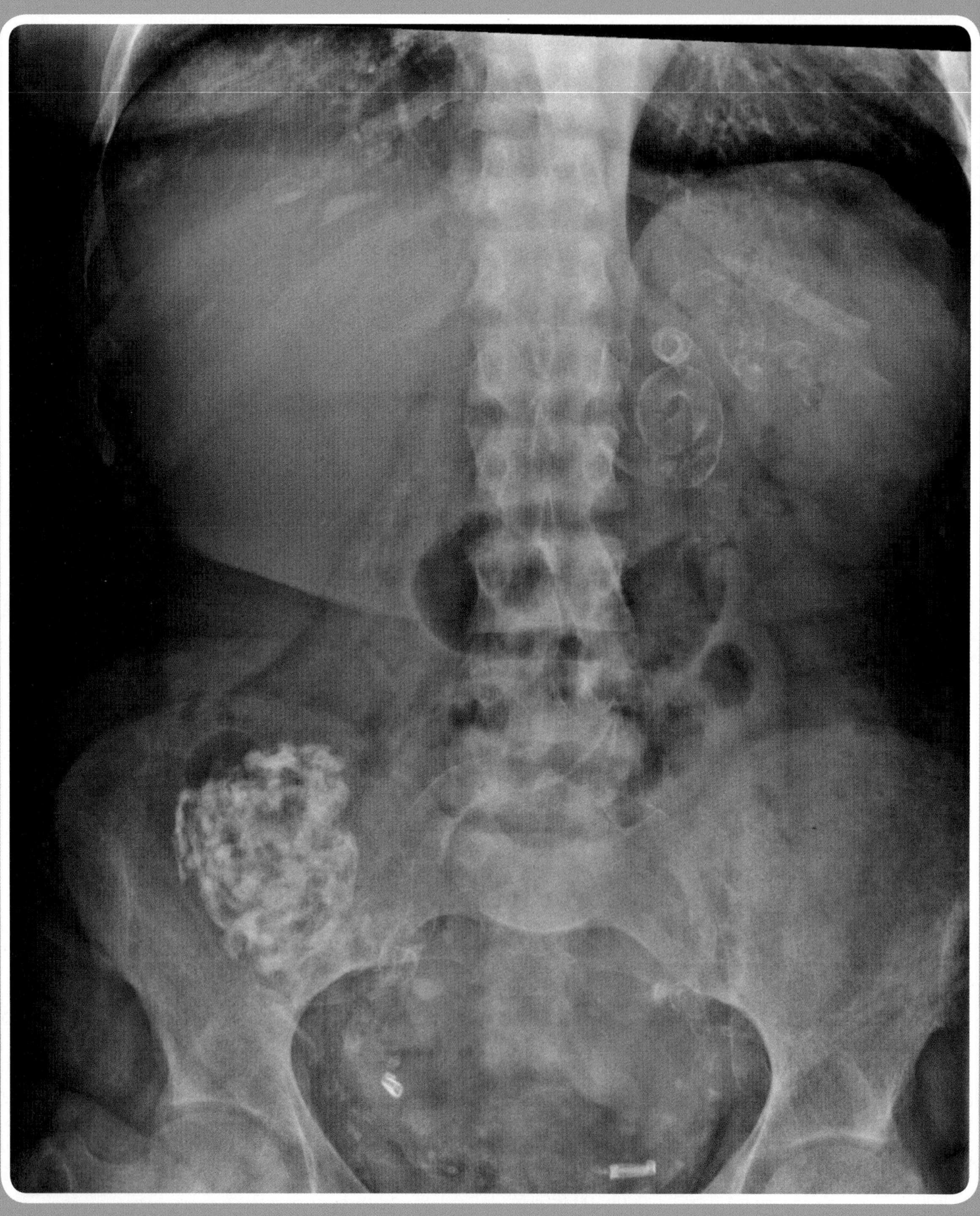

TECHNICAL INFORMATION

Patient ID: Anonymous.
Projection: AP supine.
Rotation: Adequate
Penetration: Adequate – the spinous processes are visible.
Coverage: Inadequate – the pubic symphysis and inferior pubic rami have not been included.

BOWEL GAS PATTERN

The bowel gas pattern is normal.

BOWEL WALL

There is no evidence of mural thickening or intramural gas within the large or small bowel.

PNEUMOPERITONEUM

There is no evidence of free intraabdominal gas.

SOLID ORGANS

The solid organ contours are within normal limits with no solid organ calcification.

VASCULAR

There is calcification of the abdominal aorta and iliac arteries with serpiginous calcification in the left upper quadrant in keeping with calcification.

BONES

The vertebral body endplates appear sclerotic, giving the appearance of a 'rugger jersey spine'.

No fractures or destructive bone lesions are visible in the imaged skeleton.

SOFT TISSUES

There is a well-defined radiopaque density projected over the region of the right iliac fossa, which most likely represents a calcified kidney transplant.

The psoas muscle outline is not visible on the left side, which is nonspecific.

The extraabdominal soft tissues are unremarkable.

OTHER

There are two surgical clips projected over the pelvis, possibly related to sterilization.

There are no vascular lines or drains.

REVIEW AREAS

Gallstones/renal calculi: No radiopaque calculi.
Lung bases: Normal.
Spine: Sclerotic vertebral body endplates.
Femoral heads: Normal.

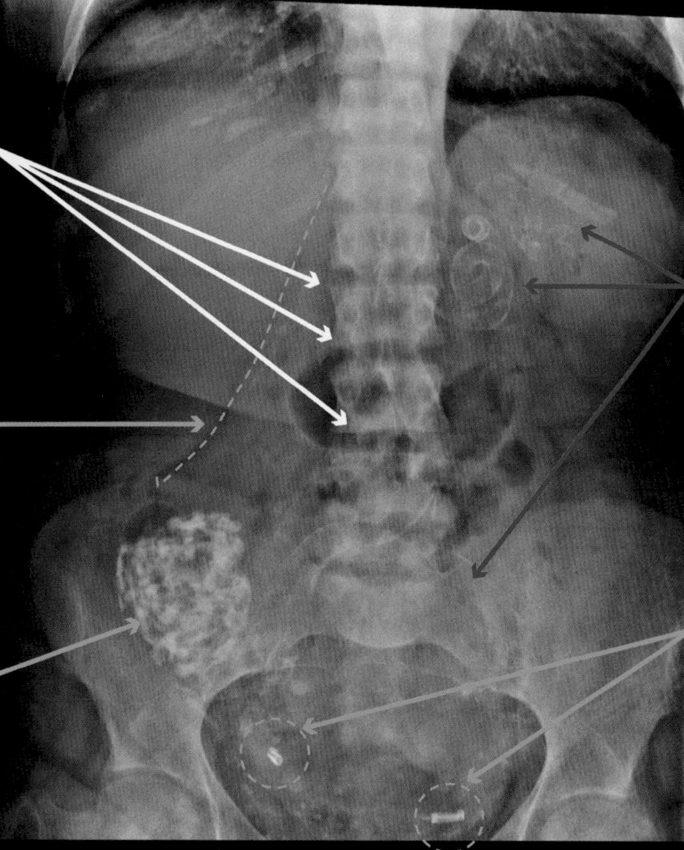

SUMMARY

This X-ray demonstrates multifocal vascular calcification as described. It also demonstrates a calcified renal transplant in the right iliac fossa with sclerotic vertebral body endplates, likely related to renal osteodystrophy.

INVESTIGATIONS AND MANAGEMENT

Adequate analgesia and hydration should be provided.

Bloods should be taken, including FBC, U&Es, LFTs, bone profile, coagulation, blood gas and CRP.

There are no clear findings on the abdominal X-ray to explain the patient's clinical presentation.

Further imaging may be considered for evaluation of the abdomen and surgical input should be sought. The renal/transplant team may also be required to optimize management of the patient's kidneys.

Case

77

A 75-year-old female presents to ED with generalized abdominal pain. Her past medical history is significant for a previous craniectomy and she is a nonsmoker. On examination, she has oxygen saturations of 95% in air and a temperature of 37.0°C. Her HR is 130 bpm, RR is 21 and blood pressure is 120/85 mmHg. There is generalized abdominal tenderness with normal bowel sounds. Urine dipstick is unremarkable.

An abdominal X-ray is requested to assess for possible bowel obstruction.

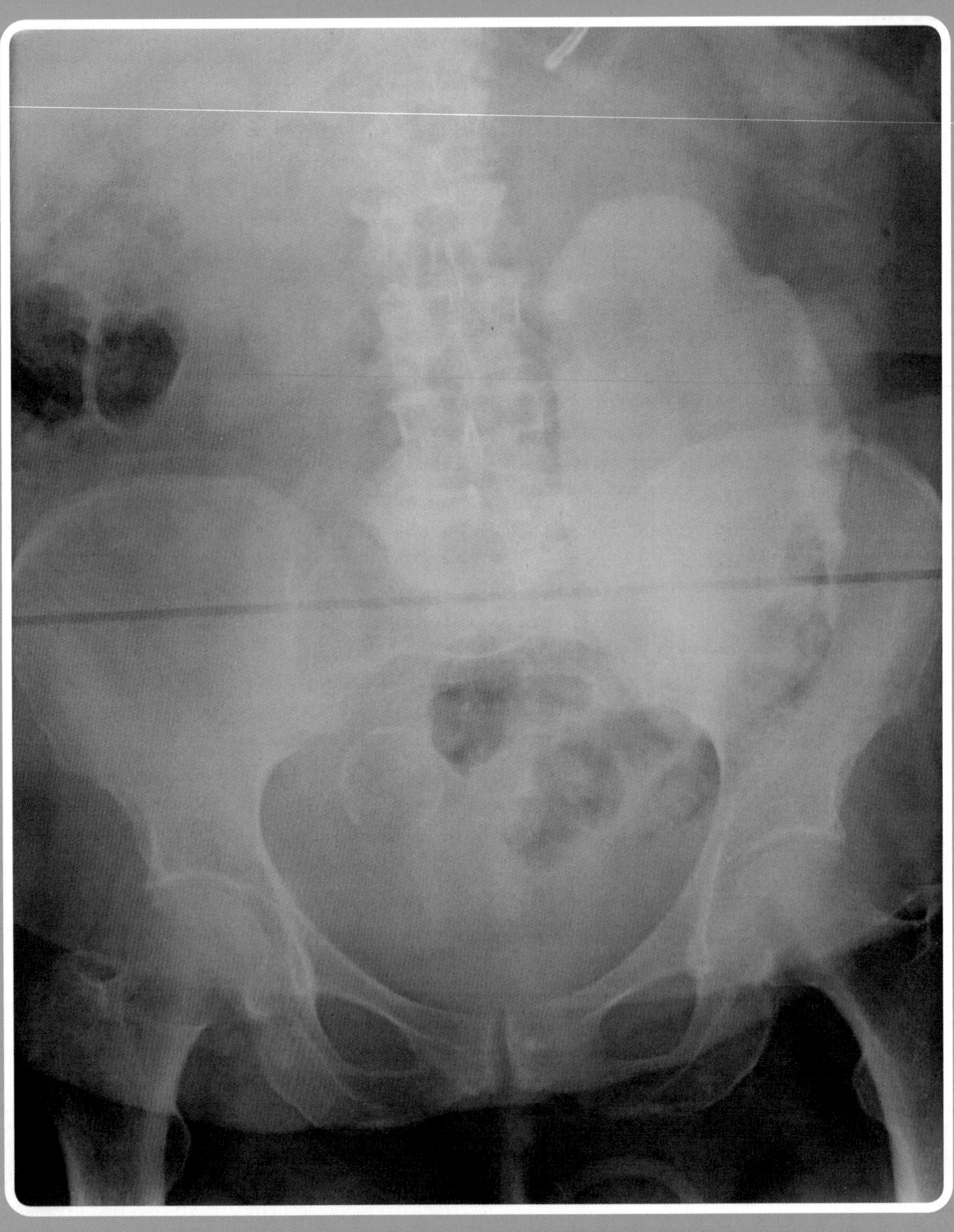

TECHNICAL INFORMATION

Patient ID: Anonymous.
Projection: AP supine.
Rotation: Adequate
Penetration: Adequate – the spinous processes are visible.
Coverage: Inadequate – the upper abdomen and right flank have not been fully imaged.

BOWEL GAS PATTERN

The bowel gas pattern is normal.

BOWEL WALL

There is no evidence of mural thickening or intramural gas within the large or small bowel.

PNEUMOPERITONEUM

There is no evidence of free intraabdominal gas.

SOLID ORGANS

The solid organ contours are within normal limits with no solid organ calcification.

VASCULAR

There is a curvilinear radiopaque density projecting over the right hemipelvis, which may represent calcification of an iliac artery aneurysm.

BONES

There is moderate degenerative change visible in the lumbar spine with bridging osteophyte formation.

No fractures or destructive bone lesions are visible in the imaged skeleton.

SOFT TISSUES

The psoas muscle outline is not visible bilaterally, which is nonspecific.

The extraabdominal soft tissues are unremarkable.

OTHER

There is an NG tube tip projected over the epigastrium likely within the stomach.

There are no vascular lines, drains or surgical clips.

There is a well-defined radiopaque density projected over the left side of the abdomen, which likely represents a craniectomy bone flap being preserved in the abdomen, given the history.

REVIEW AREAS

Gallstones/renal calculi: No radiopaque calculi.
Lung bases: Not fully included.
Spine: Degenerative change in lumbar spine.
Femoral heads: Normal.

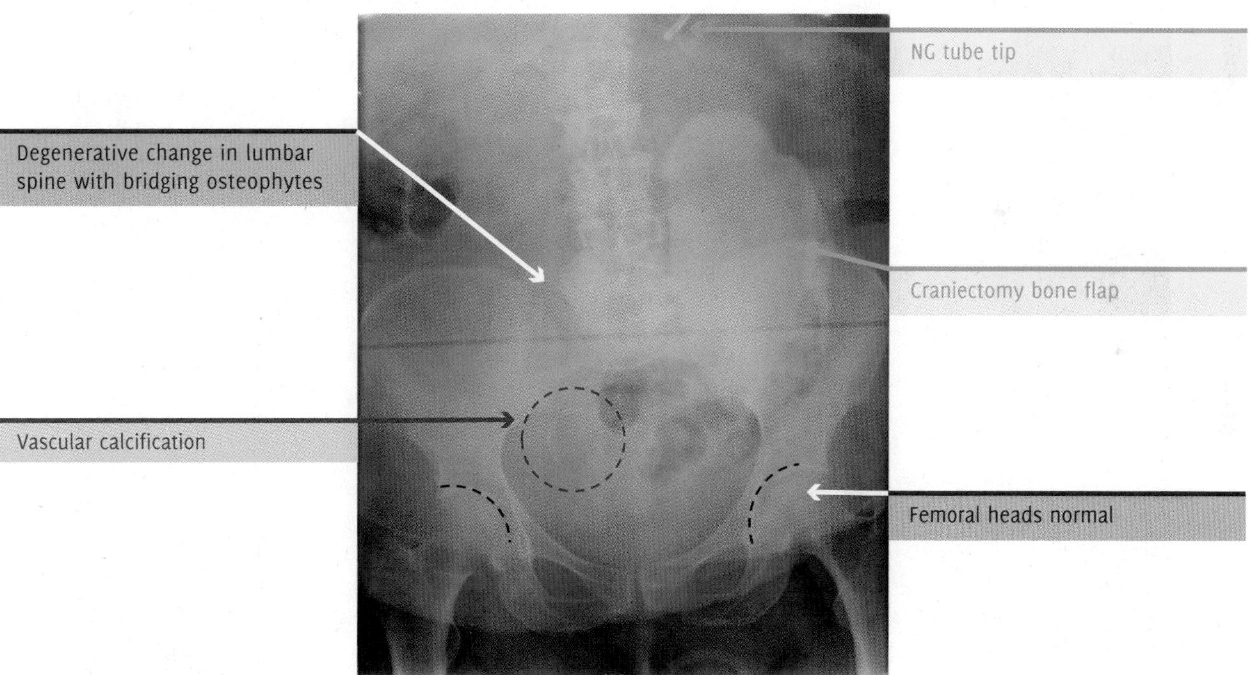

SUMMARY

This X-ray demonstrates a well-defined radiopaque density projected over the left side of the abdomen, in keeping with a craniectomy bone flap being preserved in the abdomen. There is also a radiopaque curvilinear density projecting over the right hemipelvis, which may represent calcification of an iliac artery aneurysm. There is an NG tube tip projecting likely within the stomach. The degenerative change within the lumbar spine is an incidental finding.

INVESTIGATIONS AND MANAGEMENT

The patient should be resuscitated using an ABCDE approach.

Adequate analgesia and hydration should be provided.

Urgent bloods should be taken, including FBC, U&Es, bone profile, LFTs, CRP, coagulation, blood gas, and group and save.

Broad-spectrum antibiotics should be prescribed.

A CT scan of the abdomen/pelvis with IV contrast may be considered for further evaluation of the abdomen and surgical input should be sought.

Arthritic changes in the first instance should be management with lifestyle changes and analgesia, if they are causing symptoms.

Case

78

A 50-year-old female presents to ED with vomiting, abdominal pain, palpitations and collapse. She has no significant past medical history and is a nonsmoker. On examination, she has oxygen saturations of 97% in room air and a temperature of 37.2°C. Her HR is 130 bpm, RR is 25 and blood pressure is 92/60 mmHg. Her abdomen is rigid and there is generalized tenderness with normal bowel sounds. Urine dipstick is unremarkable.

An abdominal X-ray is requested to assess for possible bowel obstruction.

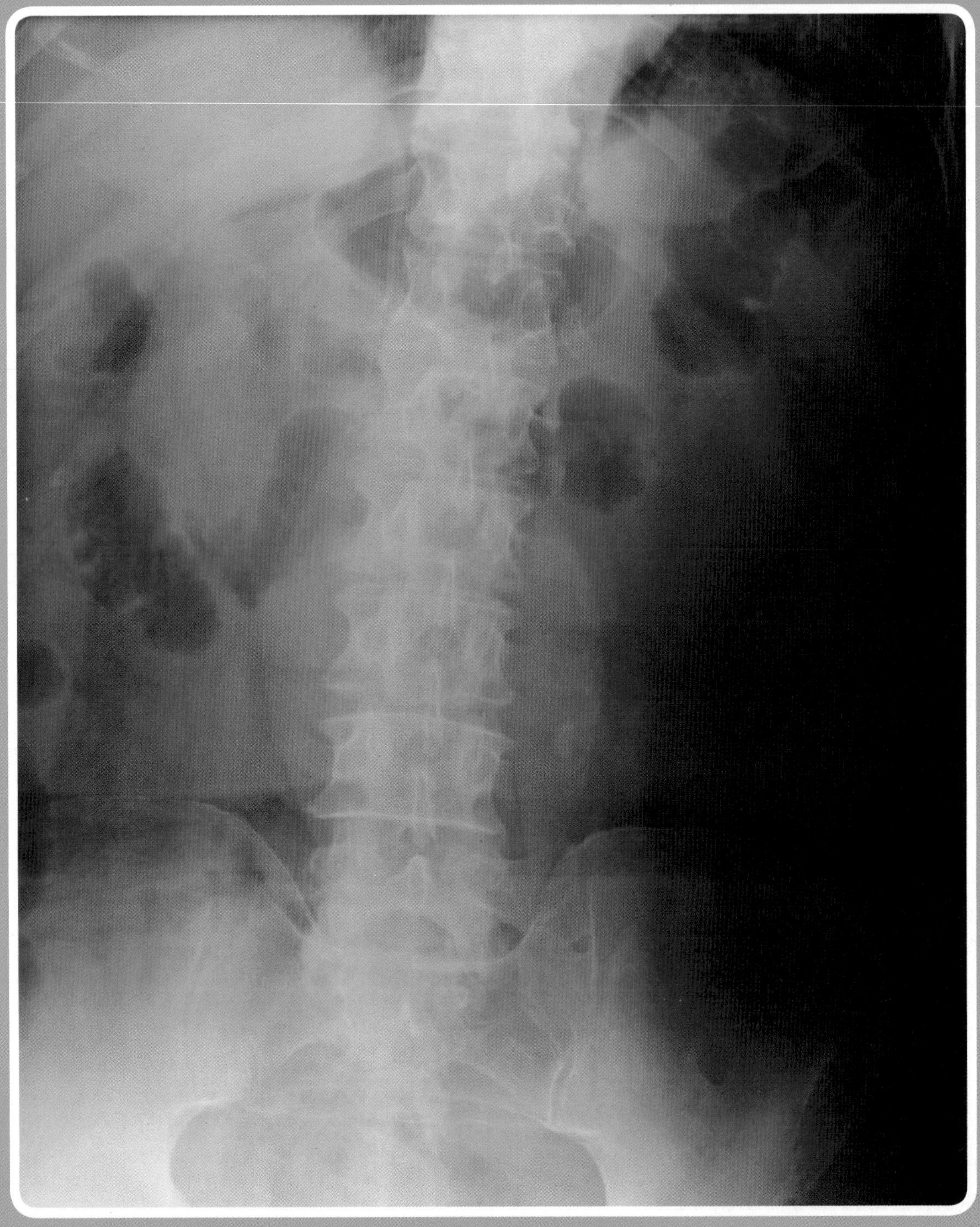

TECHNICAL INFORMATION

Patient ID: Anonymous.
Projection: AP supine.
Rotation: Adequate
Penetration: Inadequate – the left side of the X-ray is overpenetrated.
Coverage: Inadequate – the right iliac crest, pubic symphysis and inferior pubic rami have not been fully included.

BOWEL GAS PATTERN

The bowel gas pattern is normal.

BOWEL WALL

There is no evidence of mural thickening or intramural gas within the large or small bowel.

PNEUMOPERITONEUM

There is no evidence of free intraabdominal gas.

SOLID ORGANS

The right renal contour is clearly seen, which suggests the absence of fluid (haemorrhage) in this region. The left renal contour is not visualized; however, this is nonspecific.

VASCULAR

The infrarenal abdominal aorta is calcified and demonstrates fusiform aneurysmal dilatation at the level of L3 to S1.

BONES

There are no abnormalities of the imaged thoracic and lumbar spine, or within the pelvis.

SOFT TISSUES

The psoas muscle outline is not visible bilaterally, which is nonspecific but raises the possibility of an AAA leak, especially given the clinical history and low blood pressure.

The extraabdominal soft tissues are unremarkable.

OTHER

There are no radiopaque foreign bodies.

There are no vascular lines, drains or surgical clips.

REVIEW AREAS

Gallstones/renal calculi: No radiopaque calculi.
Lung bases: Not fully included.
Spine: Normal.
Femoral heads: Not visualized.

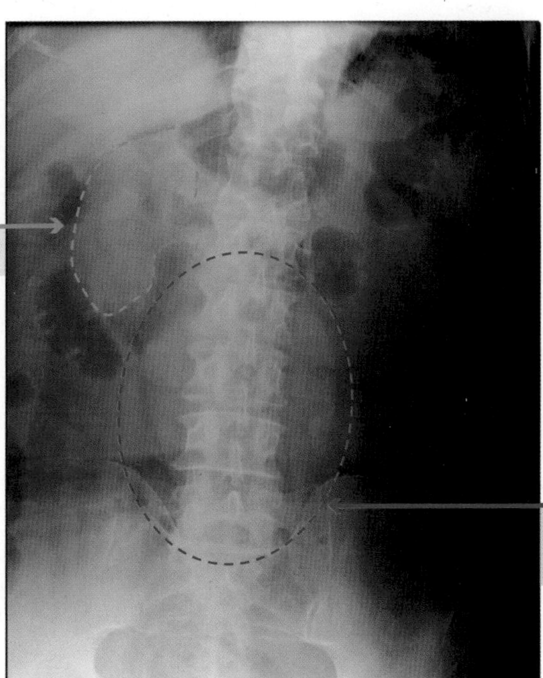

SUMMARY

This X-ray demonstrates fusiform aneurysmal dilatation of the infrarenal abdominal aorta. The psoas muscle outline is not seen bilaterally, which is nonspecific but raises the possibility of an abdominal aortic aneurysm leak given the clinical history.

INVESTIGATIONS AND MANAGEMENT

The patient should be resuscitated using an ABCDE approach.

Adequate analgesia and hydration should be provided.

Urgent bloods should be taken, including FBC, U&Es, CRP, bone profile, LFTs, coagulation, blood gas and crossmatch.

The patient should be made NBM and commenced on IV fluids.

Urgent referral to the vascular surgeons should be made for assessment of an active abdominal aortic aneurysm leak and consideration of repair. A CT scan of the aorta with IV contrast would be useful for better visualization of the anatomy and to assess for leak.

Case

79

A 69-year-old female presents to ED with worsening abdominal distension and difficulty breathing. Her past medical history is significant for treated ovarian cancer and she is a nonsmoker. On examination, she has oxygen saturations of 93% in room air and a temperature of 36.5°C. Her HR is 98 bpm, RR is 26 and blood pressure is 112/65 mmHg. The abdomen is tense and there is generalized tenderness with normal bowel sounds. Urine dipstick is unremarkable.

An abdominal X-ray is requested to assess for possible bowel obstruction.

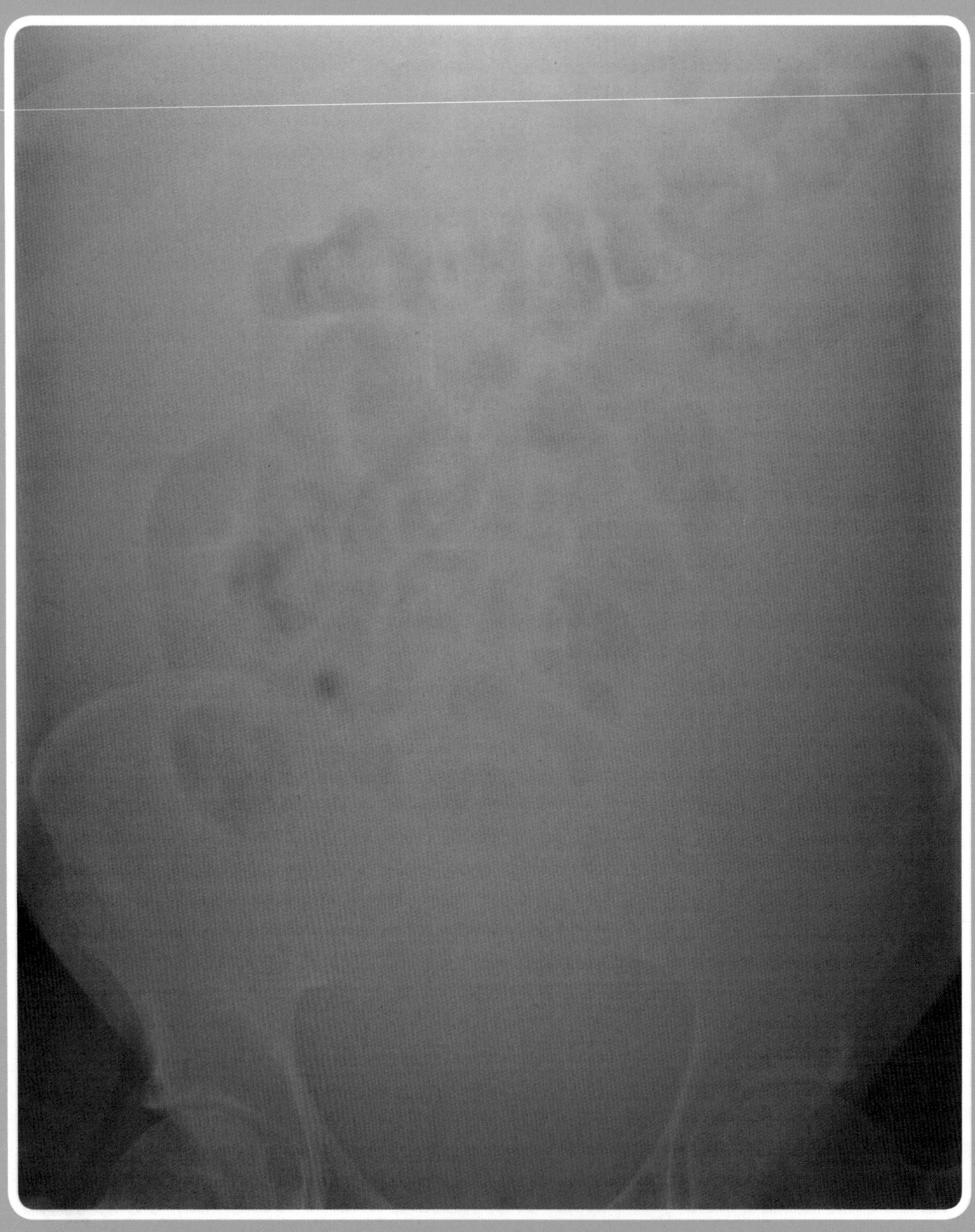

TECHNICAL INFORMATION

Patient ID: Anonymous.
Projection: AP supine.
Rotation: Adequate.
Penetration: Underpenetrated – the spinous processes are not visible.
Coverage: Inadequate – the pubic symphysis, inferior pubic rami and hemidiaphragms have not been included.

BOWEL GAS PATTERN

There are multiple loops of centrally placed bowel loops with peripheral paucity of bowel gas in the flanks and iliac fossae.

BOWEL WALL

There is no evidence of mural thickening or intramural gas within the large or small bowel.

PNEUMOPERITONEUM

There is no evidence of free intraabdominal gas.

SOLID ORGANS

There is a diffusely increased density of the abdomen with poor definition of all soft tissue shadows and solid organs.

VASCULAR

No abnormal vascular calcification.

BONES

There are no abnormalities of the imaged thoracic and lumbar spine, or within the pelvis, but the bones are not clearly visualized.

SOFT TISSUES

The psoas muscle outline is not visible bilaterally, related to the presence of ascites.

The extraabdominal soft tissues are unremarkable.

OTHER

There are no radiopaque foreign bodies. There are no vascular lines, drains or surgical clips.

REVIEW AREAS

Gallstones/renal calculi: No radiopaque calculi.
Lung bases: Normal.
Spine: Not visible.
Femoral heads: Normal.

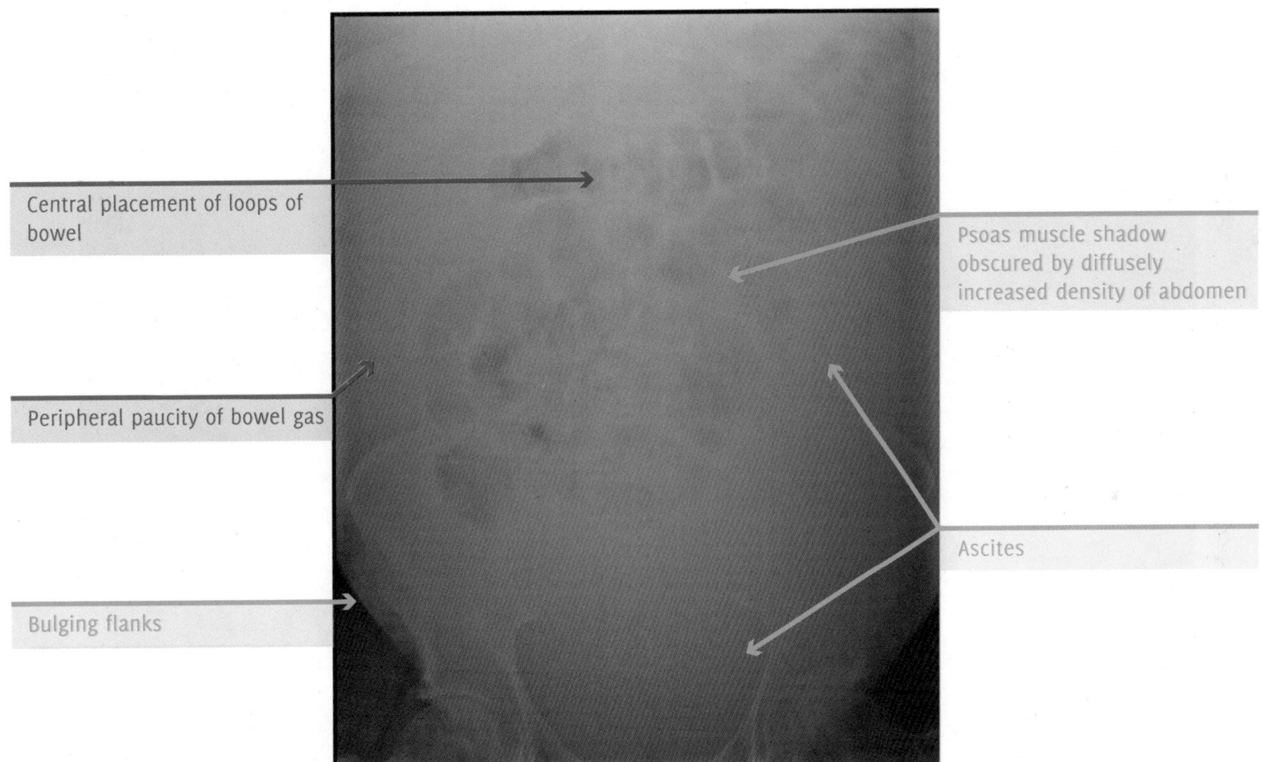

SUMMARY

This X-ray demonstrates multiple loops of centrally placed bowel within the abdomen, with peripheral paucity of bowel gas in the flanks and iliac fossae and diffusely increased density of the abdomen resulting in poor definition of soft tissues, solid organs and bones. These findings are in keeping with extensive ascites.

INVESTIGATIONS AND MANAGEMENT

The patient should be resuscitated using an ABCDE approach.

Adequate analgesia and hydration should be provided.

Urgent bloods should be taken, including FBC, U&Es, CRP, LFTs, TFTs, blood gas and bone profile.

If no recent imaging has been performed, a staging CT scan of the chest, abdomen and pelvis with IV contrast should be considered to reassess the known ovarian cancer for disease recurrence.

If the CT scan confirms disease recurrence, the patient should be referred to oncology services for further management, which may include biopsy and MDT discussion. Treatment, which may include surgery, radiotherapy, chemotherapy or palliative treatment, will depend on the outcome of the MDT investigations and the patient's wishes.

Ultrasound-guided drainage of the ascites could be performed for symptomatic relief.

Case 80

A 2-month-old baby boy presents to ED with vomiting and colicky abdominal pain. His past medical history is significant for a recent viral flu-like illness. On examination, he has oxygen saturations of 98% in room air and a temperature of 37.8°C. His HR is 170 bpm and RR 60. The abdomen is soft and a sausage-shaped mass is palpable in the right upper quadrant with tinkling bowel sounds. Urine dipstick is unremarkable.

An abdominal X-ray is requested to assess for possible bowel obstruction.

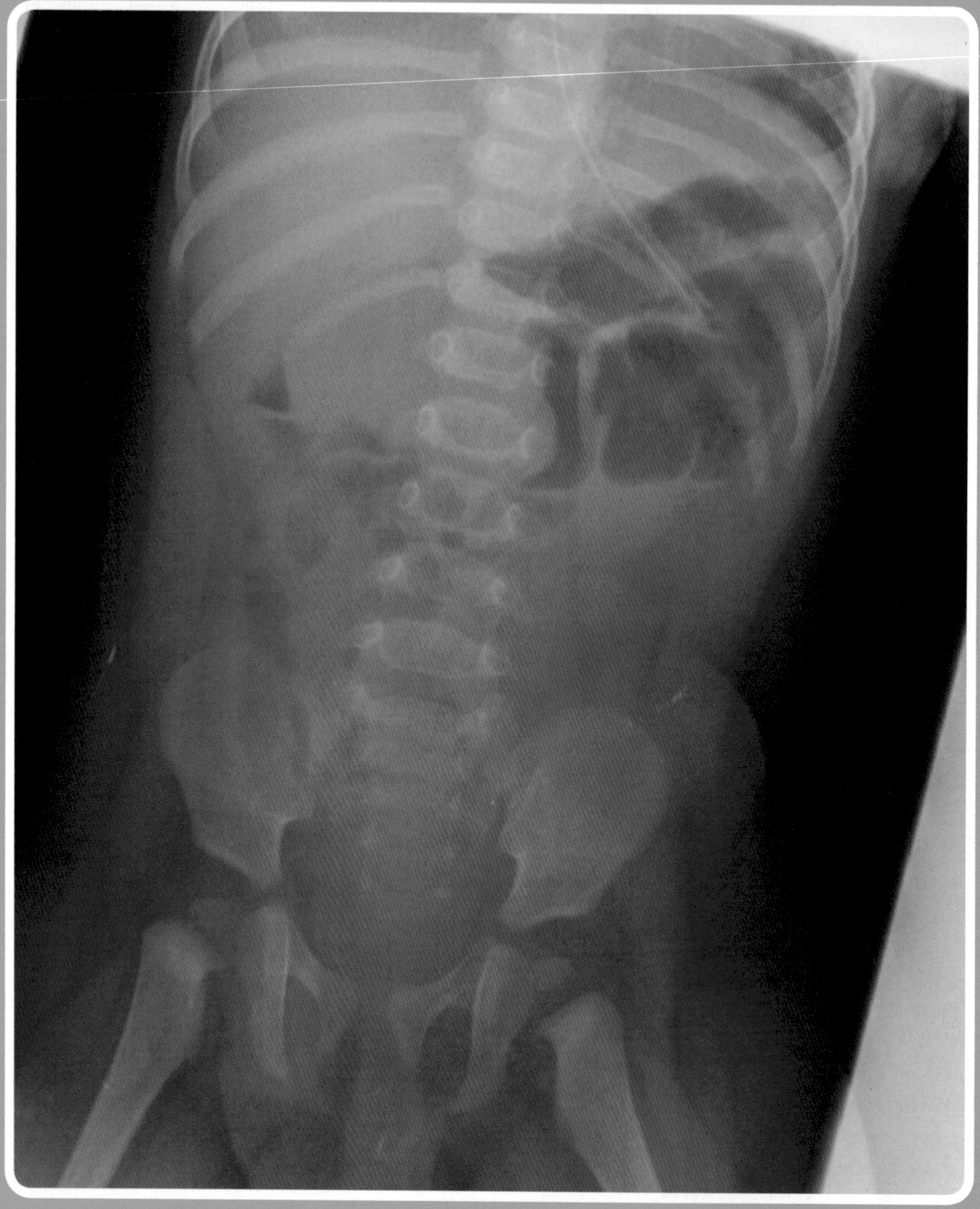

TECHNICAL INFORMATION

Patient ID: Anonymous.
Projection: AP supine.
Rotation: Adequate.
Penetration: Adequate – the spine is visible.
Coverage: Adequate – the anterior ribs are visible superiorly and the inferior pubic rami are visible.

BOWEL GAS PATTERN

There are multiple loops of dilated bowel in the left upper quadrant of the abdomen. A small volume of gas is seen within the ascending colon.

BOWEL WALL

There is no evidence of mural thickening or intramural gas within the large or small bowel.

PNEUMOPERITONEUM

There is no evidence of free intraabdominal gas.

SOLID ORGANS

The solid organ contours are within normal limits with no solid organ calcification.

VASCULAR

No abnormal vascular calcification.

BONES

There are no abnormalities of the imaged thoracic and lumbar spine, or within the pelvis.

There is cartilage present between the pelvic bones and femurs as they have not yet fused, which is a normal finding in a child of this age.

SOFT TISSUES

There is an elongated soft tissue mass seen in the right upper quadrant of the abdomen.

The psoas muscle outline is not visible bilaterally, which is nonspecific, particularly in a child of this age.

The extraabdominal soft tissues are unremarkable.

OTHER

There is an NG tube in situ, with its tip seen projecting in the left upper quadrant, likely within the stomach.

There are no vascular lines, drains or surgical clips.

REVIEW AREAS

Gallstones/renal calculi: No radiopaque calculi.
Lung bases: Right lung base not fully included.
Spine: Normal.
Femoral heads: Normal – growth plates present.

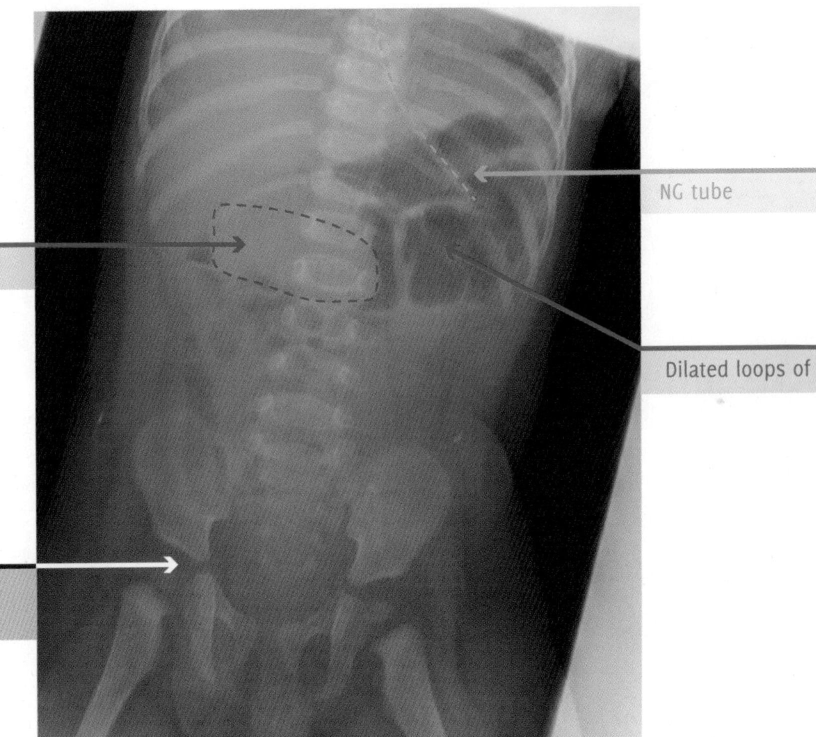

SUMMARY

This X-ray demonstrates an elongated soft tissue mass in the right upper quadrant, with dilated loops of bowel in the left upper quadrant, which given the clinical history is in keeping with intussusception. There is an NG tube in situ with the tip projecting over the stomach.

INVESTIGATIONS AND MANAGEMENT

The patient should be resuscitated using an ABCDE approach.

Adequate analgesia and hydration should be provided.

The patient should be made NBM and commenced on IV fluids.

Urgent bloods should be taken, including FBC, U&Es, blood gas, coagulation, group and save, and CRP.

An urgent abdominal USS should be performed to confirm the diagnosis of intussusception. Surgical input should be sought.

Fluoroscopic air contrast enema or water-soluble contrast enema can assist in diagnosis and in most cases can successfully reduce the intussusception.

Case

81

A 40-year-old male presents to ED with symptoms of alcohol withdrawal and abdominal pain. His past medical history is significant for alcoholism and he is a nonsmoker. On examination, he has oxygen saturations of 97% in air and a temperature of 36.8°C. His HR is 80 bpm, RR is 22 and blood pressure is 120/85 mmHg. The abdomen is soft and there is generalized tenderness with normal bowel sounds. Urine dipstick is unremarkable.

An abdominal X-ray is requested to assess for possible bowel obstruction.

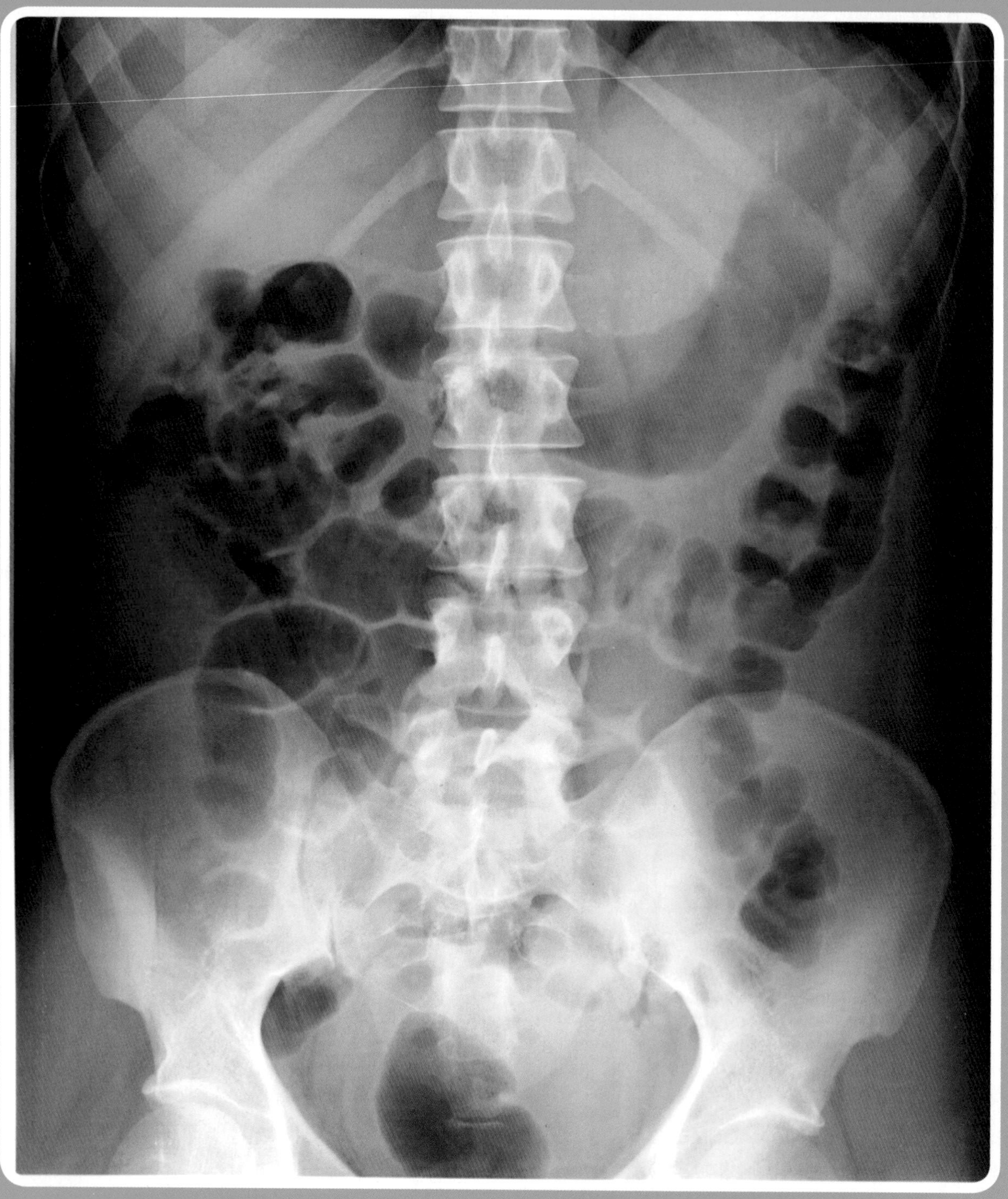

TECHNICAL INFORMATION

Patient ID: Anonymous.
Projection: AP supine.
Rotation: Adequate.
Penetration: Adequate – the spinous processes are visible.
Coverage: Inadequate – the pubic symphysis and inferior pubic rami have not been included.

BOWEL GAS PATTERN

The bowel gas pattern is normal.

BOWEL WALL

There is no evidence of mural thickening or intramural gas within the large or small bowel.

PNEUMOPERITONEUM

There is no evidence of free intraabdominal gas.

SOLID ORGANS

This X-ray demonstrates subtle speckled calcification projecting over the distribution of the pancreas, which given the clinical history may represent pancreatic calcification in keeping with chronic pancreatitis.

VASCULAR

No abnormal vascular calcification.

BONES

There are no abnormalities of the imaged thoracic and lumbar spine, or within the pelvis.

SOFT TISSUES

The psoas muscle outline is visible bilaterally.

The extraabdominal soft tissues are unremarkable.

OTHER

There are no radiopaque foreign bodies.

There are no vascular lines, drains or surgical clips.

REVIEW AREAS

Gallstones/renal calculi: No radiopaque calculi.
Lung bases: Normal.
Spine: Normal.
Femoral heads: Normal.

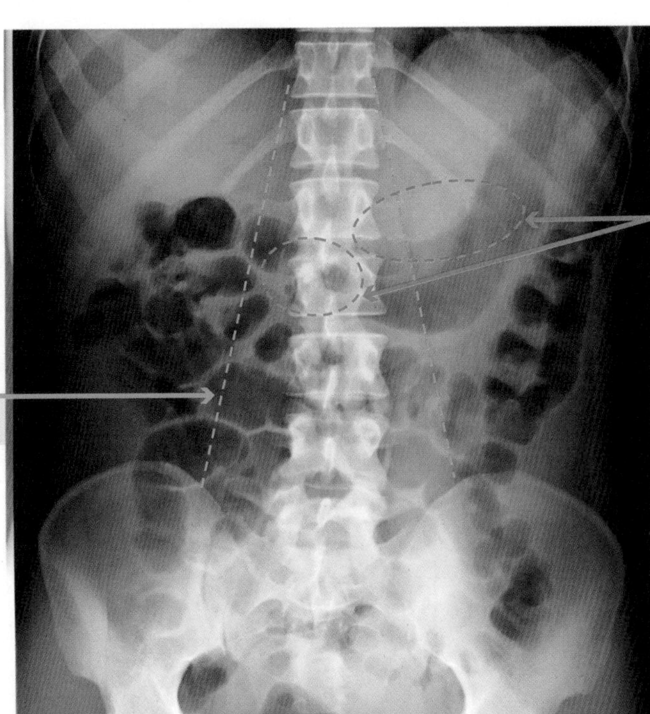

SUMMARY

This X-ray demonstrates subtle speckled calcification projecting over the distribution of the pancreas, which given the clinical history may represent pancreatic calcification in keeping with chronic pancreatitis.

INVESTIGATIONS AND MANAGEMENT

The patient should be resuscitated using an ABCDE approach.

Adequate analgesia and hydration should be provided.

Urgent bloods should be taken, including FBC, U&Es, LFTs, amylase, blood gas, bone profile and CRP.

The acute alcohol withdrawal should be treated with thiamine and benzodiazepines.

Referral to gastroenterology should be made for possible chronic pancreatitis. Management may include analgesia and enzymatic supplementation. A CT scan of the abdomen with IV contrast may be considered for further evaluation of the pancreas.

Case 82

A 52-year-old female presents to ED with generalized abdominal pain. She has a complicated past medical history, having had a previous bowel resection with a colostomy in place. She also has a long-term congenital bladder defect and she is a nonsmoker. On examination, she has oxygen saturations of 97% in room air and a temperature of 37.3°C. Her HR is 94 bpm, RR is 20 and blood pressure is 125/72 mmHg. The abdomen is soft and there is generalized tenderness with tinkling bowel sounds. Urine dipstick is unremarkable and a pregnancy test is negative.

An abdominal X-ray is requested to assess for possible bowel obstruction.

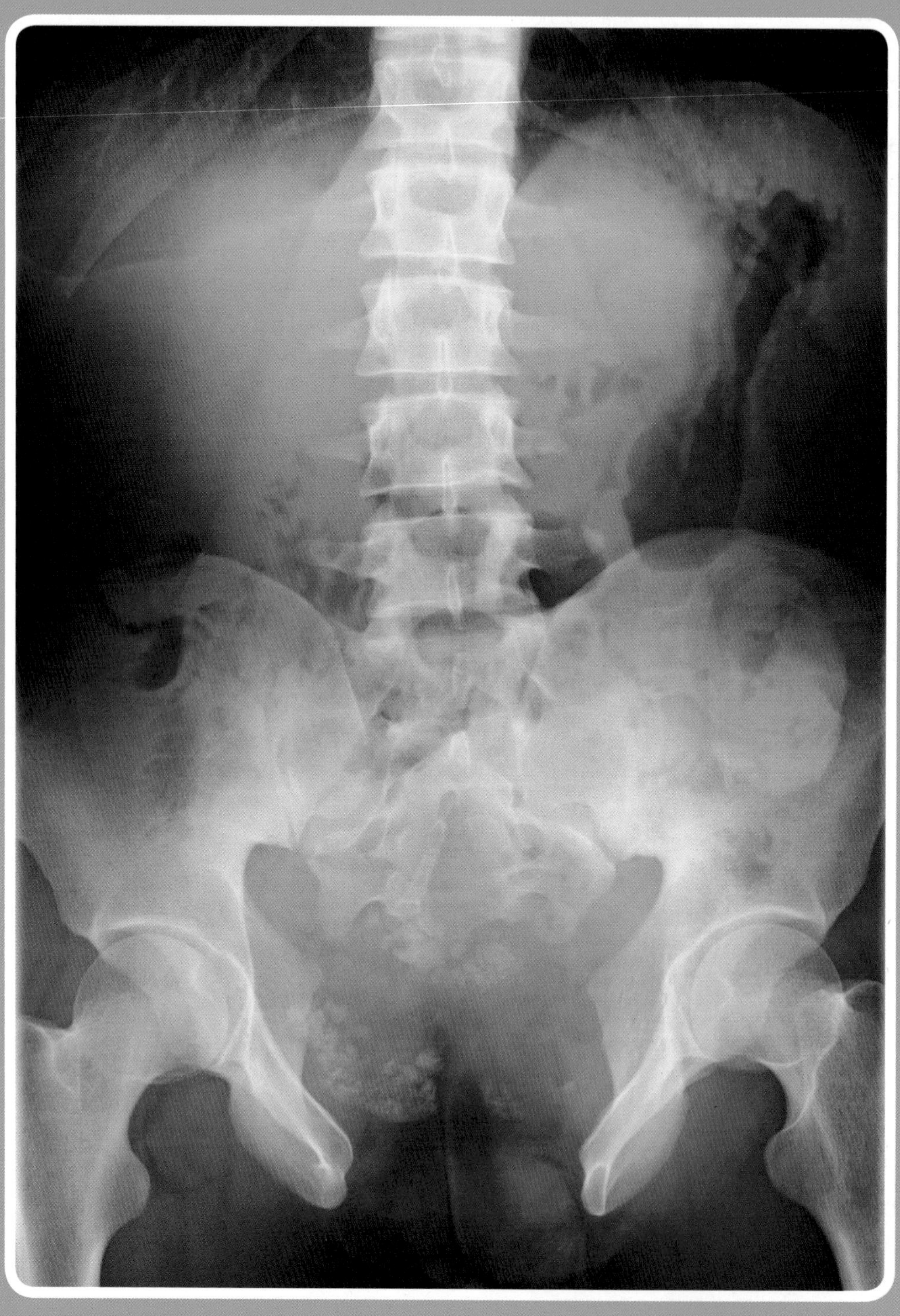

TECHNICAL INFORMATION

Patient ID: Anonymous.
Projection: AP supine.
Rotation: Adequate.
Penetration: Adequate – the spinous processes are visible.
Coverage: Adequate – the anterior ribs are visible superiorly and the inferior pubic rami are visible.

BOWEL GAS PATTERN

The bowel gas pattern is normal.

BOWEL WALL

There is no evidence of mural thickening or intramural gas within the large or small bowel.

PNEUMOPERITONEUM

There is no evidence of free intraabdominal gas.

SOLID ORGANS

The solid organ contours are within normal limits with no solid organ calcification.

VASCULAR

No abnormal vascular calcification.

BONES

There is a failure of the pubic bones to meet in the midline at the pubic symphysis, termed the 'Manta Ray sign'.

There are no abnormalities of the imaged thoracic and lumbar spine.

SOFT TISSUES

The psoas muscle outline is visible bilaterally.

There appears to be a defect in the extraabdominal soft tissues in the pelvis, overlying the region of the widened pubic symphysis.

OTHER

There is a rounded radiopaque density projected over the region of the left iliac fossa, in keeping with a colostomy bag external to the patient.

There are several radiopaque calcific densities projected over the region of the abnormally shaped bladder, which represent faceted bladder calculi.

There are no vascular lines, drains or surgical clips.

REVIEW AREAS

Gallstones/renal calculi: Multiple calculi projecting over the bladder.
Lung bases: Normal.
Spine: Normal.
Femoral heads: Normal.

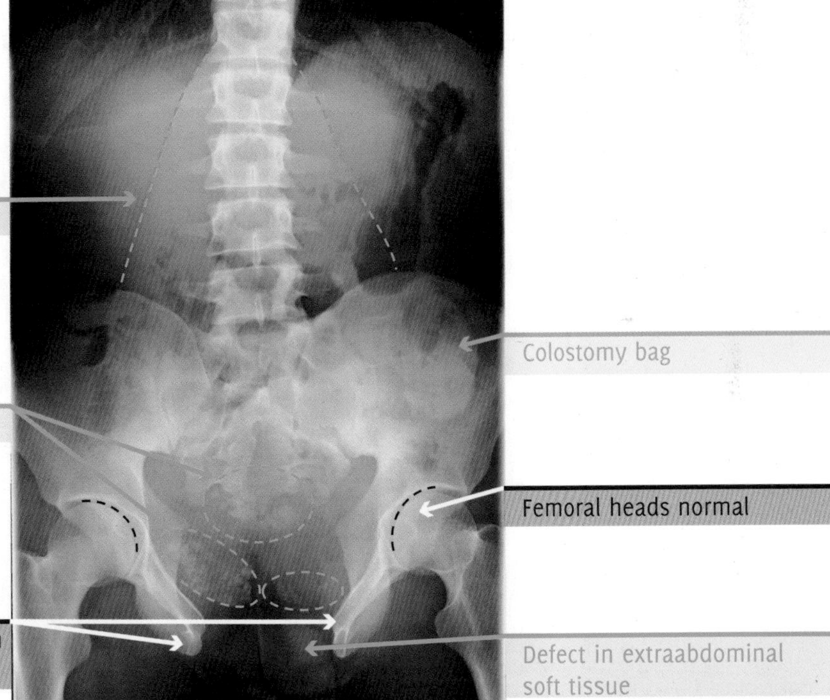

SUMMARY

This X-ray demonstrates a wide separation of the pubic bones termed the 'Manta Ray sign', and a defect in the extraabdominal soft tissues overlying this region. It also demonstrates several calcific densities projected over the region of an abnormally shaped bladder. Findings are in keeping with bladder exstrophy and vesical calculi formation. Note is also made of the left iliac fossa colostomy.

INVESTIGATIONS AND MANAGEMENT

The patient should be resuscitated using an ABCDE approach.

Adequate analgesia and hydration should be provided.

Urgent bloods should be taken, including FBC, U&Es, LFTs, amylase, bone profile, blood gas and CRP.

Vesical calculi formation is a known complication following surgery for bladder exstrophy. The patient should be referred to the urology team for further management. A CT scan of the kidneys, ureters and bladder might be useful for better visualization of the anatomy and evaluation of the abdominal pain.

Case

83

A 6-hour-old baby girl has just been admitted to NICU having been born prematurely at 28 weeks gestation. She has been intubated and had an umbilical arterial and venous catheter inserted. On examination, while intubated, she has oxygen saturations of 100% on 40% oxygen and a temperature of 36.6°C. Her HR is 176 bpm and RR is 48. The abdomen is soft with normal bowel sounds.

An abdominal X-ray is requested to assess correct positioning of lines.

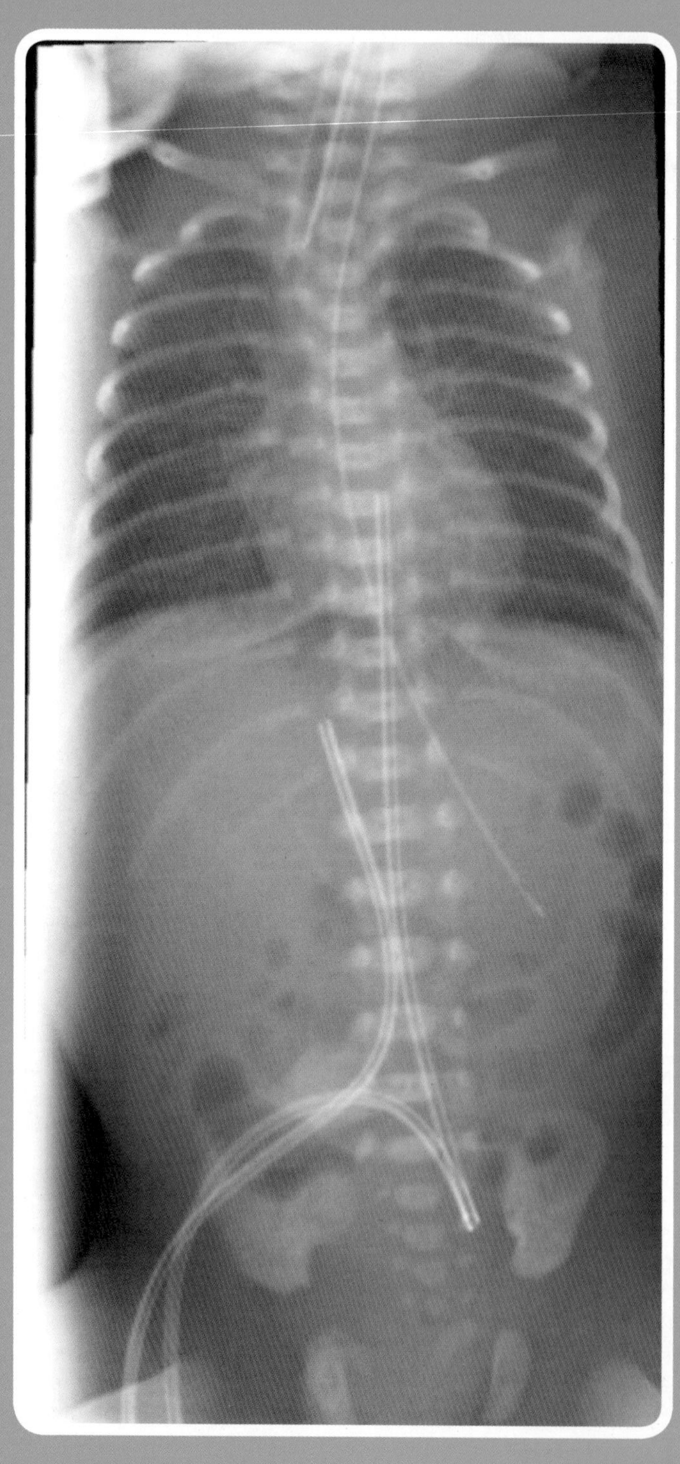

TECHNICAL INFORMATION

Patient ID: Anonymous.
Projection: AP supine 'babygram' of chest and abdomen.
Rotation: Adequate.
Penetration: Adequate – the spine is visible.
Coverage: Adequate – the anterior ribs are visible superiorly and the pubic rami are visible inferiorly.

BOWEL GAS PATTERN

The bowel gas pattern is normal.

BOWEL WALL

There is no evidence of mural thickening or intramural gas within the large or small bowel.

PNEUMOPERITONEUM

There is no evidence of free intraabdominal gas.

SOLID ORGANS

The solid organs are poorly defined due to diffusely increased density of the abdomen. The lung fields look normal.

VASCULAR

No abnormal vascular calcification.

BONES

There are no abnormalities of the imaged thoracic and lumbar spine, or within the pelvis.

There are growth plates at the femoral head, greater trochanter and acetabulum as the ossification centres have not yet fused, which is a normal finding in a child of this age.

There is cartilage seen between vertebrae, which is a normal finding in a child of this age.

SOFT TISSUES

The psoas muscle outline is not visible bilaterally, which is nonspecific, particularly in a child of this age.

The extraabdominal soft tissues are unremarkable.

OTHER

There is an NG tube in situ, with its tip projecting within the body of the stomach.

There is an ET tube in situ, with its tip at T2.

There is an umbilical artery catheter seen external to the patient, entering the umbilical artery at the umbilicus, travelling inferiorly in the umbilical artery to enter the internal iliac artery where it then travels superiorly up the common iliac artery to the aorta. Its tip is seen appropriately sited above the diaphragm, at the level of T7.

There is an umbilical venous catheter seen external to the patient, with its tip seen at the level of T11 in a slightly low position.

There are no drains or surgical clips.

REVIEW AREAS

Gallstones/renal calculi: No radiopaque calculi.
Lung bases: Normal.
Spine: Normal – cartilage between vertebrae.
Femoral heads: Normal – cartilage between femur and acetabulum.

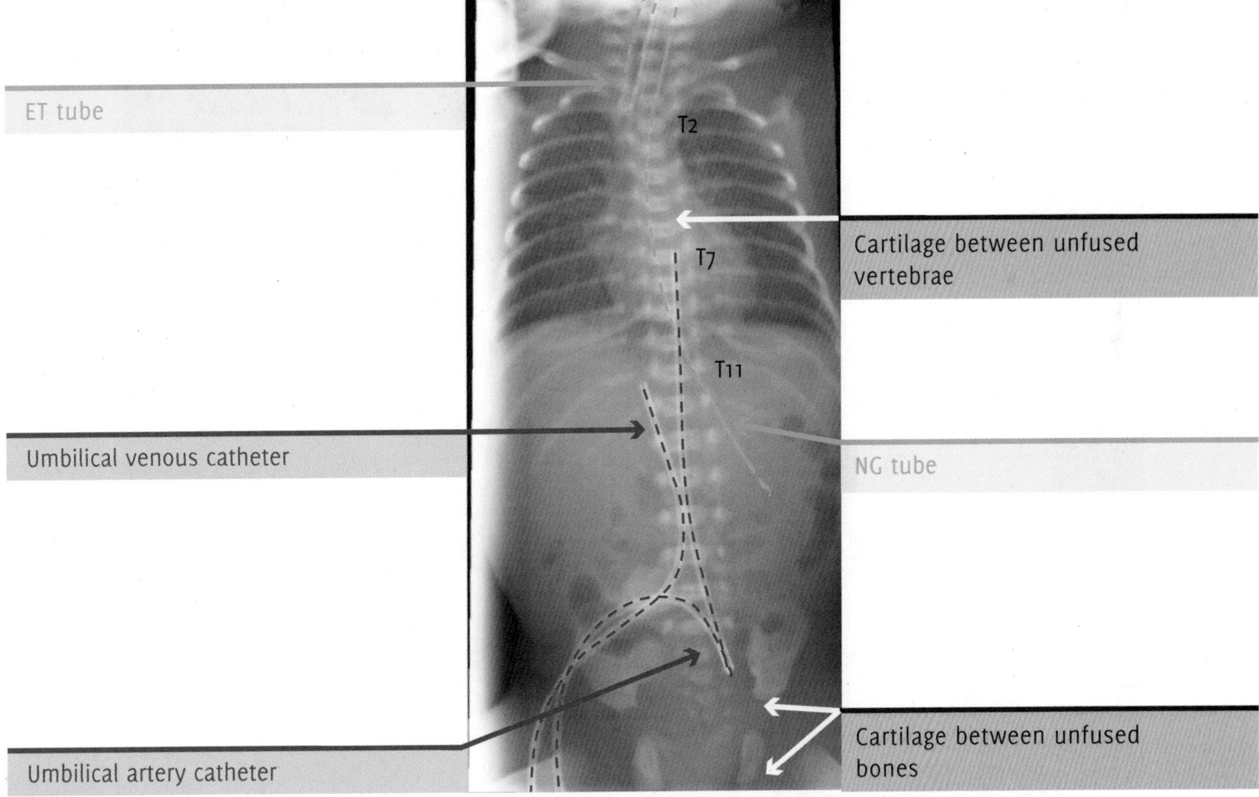

SUMMARY

This X-ray demonstrates an NG tube, ET tube and umbilical artery catheter in satisfactory positions. The umbilical venous catheter tip projects at the level of T11.

INVESTIGATIONS AND MANAGEMENT

The umbilical venous catheter is in an abnormally low position. This should be removed and replaced by another catheter advanced slightly further to approximately T10 to lie within the inferior vena cava at the level of the diaphragm.

Case

84

A 35-year-old female presents to ED with left flank pain. Her past medical history is significant for ureteric obstruction, for which she has recently undergone placement of bilateral JJ ureteric stents. She has no other significant past medical history and is a nonsmoker. On examination, she has oxygen saturations of 98% in room air and a temperature of 36.7°C. Her HR is 82 bpm, RR is 16 and blood pressure is 120/68 mmHg. The abdomen is soft and there is tenderness over the left flank with normal bowel sounds. Urine dipstick shows blood ++ and a pregnancy test is negative.

An abdominal X-ray is requested to assess for possible renal calculi.

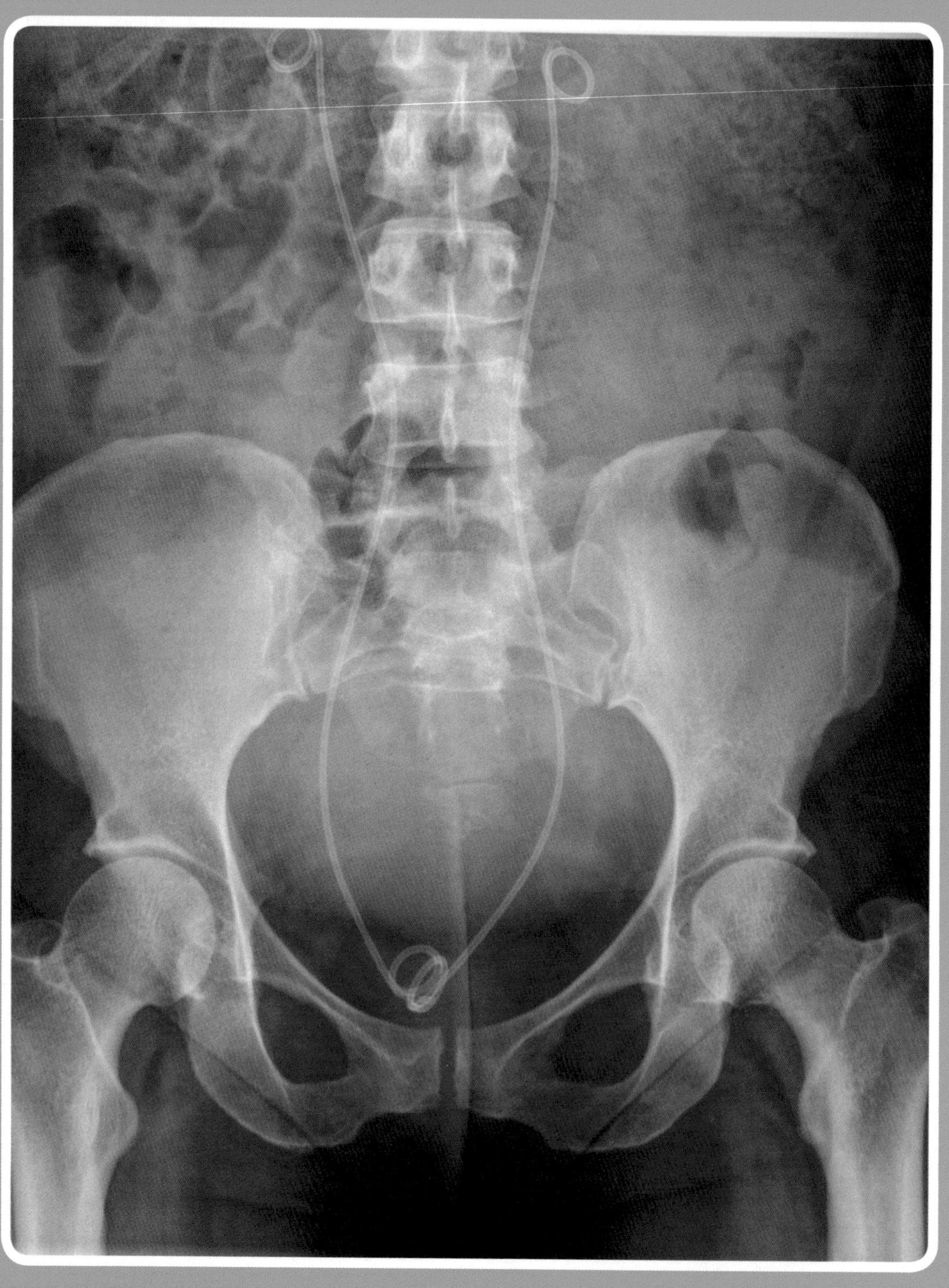

TECHNICAL INFORMATION

Patient ID: Anonymous.
Projection: AP supine.
Rotation: Adequate.
Penetration: Adequate – the spinous processes are visible.
Coverage: Inadequate – the anterior ribs have not been included.

BOWEL GAS PATTERN

The bowel gas pattern is normal.

There is a moderate volume of faecal residue present throughout the transverse and descending colon.

BOWEL WALL

There is no evidence of mural thickening or intramural gas within the large or small bowel.

PNEUMOPERITONEUM

There is no evidence of free intraabdominal gas.

SOLID ORGANS

There is medial deviation of the proximal ureters bilaterally, which contain JJ stents.

VASCULAR

No abnormal vascular calcification.

BONES

There are no abnormalities of the imaged thoracic and lumbar spine, or within the pelvis.

SOFT TISSUES

The psoas muscle outline is not visible bilaterally.

The extraabdominal soft tissues are unremarkable.

OTHER

There are bilateral JJ ureteric stents in situ. Both proximal stents are projected over the expected position of the renal pelvises, and both distal stents projected over the urinary bladder; however, both stents deviate medially.

There are no vascular lines, drains or surgical clips.

REVIEW AREAS

Gallstones/renal calculi: No radiopaque calculi.
Lung bases: Not fully included.
Spine: Normal.
Femoral heads: Normal.

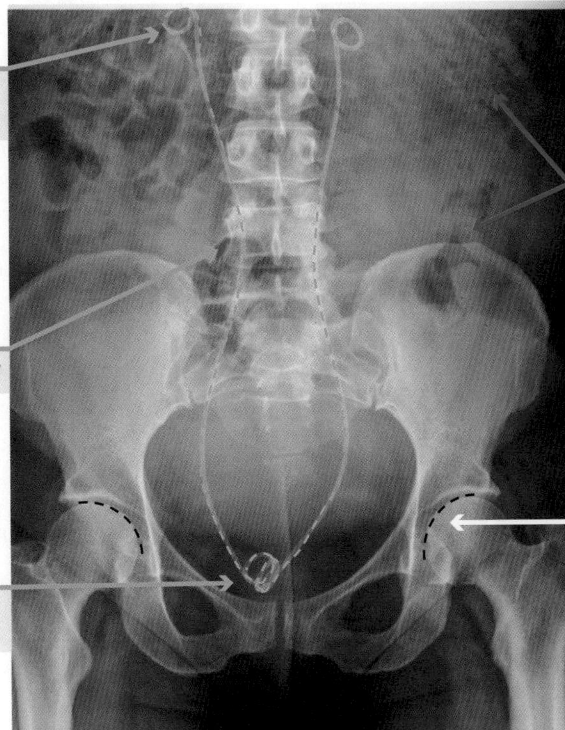

SUMMARY

This X-ray demonstrates bilateral JJ ureteric stents with medial deviation of the mid ureters, indicating that the ureteric obstruction may be due to retroperitoneal fibrosis. There is a moderate volume of faecal residue throughout the transverse and descending colon.

INVESTIGATIONS AND MANAGEMENT

The patient should be resuscitated using an ABCDE approach.

Adequate analgesia and hydration should be provided.

Referral to the renal/urology team should be made. Urgent bloods should be taken, including FBC, U&Es, CRP, ESR, LFTs, bone profile, blood gas and tumour markers.

A CT scan of the kidneys, ureters and bladder might be useful for better visualization of the anatomy, and subsequent consideration of removal/replacement of the ureteric stents if there is evidence that they are blocked.

Case

85

A 70-year-old male presents to ED with generalized abdominal pain and vomiting. His past medical history is significant for a stable abdominal aortic aneurysm and previous dynamic hip screw insertion on the right. He has no other significant past medical history and is a nonsmoker. On examination, he has oxygen saturations of 94% in air and a temperature of 37.2°C. His HR is 98 bpm, RR is 22 and blood pressure is 110/65 mmHg. The abdomen is rigid and there is generalized tenderness. Urine dipstick is unremarkable.

An abdominal X-ray is requested to assess for possible bowel obstruction.

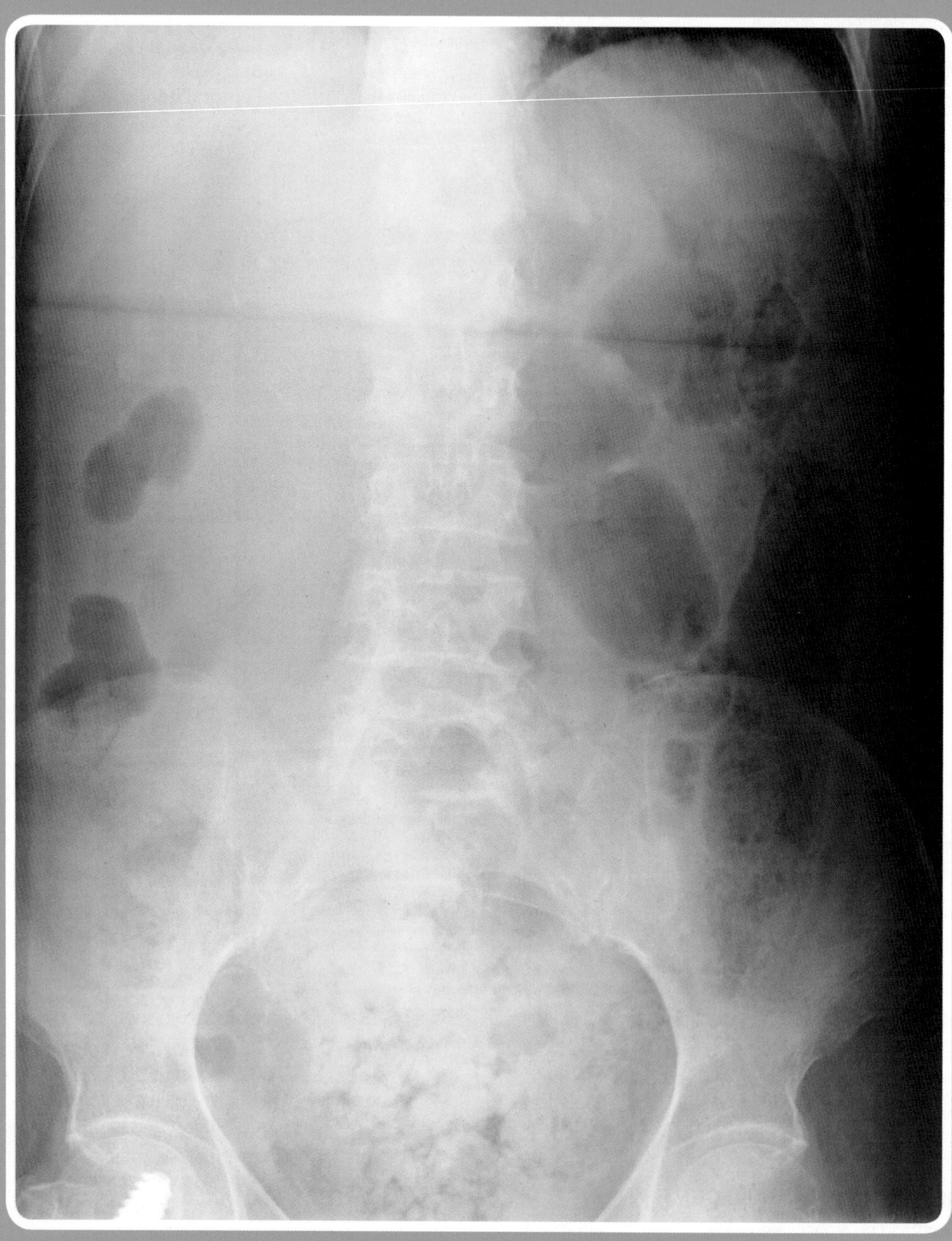

TECHNICAL INFORMATION

Patient ID: Anonymous.
Projection: AP supine.
Rotation: Adequate.
Penetration: Adequate – the spinous processes are visible.
Coverage: Inadequate – the right iliac crest, pubic symphysis and inferior pubic rami have not been fully included.

BOWEL GAS PATTERN

The bowel gas pattern is normal.

There is a significant volume of faecal residue present throughout the descending colon and prominent rectum.

BOWEL WALL

There is a prominent gaseous loop of distal large bowel on the left side of the abdomen.

There is no evidence of intramural gas.

PNEUMOPERITONEUM

There is no evidence of free intraabdominal gas.

SOLID ORGANS

The solid organ contours are within normal limits with no solid organ calcification.

VASCULAR

The abdominal aorta is calcified and demonstrates fusiform aneurysmal dilatation at the level of T12 to L4.

BONES

There are no abnormalities of the imaged thoracic and lumbar spine, or within the pelvis.

SOFT TISSUES

The right psoas muscle outline is not visible, which is nonspecific but raises the possibility of abdominal aortic aneurysm leak.

The extraabdominal soft tissues are unremarkable.

OTHER

There is a dynamic hip screw in situ in the right proximal femur. There are no other radiopaque foreign bodies.

There are no vascular lines, drains or surgical clips.

REVIEW AREAS

Gallstones/renal calculi: No radiopaque calculi.
Lung bases: The right lung base is not visualized.
Spine: Normal.
Femoral heads: Right-sided dynamic hip screw in situ.

Calcified abdominal aortic aneurysm

Left psoas muscle outline

Faecal residue throughout descending colon and dilated rectum

Dynamic hip screw

Left femoral head normal

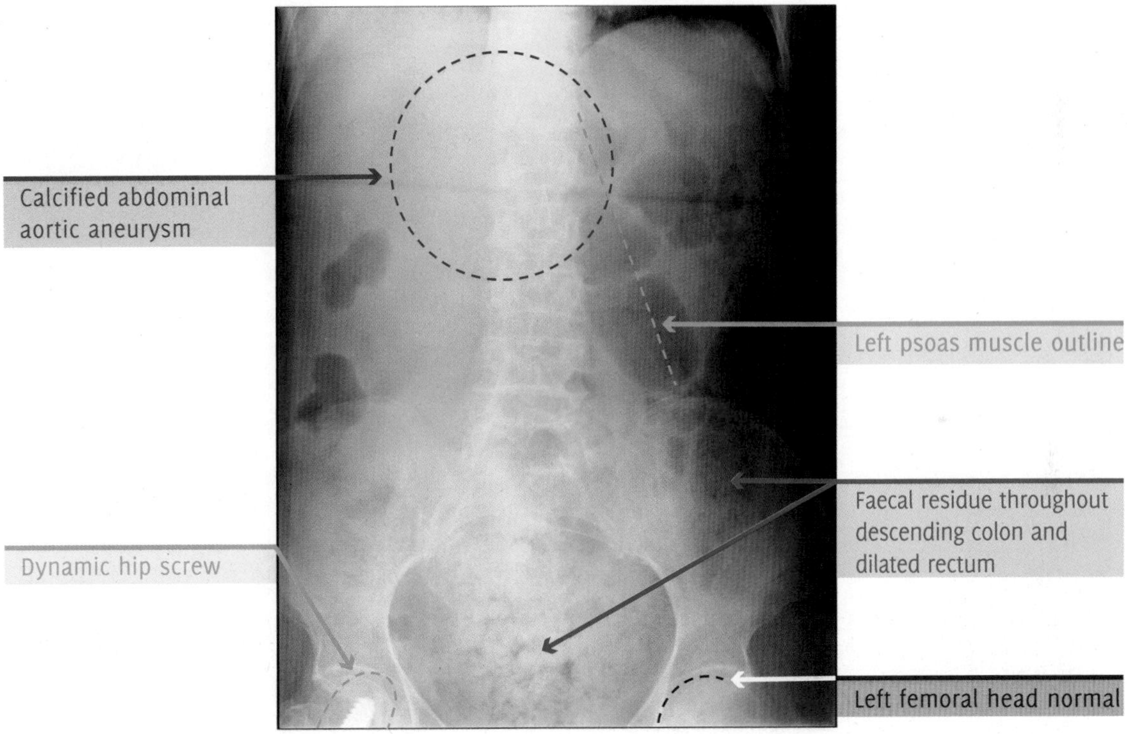

SUMMARY

This X-ray demonstrates a nonspecific prominent gaseous loop of distal large bowel and significant faecal loading of the descending colon and rectum which is dilated. The X-ray also demonstrates a longstanding large fusiform calcified abdominal aortic aneurysm. The right-sided dynamic hip screw is an incidental finding.

INVESTIGATIONS AND MANAGEMENT

The patient should be resuscitated using an ABCDE approach.

Adequate analgesia and hydration should be provided.

Urgent bloods should be taken, including FBC, U&Es, CRP, bone profile, LFTs, coagulation, blood gas and crossmatch.

The patient should be made NBM and commenced on IV fluids.

The patient should be referred urgently to vascular surgery for assessment and a CT scan of the abdomen/pelvis with IV contrast should be considered to assess for abdominal aortic aneurysm leak, which could be obscuring the psoas outline.

The general surgical team and/or the vascular team may need to be involved depending on the findings of these additional investigations and the clinical picture.

Case

86

A 60-year-old male presents to ED with generalized abdominal pain. He has no significant past medical history and is a smoker. On examination, he has oxygen saturations of 94% in air and a temperature of 36.6°C. His HR is 118 bpm, RR is 19 and blood pressure is 110/90 mmHg. The abdomen is rigid and there is generalized tenderness. Urine dipstick is unremarkable.

An abdominal X-ray is requested to assess for possible bowel obstruction.

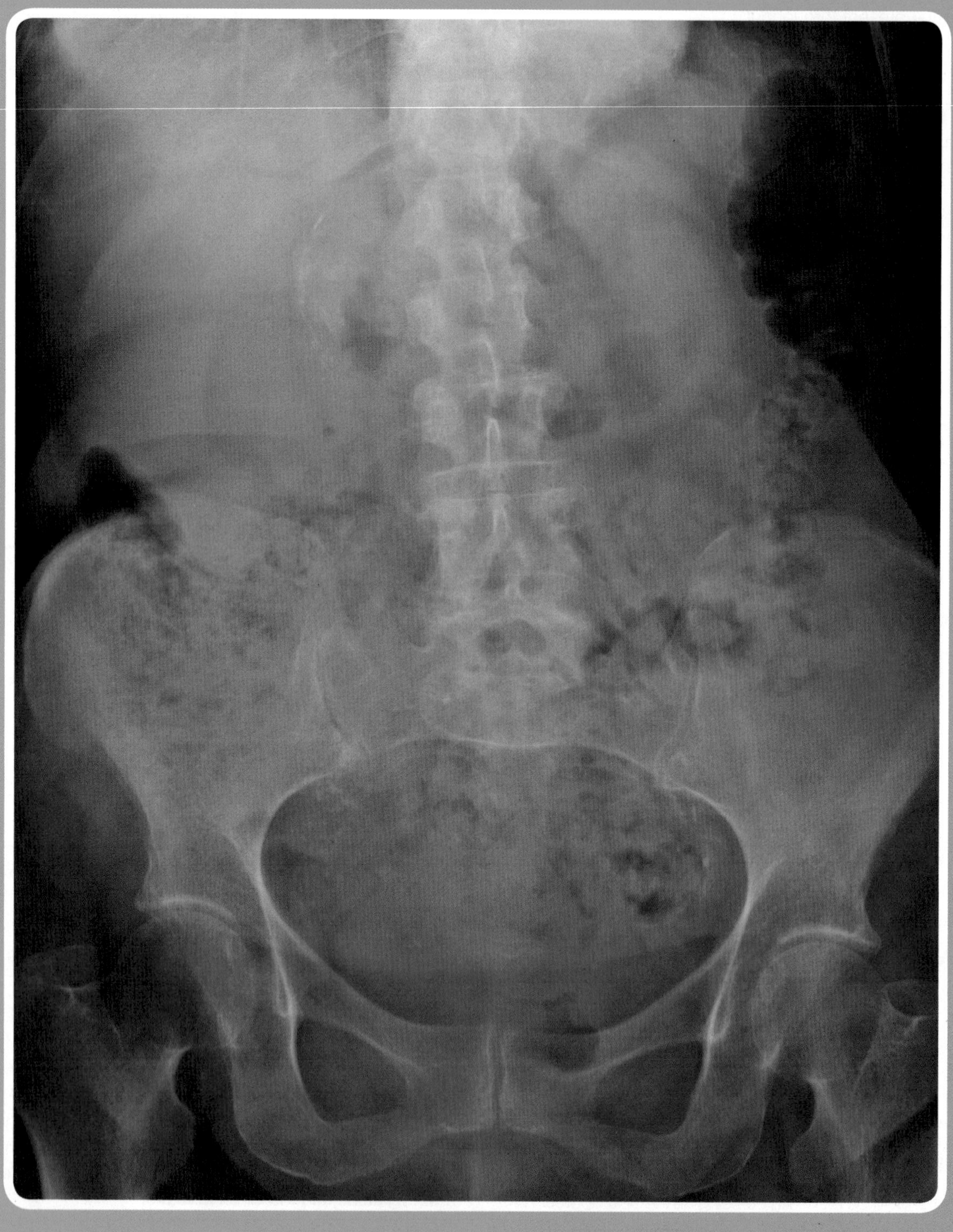

TECHNICAL INFORMATION

Patient ID: Anonymous.
Projection: AP supine.
Rotation: Adequate
Penetration: Adequate – the spinous processes are visible.
Coverage: Adequate – the anterior ribs are visible superiorly and the inferior pubic rami are visible.

BOWEL GAS PATTERN

The bowel gas pattern is normal.

There is a moderate volume of faecal residue present predominantly in the caecum, distal descending and sigmoid colon.

BOWEL WALL

There is no evidence of mural thickening or intramural gas within the large or small bowel.

PNEUMOPERITONEUM

There is no evidence of free intraabdominal gas.

SOLID ORGANS

The solid organ contours are within normal limits with no solid organ calcification.

VASCULAR

The abdominal aorta is calcified and demonstrates significant fusiform aneurysmal dilatation at the level of T12 to L3. There is calcification of the iliac arteries bilaterally.

BONES

There are no abnormalities of the imaged thoracic and lumbar spine, or within the pelvis.

SOFT TISSUES

The psoas muscle outline is visible bilaterally.

The extraabdominal soft tissues are unremarkable.

OTHER

There are no radiopaque foreign bodies.

There are no vascular lines, drains or surgical clips.

REVIEW AREAS

Gallstones/renal calculi: No radiopaque calculi.
Lung bases: Normal.
Spine: Normal.
Femoral heads: Normal.

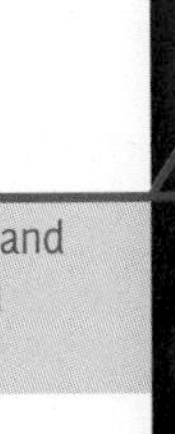

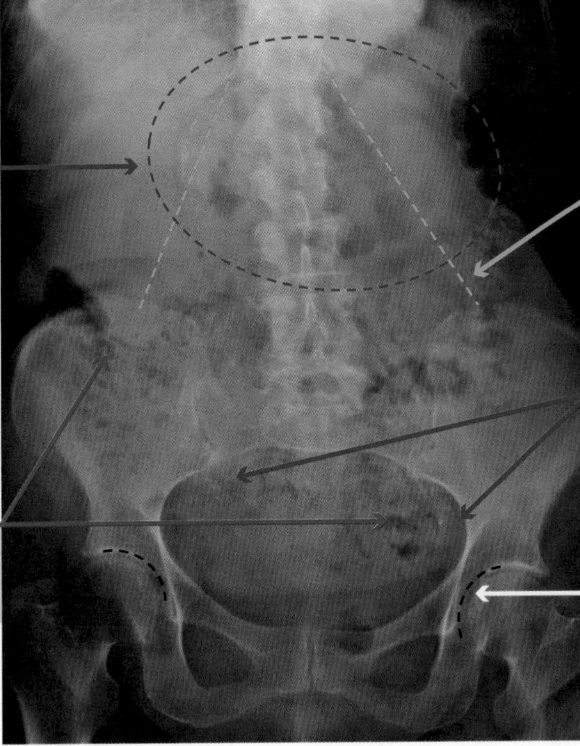

SUMMARY

This X-ray demonstrates fusiform aneurysmal dilatation of the abdominal aorta. There is a moderate volume of faecal residue present predominantly in the caecum, distal descending and sigmoid colon, however no evidence of bowel obstruction. The iliac artery calcification is an incidental finding.

INVESTIGATIONS AND MANAGEMENT

The patient should be resuscitated using an ABCDE approach.

Adequate analgesia and hydration should be provided.

Urgent bloods should be taken, including FBC, U&Es, bone profile, LFTs, CRP, coagulation, blood gas and crossmatch.

The patient should be made NBM and commenced on IV fluids.

The patient should be referred urgently to vascular surgery for assessment and a CT scan of the abdomen/pelvis with IV contrast to assess for abdominal aortic aneurysm leak should be considered.

The general surgical team and/or the vascular team may need to be involved depending on the findings of these additional investigations and the clinical picture.

Case 87

A 40-year-old female presents to ED with abdominal pain, nausea and vomiting. She has not opened her bowels for 5 days. She has a complex past medical history having had a previous bowel resection with formation of an ileostomy for Crohn's disease. She is a nonsmoker. On examination, she has oxygen saturations of 98% in room air and a temperature of 36.5°C. Her HR is 100 bpm, RR is 24 and blood pressure is 118/64 mmHg. The abdomen is rigid and there is generalized tenderness with normal bowel sounds. Urine dipstick is unremarkable and a pregnancy test is negative.

An abdominal X-ray is requested to assess for possible bowel obstruction.

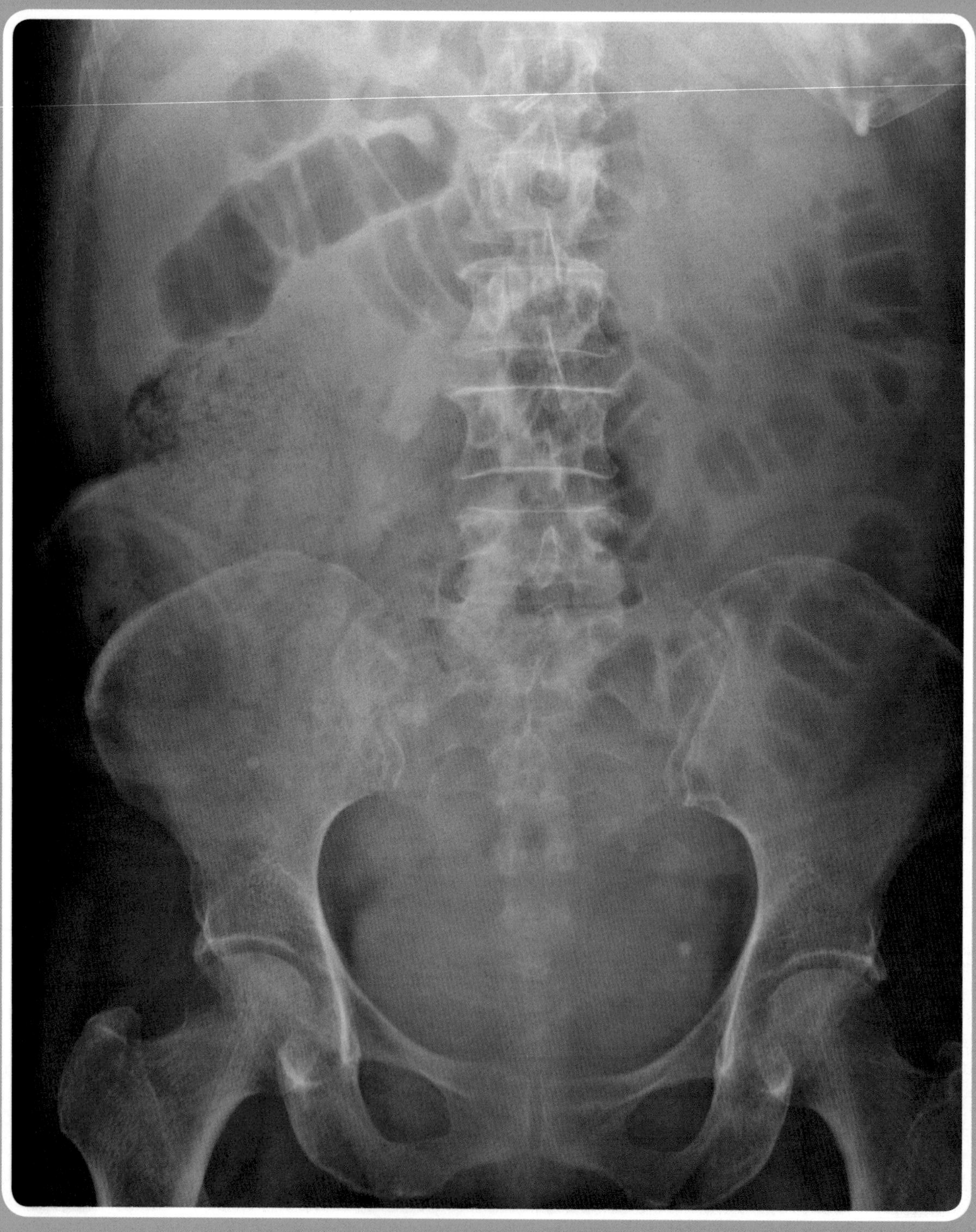

TECHNICAL INFORMATION

Patient ID: Anonymous.
Projection: AP supine.
Rotation: Adequate.
Penetration: Adequate – the spinous processes are visible.
Coverage: Adequate – the anterior ribs are visible superiorly and the pubic rami are visible inferiorly.

BOWEL GAS PATTERN

There are multiple loops of dilated bowel seen predominantly centrally in the abdomen. Valvulae conniventes are present, which appear separated with trapped gas in between in keeping with small bowel dilatation.

BOWEL WALL

There is no evidence of mural thickening or intramural gas within the large or small bowel.

PNEUMOPERITONEUM

There is no evidence of free intraabdominal gas.

SOLID ORGANS

The solid organ contours are within normal limits with no solid organ calcification.

VASCULAR

No abnormal vascular calcification.

BONES

There are mild degenerative changes in the hip joints with osteophyte formation.

SOFT TISSUES

The psoas muscle outline is visible bilaterally.

The extraabdominal soft tissues are unremarkable.

OTHER

There is a rounded radiopaque density seen projected over the region of the right iliac fossa, in keeping with an ileostomy bag external to the patient. There is a moderate volume of faecal material in the area surrounding the ileostomy bag.

There is a small rounded radiopaque density projected over the region of the pelvis, which most likely represents a phlebolith.

There are surgical clips projected over the epigastrium.

There are no vascular lines or drains.

REVIEW AREAS

Gallstones/renal calculi: No radiopaque calculi.
Lung bases: Not fully included.
Spine: Normal.
Femoral heads: Normal.

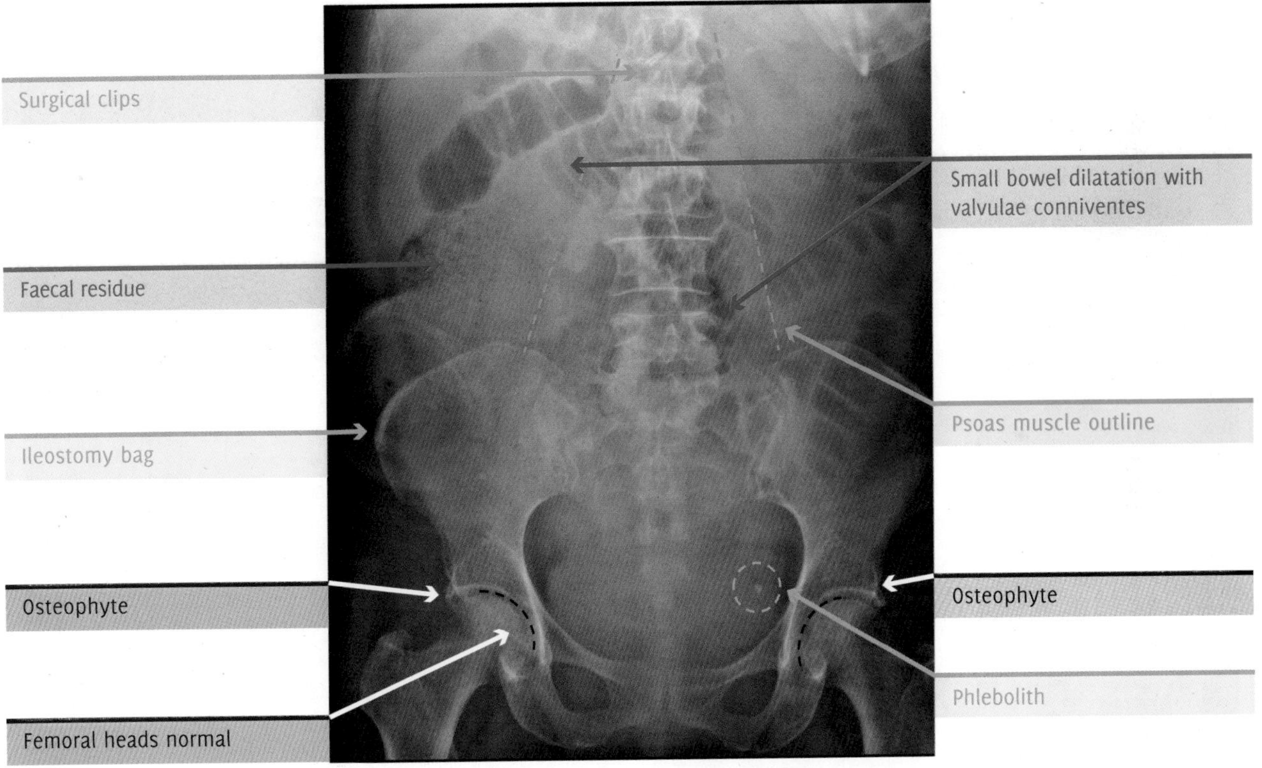

SUMMARY

This X-ray demonstrates predominantly centrally located bowel dilatation with valvulae conniventes, in keeping with small bowel obstruction. It also demonstrates an ileostomy bag projecting over the right iliac fossa with moderate volume faecal material seen in and surrounding the bag. Findings may be related to adhesions, recurrence of a Crohn's stricture or faecal impaction.

INVESTIGATIONS AND MANAGEMENT

The patient should be resuscitated using an ABCDE approach.

Adequate analgesia and hydration should be provided. The stoma should be assessed for patency.

The patient should be kept NBM, with an NG tube inserted on free drainage to relieve the pressure in the small bowel and IV fluids started.

Urgent bloods should be taken, including FBC, U&Es, CRP, LFTs, coagulation, blood gas, and group and save.

The general surgical team should be contacted urgently and a CT scan of the abdomen/pelvis with IV contrast considered.

Case

88

A 27-year-old male presents to the gastroenterology outpatient clinic with worsening abdominal pain and a recent history of loss of weight. He has no significant past medical history and is a nonsmoker. On examination, he has oxygen saturations of 97% in room air and a temperature of 39.2°C. His HR is 112 bpm, RR is 26 and blood pressure is 140/78 mmHg. He has severe generalized tenderness and guarding with normal bowel sounds. Urine dipstick is unremarkable.

An abdominal X-ray is requested to assess for possible perforation.

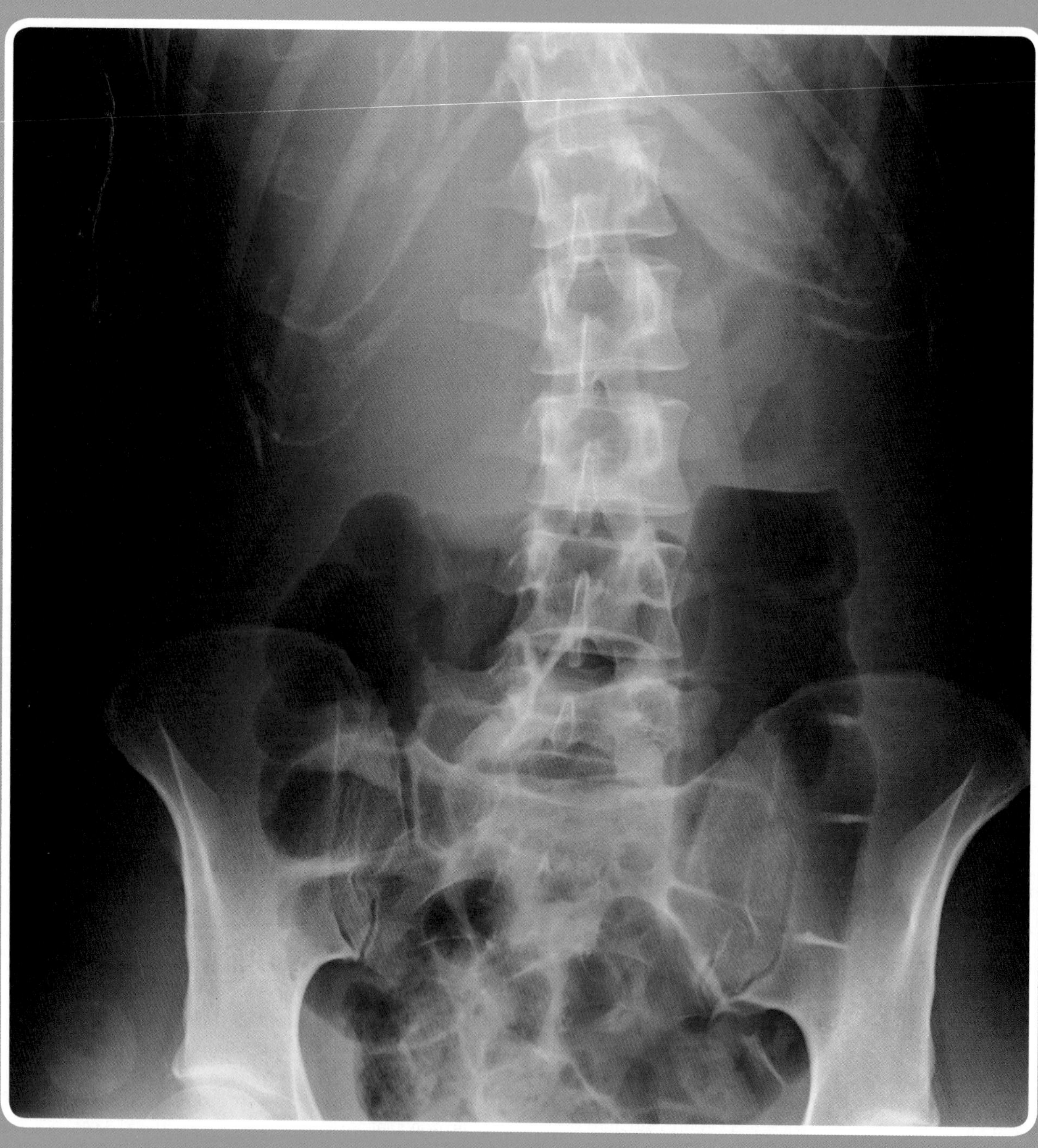

TECHNICAL INFORMATION

Patient ID: Anonymous.
Projection: AP supine.
Rotation: Adequate.
Penetration: Adequate – the spinous processes are visible.
Coverage: Inadequate – the pubic symphysis, inferior pubic rami and hip joints have not been fully included.

BOWEL GAS PATTERN

The large bowel is displaced inferiorly towards the pelvis, implying there is possibly a large soft tissue mass in the upper abdomen.

BOWEL WALL

There is no evidence of mural thickening or intramural gas within the large or small bowel.

PNEUMOPERITONEUM

There is no evidence of free intraabdominal gas.

SOLID ORGANS

The solid organ contours are within normal limits with no solid organ calcification.

VASCULAR

No abnormal vascular calcification.

BONES

There is mild lumbar scoliosis convex to the left, centred at the L2/L3 level.

There are no other abnormalities of the imaged thoracic and lumbar spine, or within the pelvis.

SOFT TISSUES

The psoas muscle outline is not preserved on the right side, which may relate to the presence of an abdominal mass.

The extraabdominal soft tissues are unremarkable.

OTHER

There is a large homogeneous opacification seen in the upper abdomen, which is displacing the large bowel down into the pelvis.

There are no vascular lines, drains or surgical clips.

REVIEW AREAS

Gallstones/renal calculi: No radiopaque calculi.
Lung bases: Normal.
Spine: Lumbar scoliosis seen convex to the left, centred on the L2/L3 vertebral bodies.
Femoral heads: Not visible.

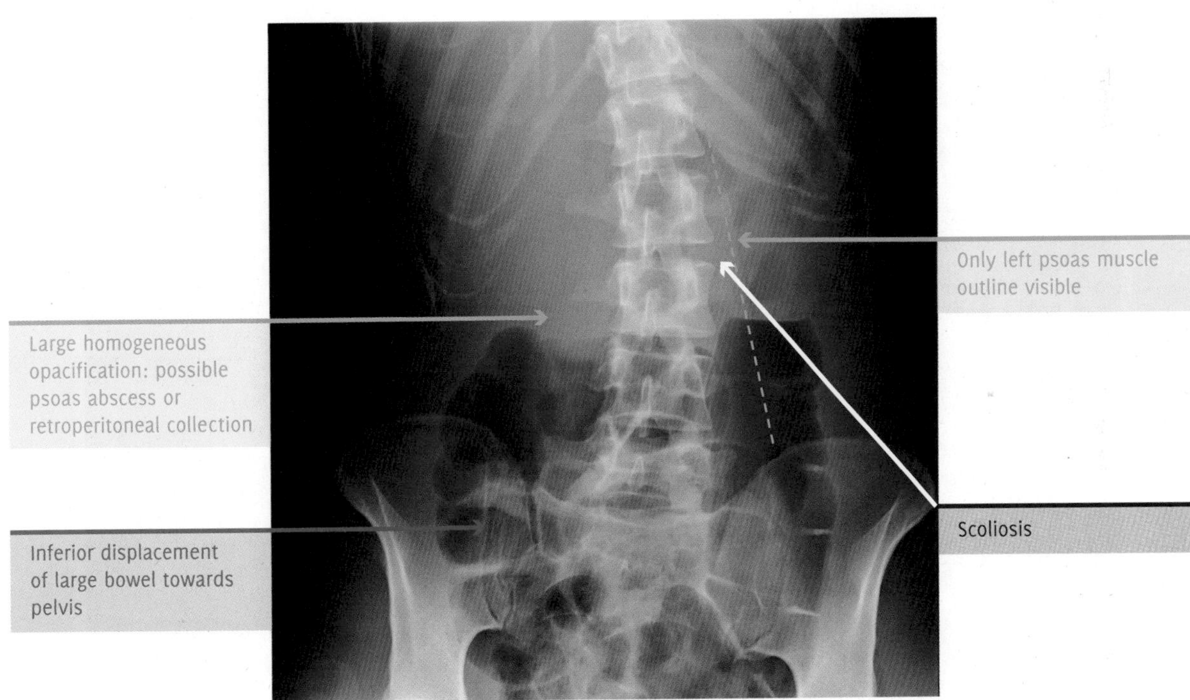

SUMMARY

This X-ray demonstrates a large homogeneous opacification in the upper abdomen, which is displacing the large bowel inferiorly into the pelvis and obscuring the right psoas muscle outline. Given the clinical history, findings are suggestive of a large abdominal mass, which is probably retroperitoneal due to the loss of the right psoas muscle outline. The mild lumbar scoliosis is likely relative to this.

INVESTIGATIONS AND MANAGEMENT

The patient is clinically unwell and should be resuscitated using an ABCDE approach.

Adequate analgesia and hydration should be provided.

Urgent bloods should be taken, including FBC, U&Es, LFTs, amylase, bone profile, CRP, blood gas and blood cultures.

The Sepsis 6 pathway should be started immediately, including administration of oxygen, IV broad-spectrum antibiotics and consideration of a fluid bolus as well as measurement of lactate and urinary output and blood cultures.

A CT scan of the abdomen/pelvis with IV contrast would be useful for better visualization of the anatomy and the general surgical team should be involved.

Case

89

A 52-year-old male is currently admitted to the surgical ward following cardiothoracic surgery. He has not opened his bowels for 5 days. His past medical history is significant for aortic stenosis and type II diabetes mellitus. He is an ex-smoker. On examination, he has oxygen saturations of 98% in room air and a temperature of 37.1°C. His HR is 75 bpm, RR is 13 and blood pressure is 120/65 mmHg. The abdomen is soft and there is no tenderness with normal bowel sounds. Urine dipstick is unremarkable.

An abdominal X-ray is requested to assess for possible bowel obstruction.

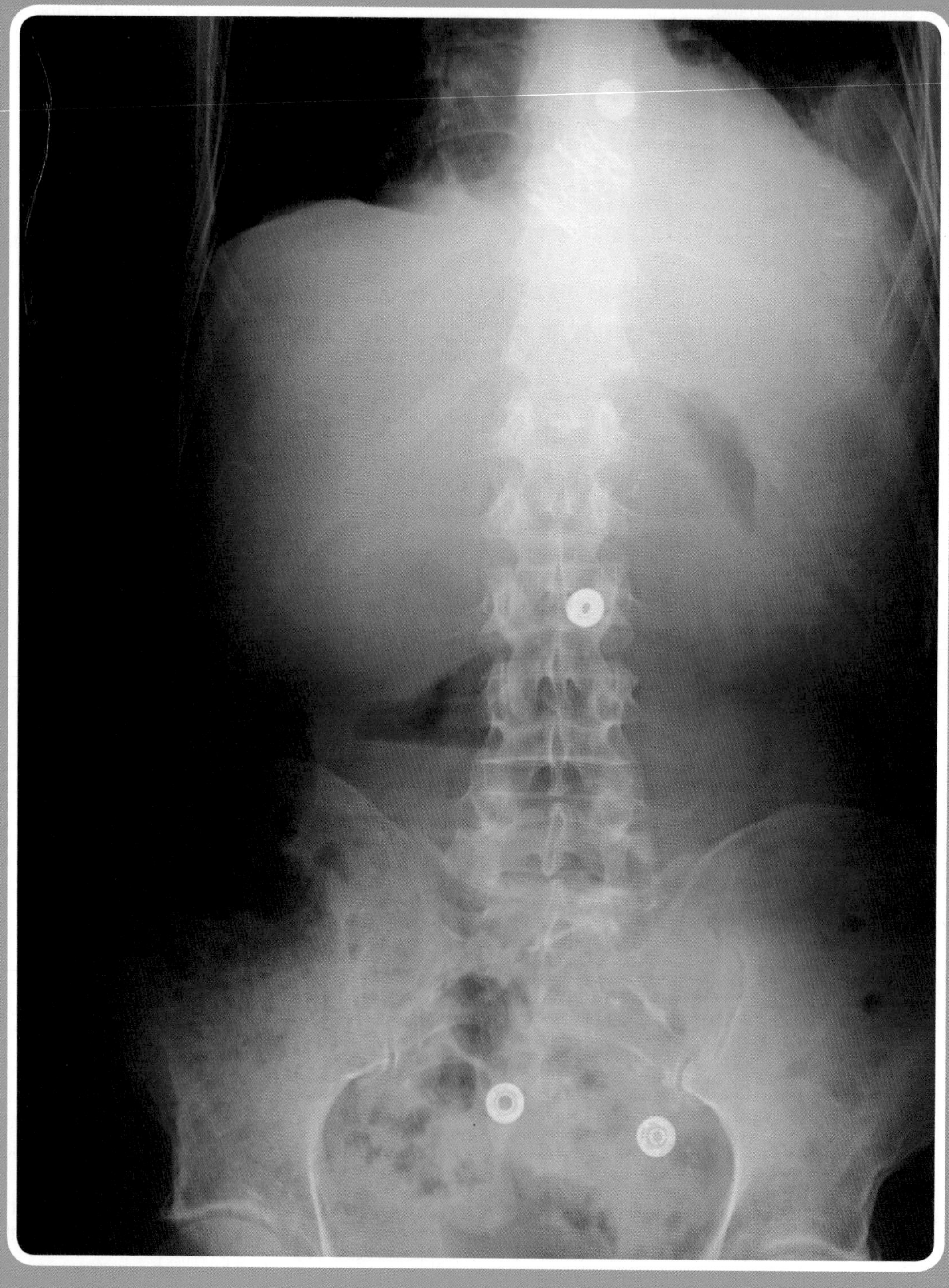

TECHNICAL INFORMATION

Patient ID: Anonymous.
Projection: AP supine.
Rotation: Adequate.
Penetration: Adequate – the spinous processes are visible.
Coverage: Inadequate – the pubic symphysis, inferior pubic rami and hip joints have not been fully included.

BOWEL GAS PATTERN

The bowel gas pattern is normal. There is a moderate volume of faecal residue in the caecum.

BOWEL WALL

There is no evidence of mural thickening or intramural gas within the large or small bowel.

PNEUMOPERITONEUM

There is no evidence of free intraabdominal gas.

SOLID ORGANS

There is a triangular opacity projecting in the left retrocardiac area in keeping with left lower lobe collapse.

There is also heterogeneous opacification at the base of the left lung in keeping with possible consolidation/effusion.

VASCULAR

No abnormal vascular calcification.

BONES

There are no abnormalities of the imaged thoracic and lumbar spine, or within the pelvis.

SOFT TISSUES

The psoas muscle outline is not visible bilaterally, which is nonspecific.

The extraabdominal soft tissues are unremarkable.

OTHER

There are two surgical clips projecting over the left cardiac border with a further surgical clip projecting over the mediastinum.

There is a radiopaque density projected over the mediastinum in the midline, in keeping with a transcatheter aortic valve implantation.

There are four small rounded radiopaque densities projected in the midline from the chest to the pelvis external to the patient, most likely popper fastenings on a cardigan.

There are no vascular lines or drains.

REVIEW AREAS

Gallstones/renal calculi: No radiopaque calculi.
Lung bases: Left lower lobe collapse with possible consolidation/effusion.
Spine: Normal.
Femoral heads: Normal.

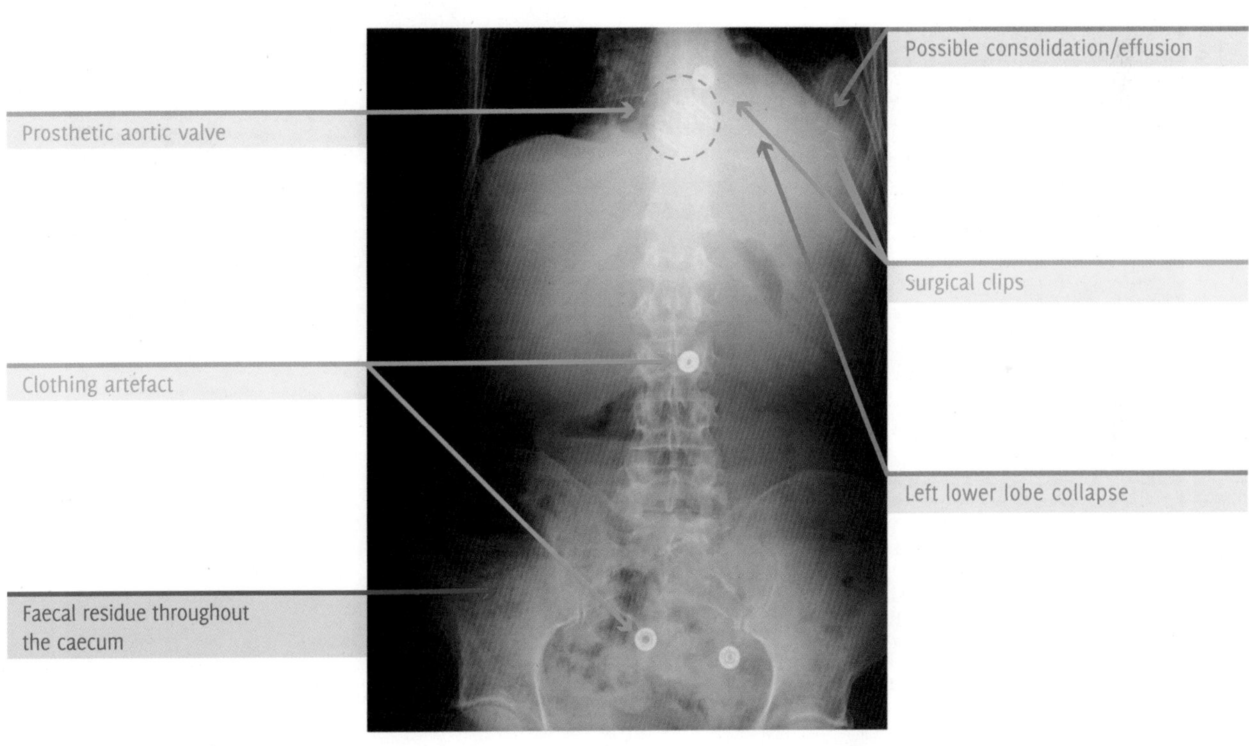

SUMMARY

This X-ray demonstrates a prosthetic aortic valve in situ. There is left lower lobe collapse with possible left basal consolidation/effusion. There is a moderate volume of faecal residue in the caecum.

INVESTIGATIONS AND MANAGEMENT

Adequate analgesia and hydration should be provided.

A formal CXR would be helpful, as would an ultrasound to quantify the size of any effusion.

Urgent bloods should be taken, including FBC, U&Es, LFTs, blood gas, blood culture and CRP.

The patient should be commenced on antibiotics for a hospital-acquired pneumonia. Laxatives should be considered for constipation.

Case

90

A 6-hour-old newborn currently admitted to the postnatal ward develops vomiting and abdominal distension. His past medical history is significant for Down syndrome. On examination, he has oxygen saturations of 98% in room air and a temperature of 36.9°C. His HR is 170 bpm and RR is 60. The abdomen is grossly distended and bowel sounds are absent.

An abdominal X-ray is requested to assess for possible bowel obstruction.

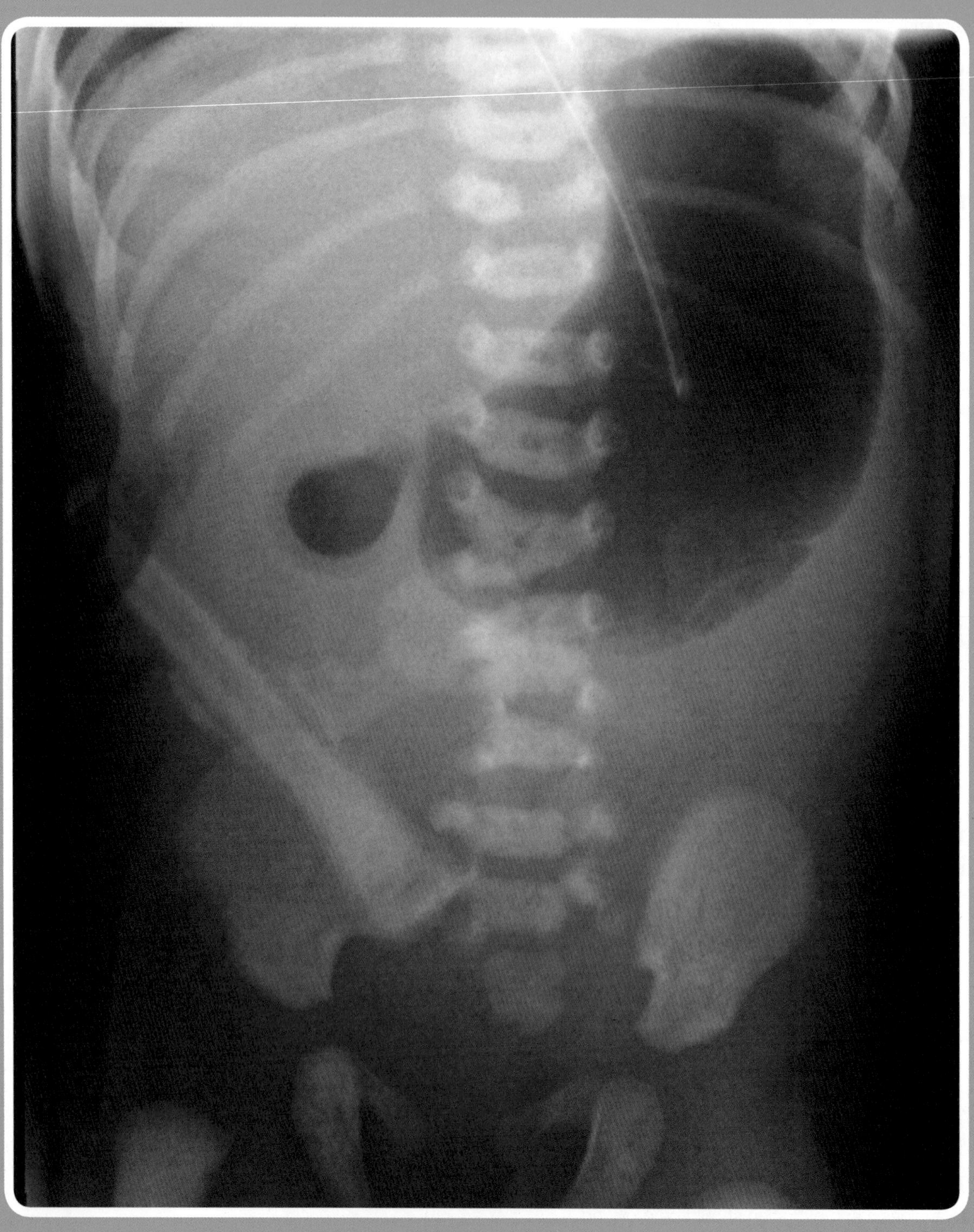

TECHNICAL INFORMATION

Patient ID: Anonymous.
Projection: AP supine.
Rotation: Asymmetrical appearance of the pelvis due to patient rotation to the right.
Penetration: Adequate – the spine is visible.
Coverage: Adequate – the anterior ribs are visible superiorly and the inferior pubic rami are visible.

BOWEL GAS PATTERN

There is distension of the stomach and proximal duodenum which are filled with gas and separated by the pyloric sphincter, creating a 'double-bubble' sign.

There is absence of bowel gas seen distal to the duodenum.

BOWEL WALL

There is no evidence of mural thickening or intramural gas within the large or small bowel.

PNEUMOPERITONEUM

There is no evidence of free intraabdominal gas.

SOLID ORGANS

The solid organ contours are within normal limits with no solid organ calcification.

VASCULAR

No abnormal vascular calcification.

BONES

There are segmentation abnormalities of the lumbar spine, which may be part of an underlying syndrome.

SOFT TISSUES

The psoas muscle outline is not visible bilaterally, which is nonspecific, particularly in a child of this age.

The extraabdominal soft tissues are unremarkable.

OTHER

There is an NG tube in situ, with its tip seen in the left upper quadrant, within the body of the stomach.

There is a clamp seen projecting external to the patient on the right side of the abdomen in keeping with an umbilical cord clamp.

There are no vascular lines, drains or surgical clips.

REVIEW AREAS

Gallstones/renal calculi: No radiopaque calculi.
Lung bases: Not fully included.
Spine: Normal – cartilage between vertebrae.
Femoral heads: Normal – growth plates present.

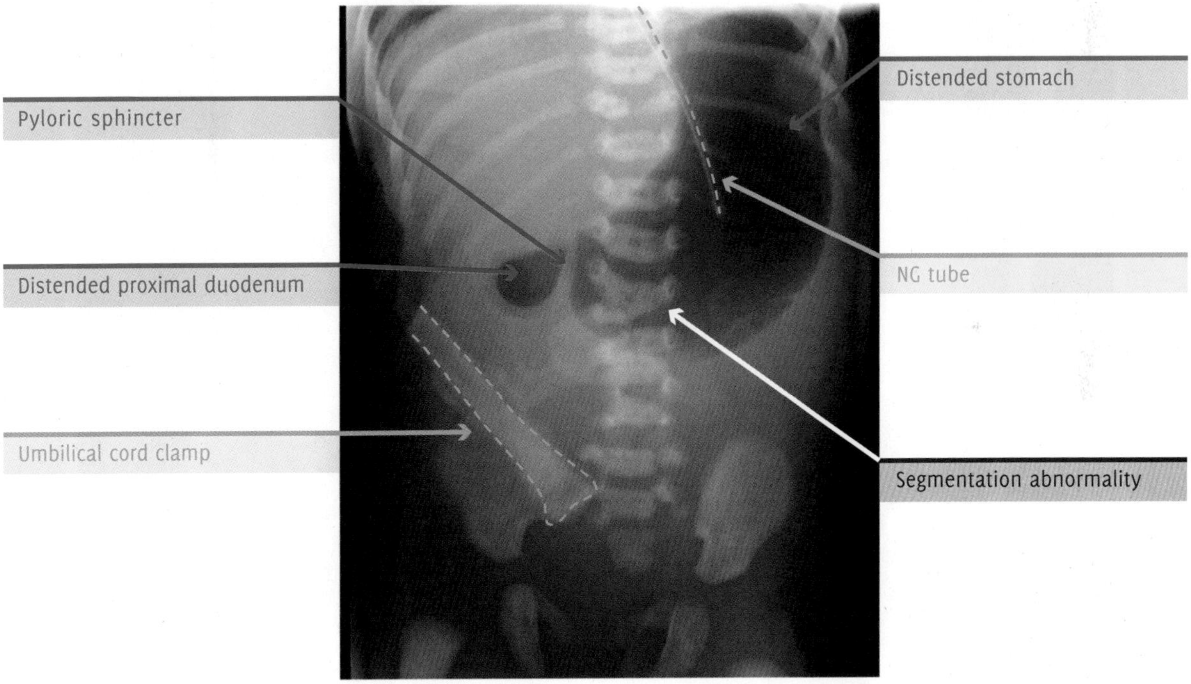

Pyloric sphincter

Distended proximal duodenum

Umbilical cord clamp

Distended stomach

NG tube

Segmentation abnormality

SUMMARY

This X-ray demonstrates gaseous distension of the stomach and proximal duodenum with absence of bowel gas distal to this point, in keeping with duodenal atresia. There is an NG tube in situ in satisfactory position within the stomach and the umbilical cord is clamped.

INVESTIGATIONS AND MANAGEMENT

The baby should be resuscitated using an ABCDE approach.

The baby should be commenced on broad-spectrum antibiotics, IV fluids and be made NBM.

Urgent bloods should be taken, including FBC, U&Es, blood culture, blood gas and CRP.

The patient should be referred urgently to the neonatal surgeons for operative intervention. Given the vertebral abnormalities, associated defects should be looked for, i.e. VACTERL (anal atresia, cardiac defects, tracheo-esophageal fistula, renal anomalies and limb abnormalities).

Case

91

A 21-day-old baby boy, currently admitted to NICU after being born at 29 weeks, develops abdominal distension, bile-stained vomitus and is feeding poorly. On examination, he has oxygen saturations of 100% while intubated on 40% oxygen, and a temperature of 37.8°C. His HR is 180 bpm and RR is 65. The abdomen is rigid and bowel sounds are absent.

An abdominal X-ray is requested to assess for possible necrotizing enterocolitis.

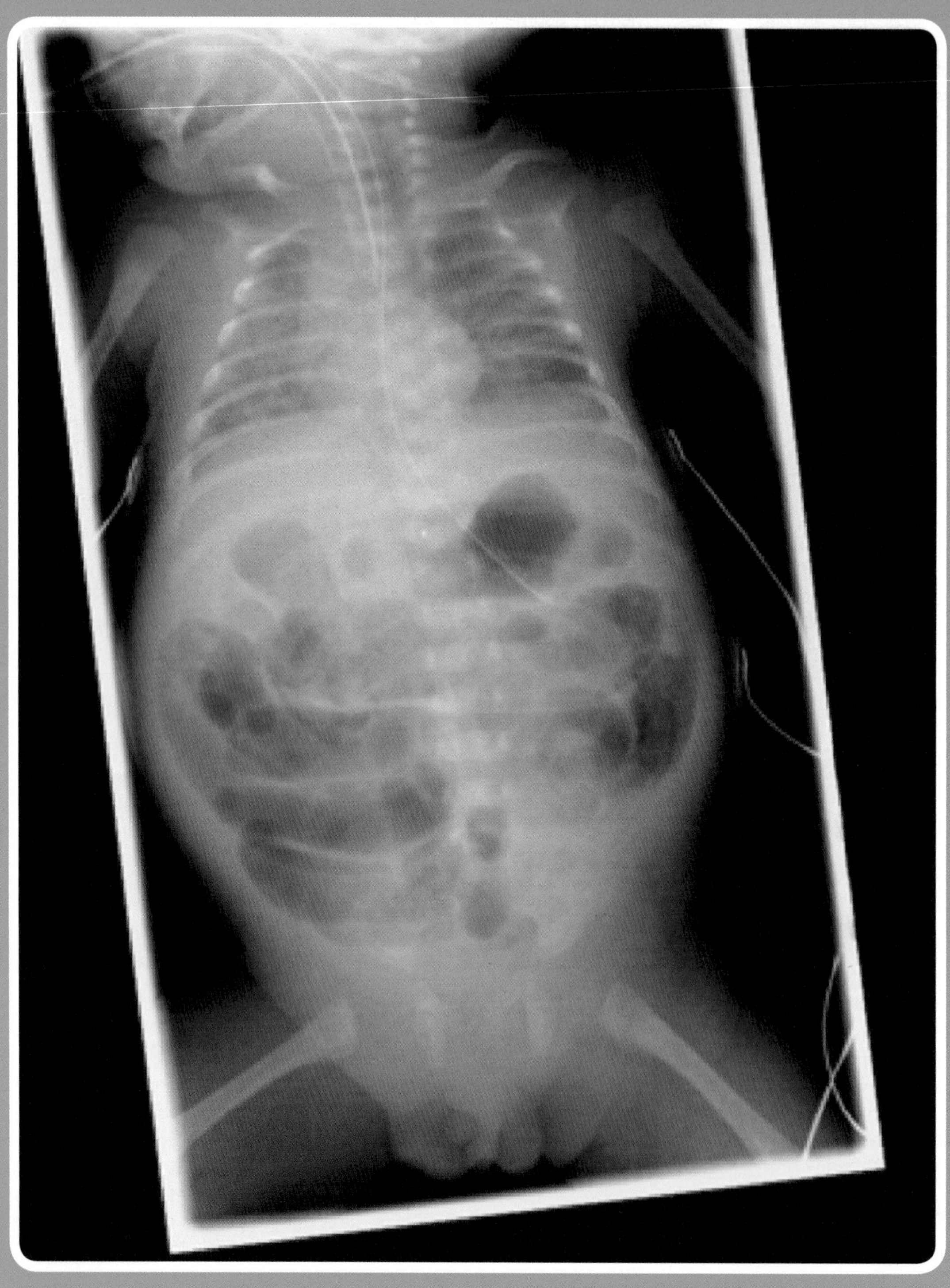

TECHNICAL INFORMATION

Patient ID: Anonymous.
Projection: AP supine 'babygram' of chest and abdomen.
Rotation: Asymmetrical appearances of the pelvis with deviation of the spine to the left due to patient rotation to the right.
Penetration: Adequate – the spine is visible.
Coverage: Adequate – the anterior ribs are visible superiorly and the inferior pubic rami are visible.

BOWEL GAS PATTERN

There are multiple, predominantly small bowel loops of dilated bowel seen throughout the abdomen. These demonstrate a 'featureless' appearance in keeping with inflammation.

BOWEL WALL

There is no evidence of mural thickening or intramural gas within the large or small bowel.

PNEUMOPERITONEUM

There is evidence of free intraabdominal gas, in keeping with pneumoperitoneum. Rigler's sign can be seen (double-wall sign), in keeping with air present on both the luminal and peritoneal sides of the bowel wall.

SOLID ORGANS

Lung fields show bilateral heterogeneous opacification. Abdominal organs are difficult to visualize.

VASCULAR

No abnormal vascular calcification.

BONES

There are no abnormalities of the imaged thoracic and lumbar spine, or within the pelvis.

There is cartilage present between the pelvic bones and femurs as they have not yet fused, which is a normal finding in a child of this age.

SOFT TISSUES

The psoas muscle outline is not visible bilaterally, which is nonspecific, particularly in a child of this age.

The extraabdominal soft tissues are unremarkable.

OTHER

There is an NG tube in situ, with its tip seen in the left upper quadrant of the abdomen, within the body of the stomach.

There is an ET tube in situ, with its tip seen in the midline, just proximal to the carina.

There are three electrodes and leads external to the patient, in keeping with cardiopulmonary monitoring.

There are no vascular lines, drains or surgical clips.

REVIEW AREAS

Gallstones/renal calculi: No radiopaque calculi.
Lung bases: Normal.
Spine: Normal.
Femoral heads: Normal – growth plates present.

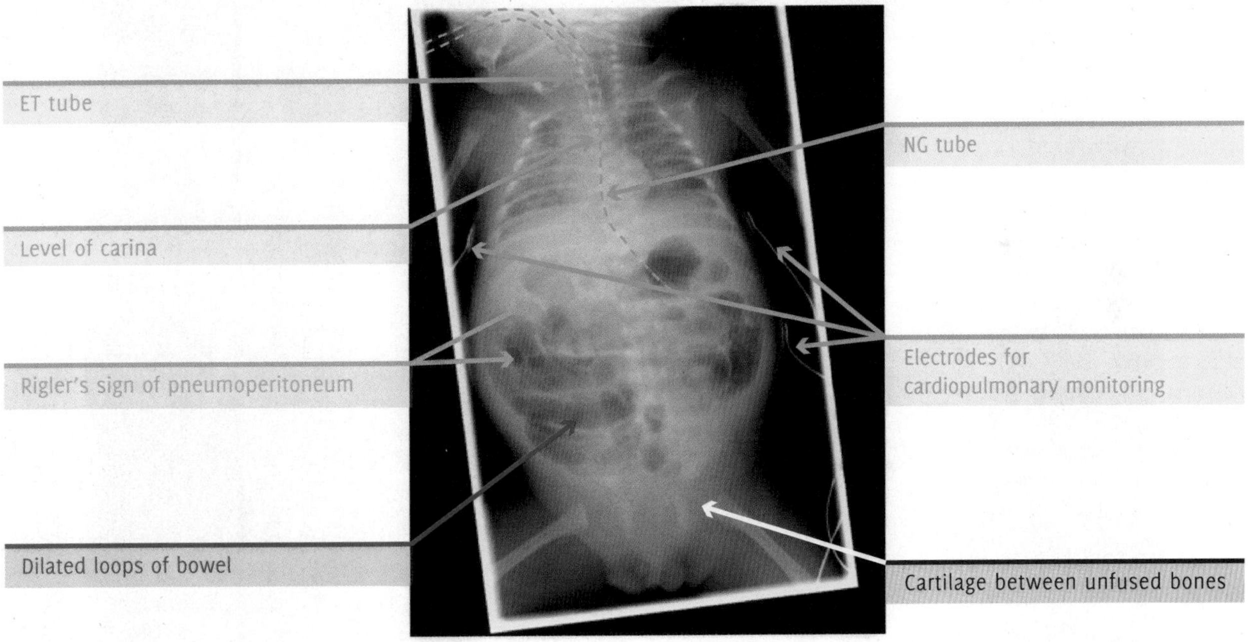

SUMMARY

This X-ray demonstrates multiple loops of dilated featureless bowel throughout the abdomen with evidence of pneumoperitoneum. Given the clinical history, findings are in keeping with bowel obstruction and secondary bowel perforation. There is likely respiratory distress syndrome in keeping with prematurity. The NG tube is in a satisfactory position, but the ET tube will need to be pulled back slightly.

INVESTIGATIONS AND MANAGEMENT

The patient should be resuscitated using an ABCDE approach. Adequate analgesia and hydration should be provided.

The baby should be started on broad-spectrum antibiotics and IV fluids and be made NBM.

Urgent bloods should be taken, including FBC, U&Es, CRP, bone profile, LFTs, coagulation, blood cultures, blood gas, and group and save. A lateral shoot through X-ray would be helpful for confirmation of perforation.

The patient should be referred urgently to the neonatal surgeons for ongoing management.

Case

92

A 31-year-old male is admitted to the general surgical ward following surgery for a stabbing injury. On examination, he has oxygen saturations of 98% in room air and a temperature of 37.2°C. His HR is 86 bpm, RR is 28 and blood pressure is 112/58 mmHg. The abdomen is tender and bowel sounds are present.

An abdominal X-ray is requested to assess the positions of the surgical drains.

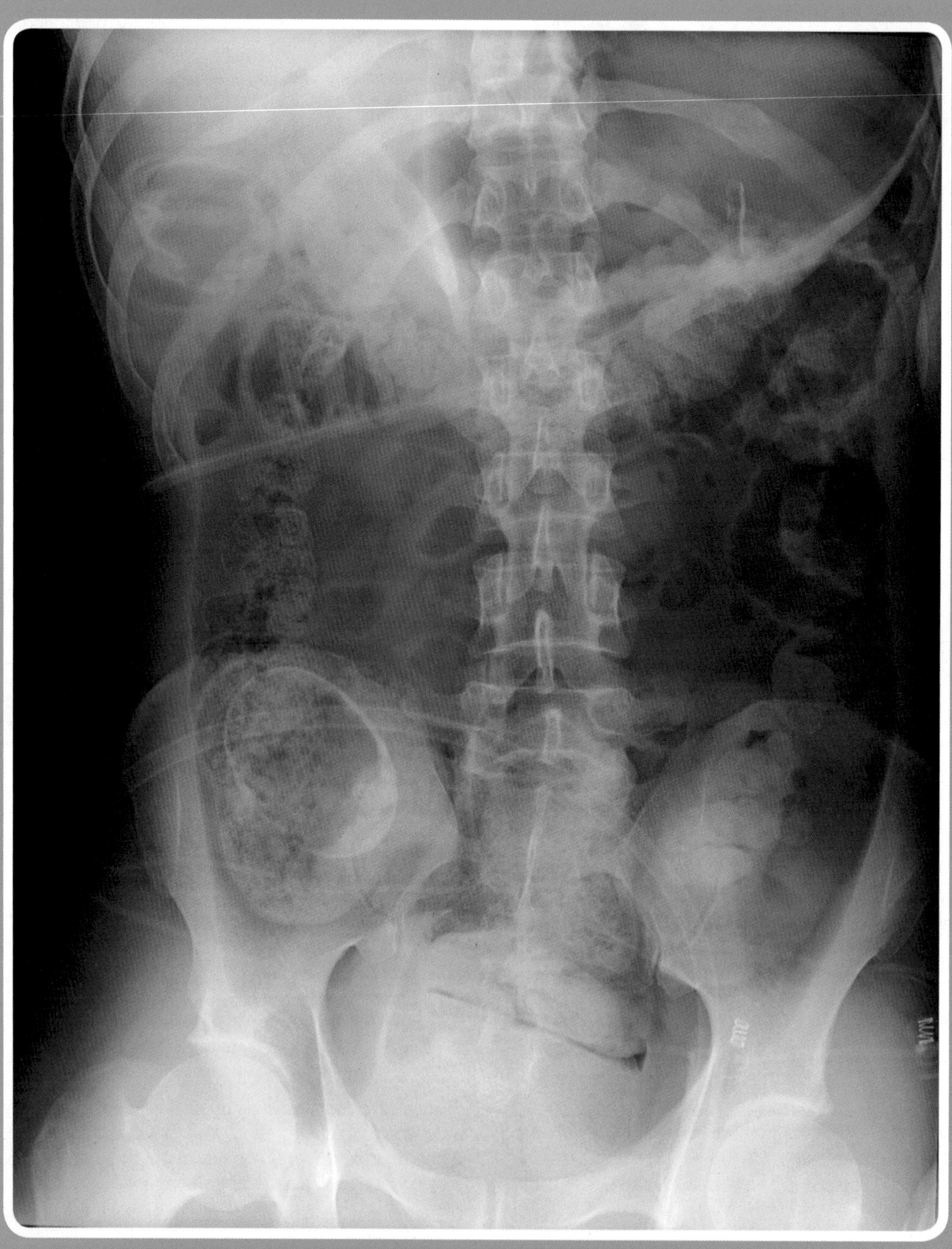

TECHNICAL INFORMATION

Patient ID: Anonymous.
Projection: AP supine.
Rotation: The spine is deviated to the left in keeping with mild patient rotation to the right.
Penetration: Adequate – the spinous processes are visible.
Coverage: Inadequate – the inferior pubic rami and left neck of femur have not been included.

BOWEL GAS PATTERN

The bowel gas pattern is normal.

There is a mild to moderate volume of faecal material present throughout the large bowel.

BOWEL WALL

There is no evidence of mural thickening or intramural gas within the large or small bowel.

PNEUMOPERITONEUM

There is evidence of extensive free intraabdominal gas, in keeping with pneumoperitoneum.

Rigler's sign (double-wall sign) can be seen, in keeping with air present on both the luminal and peritoneal sides of the bowel wall.

The falciform ligament sign can be seen, in keeping with air present within the abdomen outlining the falciform ligament.

SOLID ORGANS

The solid organ contours are within normal limits with no solid organ calcification.

VASCULAR

No abnormal vascular calcification.

BONES

There are no abnormalities of the imaged thoracic and lumbar spine, or within the pelvis.

SOFT TISSUES

The right psoas muscle outline is preserved. The left psoas muscle outline is not preserved, which is nonspecific.

The extraabdominal soft tissues are unremarkable.

OTHER

There is a surgical drain in situ projecting over the right upper quadrant with its tip projecting over the right L2 transverse process. There is a second surgical drain in situ projecting over the right lower quadrant with its tip projecting over the left pelvic ring.

There are further radiopaque lines projecting over the lower abdomen which likely represent external lines. There is an external artefact in the right lower quadrant as well, which may represent a dressing, although this should be correlated with clinical assessment.

There are no vascular lines or surgical clips.

REVIEW AREAS

Gallstones/renal calculi: No radiopaque calculi.
Lung bases: Not fully included.
Spine: Normal.
Femoral heads: Normal.

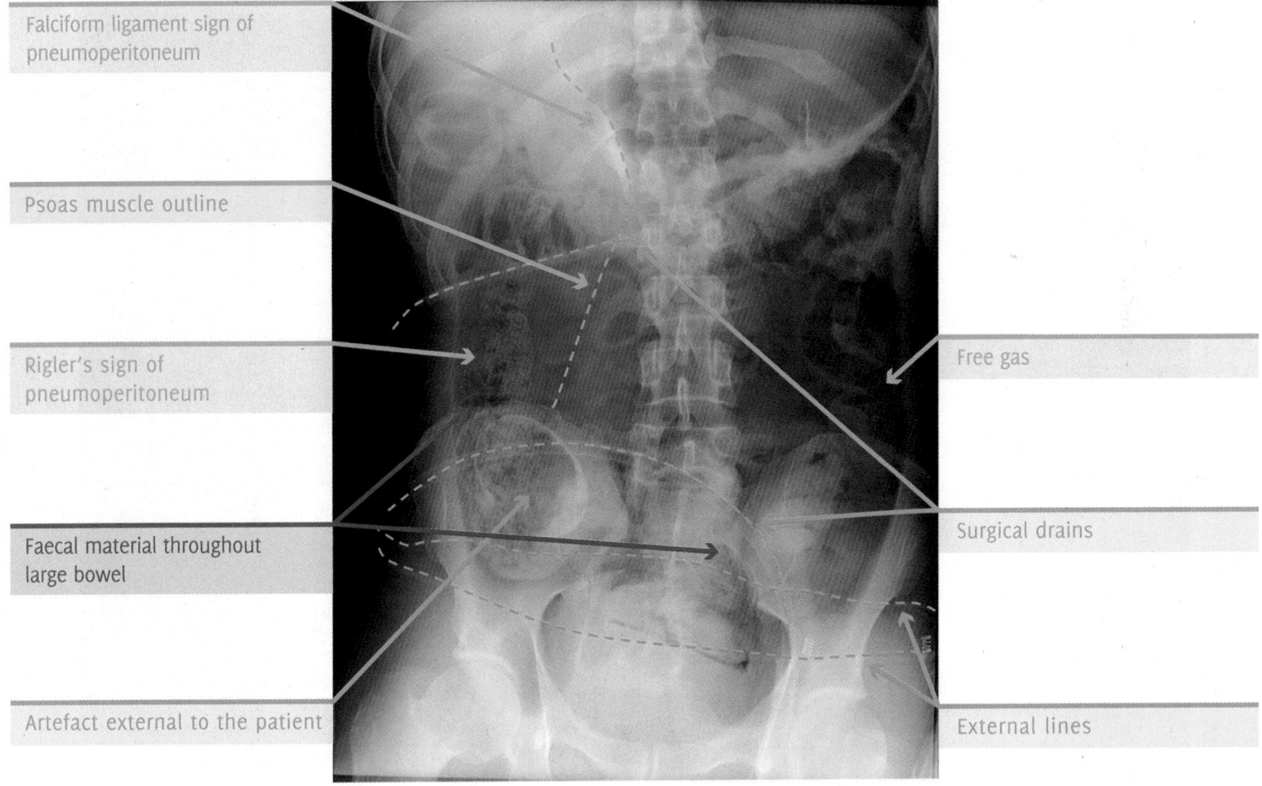

SUMMARY

This X-ray demonstrates two surgical drains in situ as described. There is evidence of pneumoperitoneum, which is likely related to the recent surgery and penetrating trauma injury.

INVESTIGATIONS AND MANAGEMENT

The patient should undergo regular review by the general surgical team. The drain outputs should be monitored and removed at the discretion of the general surgical team.

Case

93

An 18-year-old female presents to ED with abdominal distension and increasing frequency of diarrhoea and passing mucus. She has a background of ulcerative colitis and is a nonsmoker. On examination, she has oxygen saturations of 96% in room air and a temperature of 37.8°C. Her HR is 94 bpm, RR is 28 and blood pressure is 110/60 mmHg. The abdomen is soft and there is generalized tenderness with frequent normal bowel sounds. Urine dipstick is unremarkable and a pregnancy test is negative.

An abdominal X-ray is requested to assess for possible active colitis.

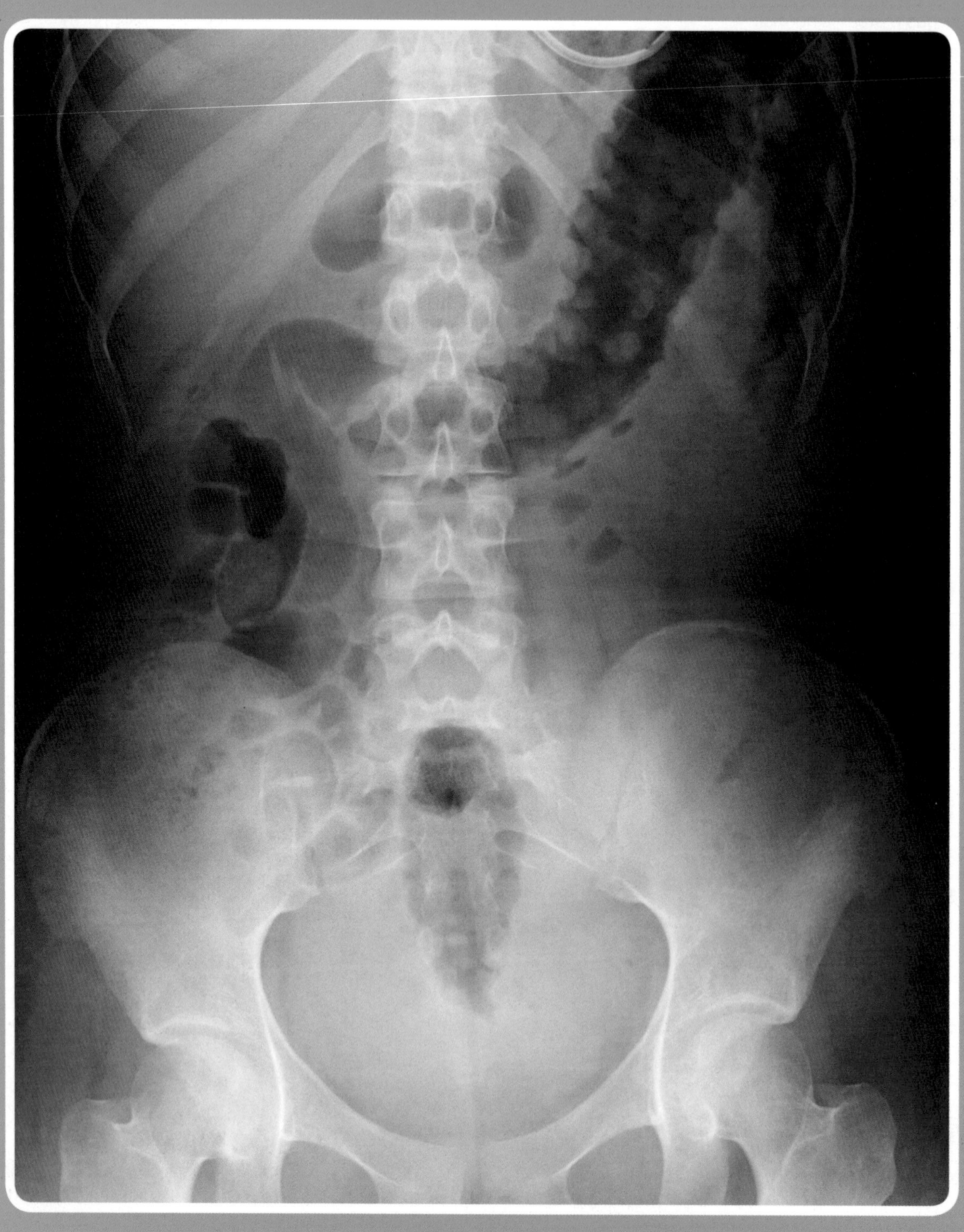

TECHNICAL INFORMATION

Patient ID: Anonymous.
Projection: AP supine.
Rotation: Adequate.
Penetration: Adequate – the spinous processes are visible.
Coverage: Inadequate – the inferior pubic rami and hemidiaphragms have not been fully included.

BOWEL GAS PATTERN

There is dilatation of the transverse colon.

BOWEL WALL

There is evidence of mural thickening of the distal transverse colon in the left upper quadrant, with evidence of 'thumbprinting', in keeping with mural oedema.

There are multiple rounded areas of hyperdensity within the distal transverse colon, which may represent inflammatory pseudopolyps.

There is no evidence of intramural gas within the large or small bowel.

PNEUMOPERITONEUM

There is no evidence of free intraabdominal gas.

SOLID ORGANS

The solid organ contours are within normal limits with no solid organ calcification.

VASCULAR

No abnormal vascular calcification.

BONES

There are no abnormalities of the imaged thoracic and lumbar spine, or within the pelvis.

SOFT TISSUES

The psoas muscle outline is visible bilaterally.

The extraabdominal soft tissues are unremarkable.

OTHER

There is a radiopaque line seen in the upper left quadrant in keeping with an NG tube. The tip is not visualized.

There are no vascular lines, drains or surgical clips.

REVIEW AREAS

Gallstones/renal calculi: No radiopaque calculi.
Lung bases: Not fully included.
Spine: Normal.
Femoral heads: Normal.

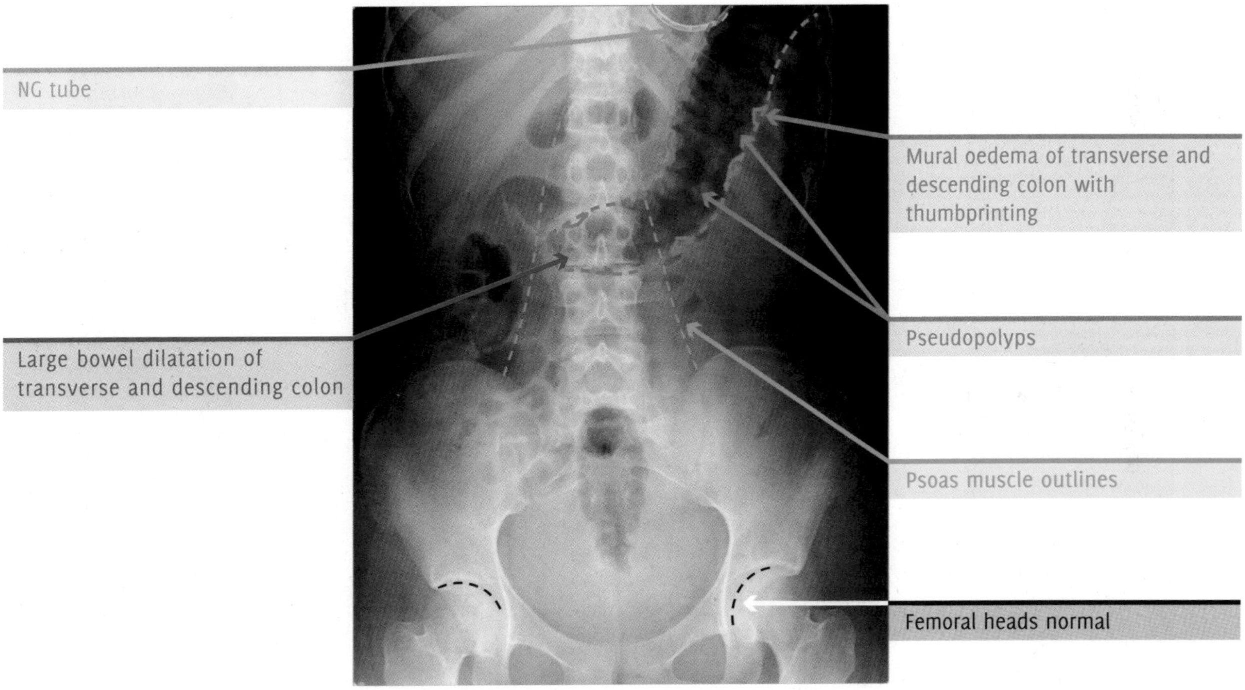

SUMMARY

This X-ray demonstrates dilatation and mural oedema of the distal transverse and proximal descending colon with evidence to suggest possible inflammatory pseudopolyposis. Given the clinical history, findings are in keeping with an acute exacerbation of ulcerative colitis.

INVESTIGATIONS AND MANAGEMENT

The patient should be resuscitated using an ABCDE approach.

Adequate analgesia and hydration should be provided.

Urgent bloods should be taken, including FBC, U&Es, LFTs, ESR, CRP, iron studies, folate, coagulation, blood gas, and group and save. A stool sample should be sent.

Urgent referral to both the general surgeons and gastroenterology team should be considered.

A CT scan of the abdomen/pelvis with IV contrast should be considered for better visualization of the anatomy and to assess for the extent of the disease.

Treatment will depend on the results of further investigations as well as the clinical state of the patient.

Case

94

A 9-month-old baby boy, born at 28 weeks' gestation, develops worsening abdominal distension and vomiting. He has a PEG-J tube in situ due to severe reflux. On examination, he has oxygen saturations of 98% in room air and a temperature of 37.9°C. His HR is 180 bpm and RR is 62. The abdomen is rigid and bowel sounds are tinkling.

An urgent abdominal X-ray is requested to assess for possible bowel obstruction.

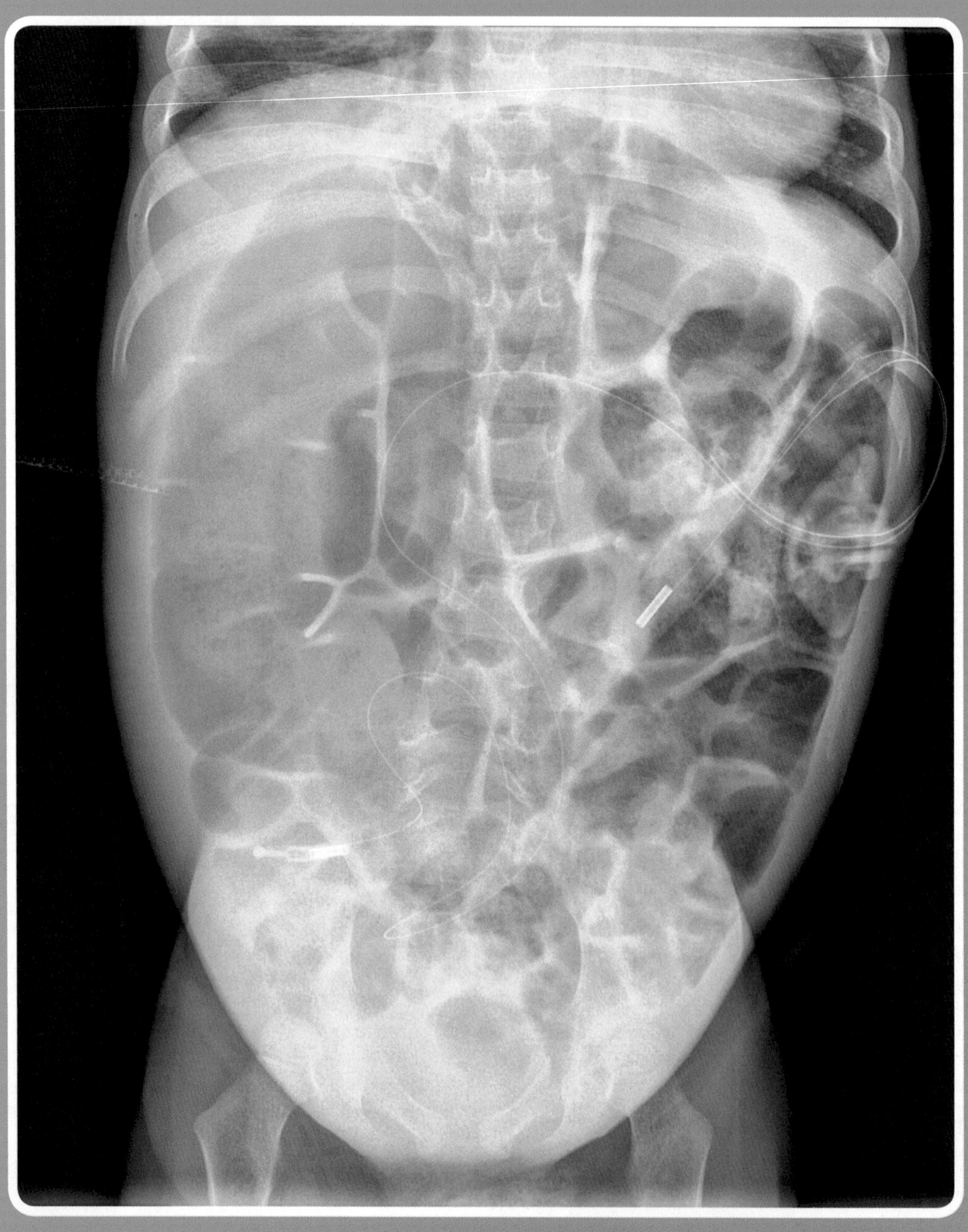

TECHNICAL INFORMATION

Patient ID: Anonymous.
Projection: AP supine.
Rotation: Adequate.
Penetration: Adequate – the spine is visible.
Coverage: Adequate – the anterior ribs are visible superiorly and the inferior pubic rami are visible.

BOWEL GAS PATTERN

There are multiple loops of dilated predominantly large bowel seen throughout the abdomen.

BOWEL WALL

There is no evidence of mural thickening or intramural gas within the large or small bowel.

PNEUMOPERITONEUM

There is no evidence of free intraabdominal gas.

SOLID ORGANS

The solid organ contours are within normal limits with no solid organ calcification.

VASCULAR

No abnormal vascular calcification.

BONES

There are no abnormalities of the imaged thoracic and lumbar spine, or within the pelvis.

SOFT TISSUES

The psoas muscle outline is not visible bilaterally, which is nonspecific, particularly in a child of this age.

The extraabdominal soft tissues are unremarkable.

OTHER

There is a radiopaque internal–external line seen coiled across the abdomen, crossing the midline, with its tip seen in the right lower quadrant in keeping with a PEG-J tube. The PEG terminates within the stomach and the PEJ in the right lower quadrant likely within the distal jejunum. This follows an abnormal contour at the region of the duodenojejunal flexure, which is likely to represent underlying malrotation.

There are no vascular lines, drains or surgical clips.

REVIEW AREAS

Gallstones/renal calculi: No radiopaque calculi.
Lung bases: Normal.
Spine: Normal.
Femoral heads: Normal – growth plates present.

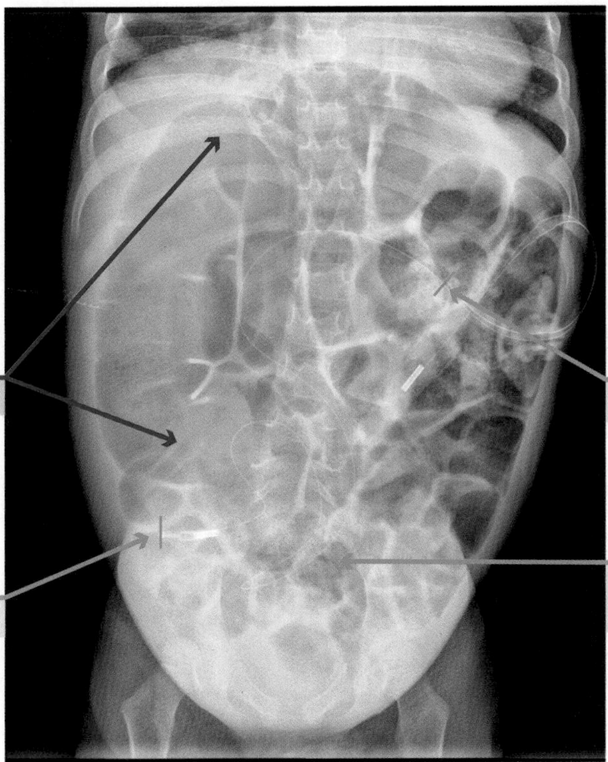

SUMMARY

This X-ray demonstrates multiple loops of dilated predominantly large bowel seen throughout the abdomen. There is a PEG-J line in situ, which follows an abnormal contour at the region of the duodenojejunal flexure, which is likely to represent underlying malrotation.

INVESTIGATIONS AND MANAGEMENT

The baby should be resuscitated using an ABCDE approach.

Adequate analgesia and hydration should be provided.

The baby should be started on broad-spectrum antibiotics, be made NBM and be started on IV fluids. The gastrostomy limb of the PEG-J should be put on free drainage.

Urgent bloods should be taken, including FBC, U&Es, CRP, bone profile, LFTs, coagulation, blood cultures, blood gas and crossmatch.

The baby should be referred urgently to the surgeons for assessment and consideration of possible surgery. A contrast study would be helpful in assessing for possible malrotation.

Case

95

An 81-year-old male presents to ED with weight loss and lethargy. He reports nausea, but has not vomited, and has significantly reduced urine output. He has no significant past medical history but complains of frequent aches and pains. He is a nonsmoker. On examination, he has oxygen saturations of 95% in air and a temperature of 36.5°C. His HR is 86 bpm, RR is 18 and blood pressure is 115/66 mmHg. The abdomen is soft and there is diffuse tenderness with normal bowel sounds. Urine dipstick is unremarkable. Early blood tests show markedly raised serum urea and creatinine, and a diagnosis of severe acute renal failure is made.

An abdominal X-ray is requested to assess for any possible bowel obstruction or abdominal lesions.

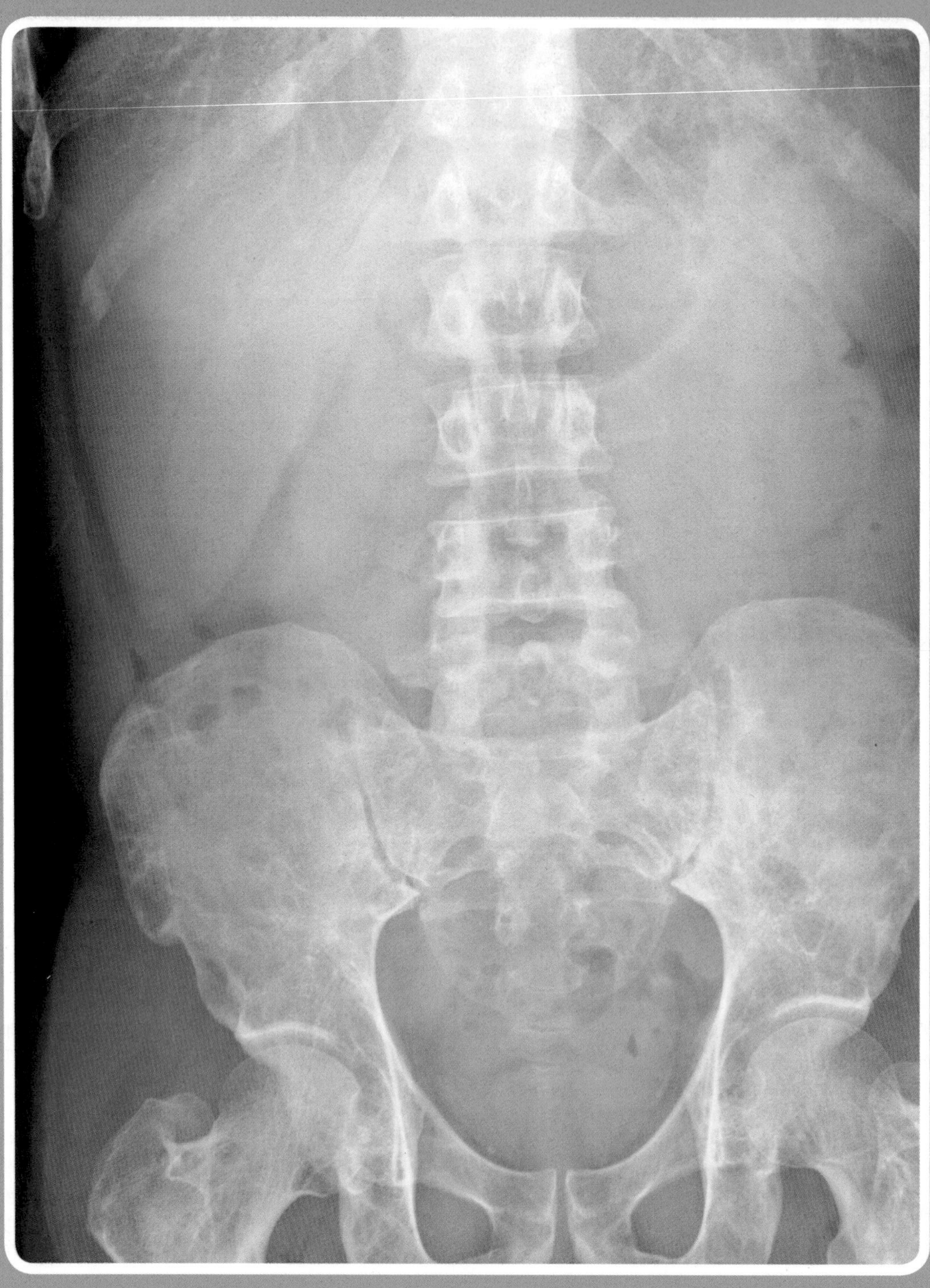

TECHNICAL INFORMATION

Patient ID: Anonymous.
Projection: AP supine.
Rotation: Adequate.
Penetration: Adequate – the spinous processes are visible.
Coverage: Adequate – the anterior ribs are visible superiorly and the inferior pubic rami are visible.

BOWEL GAS PATTERN

There is a paucity of bowel gas, which is nonspecific.

BOWEL WALL

There is no evidence of mural thickening or intramural gas within the large or small bowel.

PNEUMOPERITONEUM

There is no evidence of free intraabdominal gas.

SOLID ORGANS

The solid organ contours are within normal limits with no solid organ calcification.

VASCULAR

No abnormal vascular calcification.

BONES

There are no abnormalities of the imaged thoracic and lumbar spine.

There are multiple lytic lesions, some of which have sclerotic borders throughout the pelvis and both femoral heads. The zones of transition are narrow, they are not expansile, there is no obvious soft tissue component, and no periosteal reaction.

SOFT TISSUES

The psoas muscle outline is not visible bilaterally, which is nonspecific.

The extraabdominal soft tissues are unremarkable.

OTHER

There are no radiopaque foreign bodies.

There are no vascular lines, drains or surgical clips.

REVIEW AREAS

Gallstones/renal calculi: No radiopaque calculi.
Lung bases: Not fully included.
Spine: Normal.
Femoral heads: Multiple lytic bone lesions.

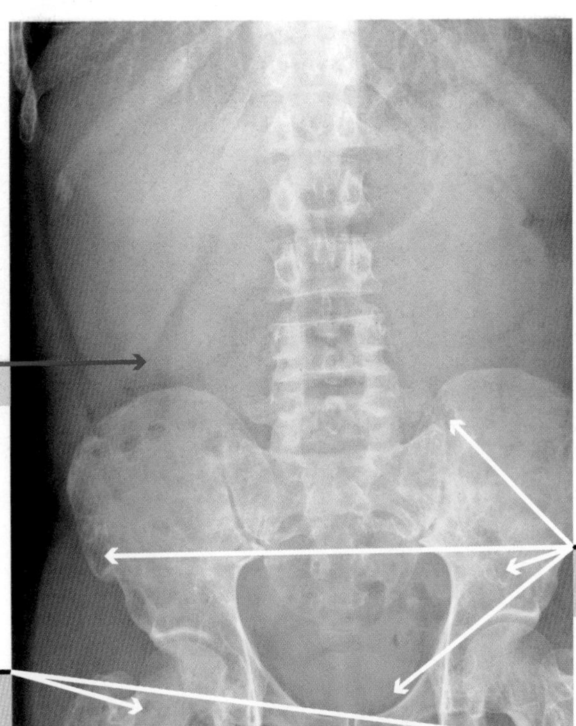

SUMMARY

This X-ray demonstrates multiple lytic bone lesions, some of which have sclerotic borders, throughout the pelvis and both femoral heads, which given the clinical history is suspicious for either metastatic deposits from an underlying primary tumour or possible multiple myeloma.

INVESTIGATIONS AND MANAGEMENT

The patient should be resuscitated using an ABCDE approach.

Adequate analgesia and hydration should be provided.

Bloods should be taken, including FBC, repeat U&Es, CRP, LFTs, bone profile, blood gas and tumour markers.

A staging CT scan of the chest, abdomen and pelvis with IV contrast should be considered, once the acute renal failure has resolved, to identify any underlying malignancy.

Serum or urine electrophoresis should be performed to assess the presence of immunoglobulin light chains, as a diagnostic test for myeloma.

The patient should be referred to oncology services for further management, which may include biopsy and MDT discussion. Treatment, which may include surgery, radiotherapy, chemotherapy or palliative treatment, will depend on the outcome of the MDT investigations and the patient's wishes.

Case 96

A 60-year-old female presents to ED following a collapse at home. Her past medical history is significant for advanced nasopharyngeal cancer and she is an ex-smoker. A radiologically inserted gastrostomy tube was recently inserted for long-term nutrition administration. On examination, she has oxygen saturations of 97% in room air and a temperature of 39°C. Her HR is 102 bpm, RR is 17 and blood pressure is 110/60 mmHg. The abdomen is rigid and there is widespread tenderness. Urine dipstick is unremarkable.

An abdominal X-ray is requested to assess for possible obstruction.

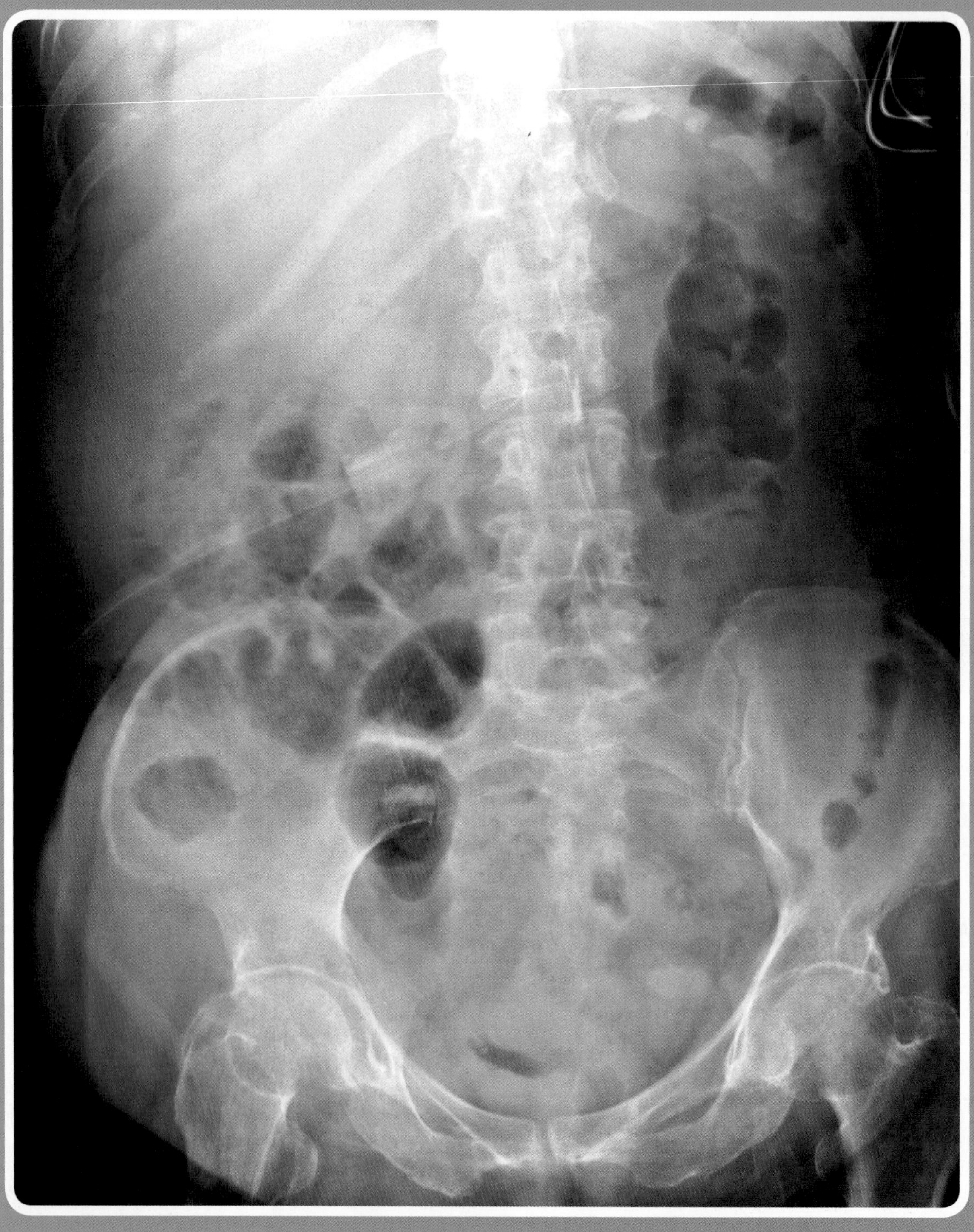

TECHNICAL INFORMATION

Patient ID: Anonymous.
Projection: AP supine.
Rotation: Adequate.
Penetration: Adequate – the spinous processes are visible.
Coverage: Adequate – the anterior ribs are visible superiorly and the inferior pubic rami are visible.

BOWEL GAS PATTERN

The bowel gas pattern is normal.

BOWEL WALL

There is mural thickening of the descending colon.

PNEUMOPERITONEUM

There is no evidence of free intraabdominal gas.

SOLID ORGANS

The solid organ contours are within normal limits with no solid organ calcification.

VASCULAR

There is linear serpiginous calcification projecting over the left upper quadrant in keeping with splenic artery calcification.

BONES

There is mild lumbar scoliosis seen convex to the left, centred on the L3 vertebral body.

There is severe bilateral degenerative change in the hip joints.

SOFT TISSUES

The psoas muscle outline is visible bilaterally.

The extraabdominal soft tissues are unremarkable.

OTHER

There is a radiopaque tube projected over the region of the central abdomen with a triangular fixation device seen to the right of the midline. This is most likely a radiologically inserted gastrostomy tube.

There are no vascular lines, drains or surgical clips.

REVIEW AREAS

Gallstones/renal calculi: No radiopaque calculi.
Lung bases: Normal.
Spine: Lumbar scoliosis seen convex to the left, centred on the L3 vertebral body.
Femoral heads: Both femoral heads flattened, particularly the right femoral head suggestive of previous avascular necrosis. Right femoral neck is shortened, in keeping with an old right neck of femur fracture.

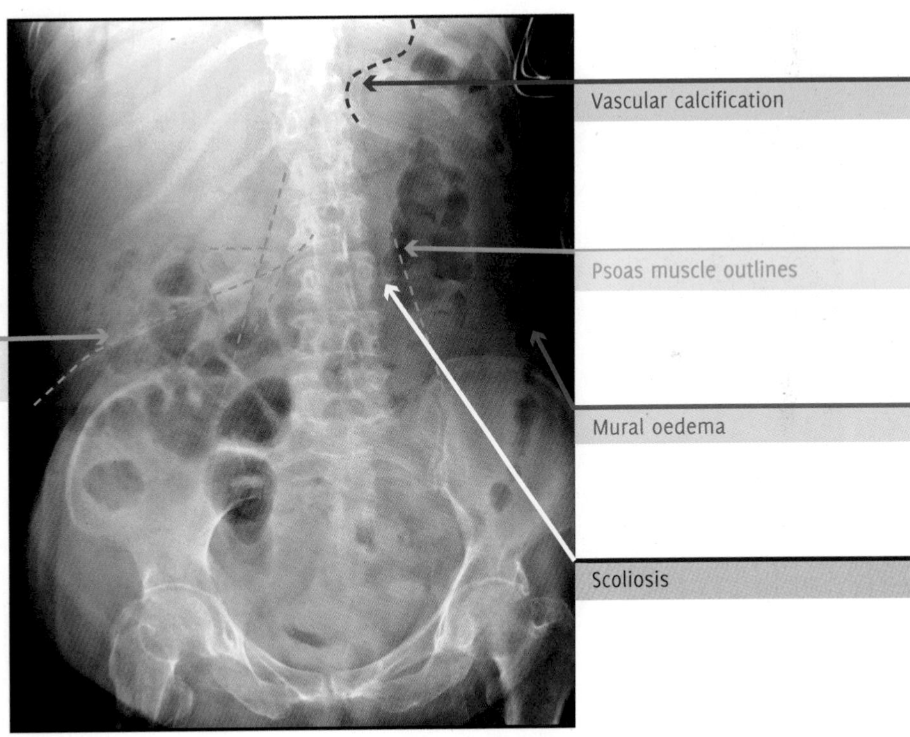

SUMMARY

This X-ray demonstrates an appropriately positioned RIG. There is no evidence of pneumoperitoneum. There is some mural oedema, which is nonspecific, but may be related to the collapsed descending colon. It also demonstrates severe degenerative changes of the hip joints bilaterally.

INVESTIGATIONS AND MANAGEMENT

The patient should be resuscitated using an ABCDE approach.

Adequate analgesia and hydration should be provided.

Urgent bloods should be taken, including FBC, U&Es, LFTs, bone profile, CRP, coagulation, blood culture, blood gas, blood cultures, and group and save.

Broad-spectrum antibiotics should be prescribed, the patient should be made NBM and started on IV fluids.

A CT scan of the abdomen/pelvis with IV contrast may be considered for further evaluation of the abdomen and surgical input should be sought.

Case

97

A non-binary 40-year-old presents to ED with worsening abdominal pain and 19 episodes of diarrhoea and passing mucus in the past 36 hours. They have no significant past medical history and are a nonsmoker. On examination, they have oxygen saturations of 96% in room air and a temperature of 39.1°C. Their HR is 103 bpm, RR is 23 and blood pressure is 140/80 mmHg. The abdomen is tender in the left upper quadrant with normal bowel sounds. Urine dipstick is unremarkable.

An abdominal X-ray is requested to assess for possible obstruction.

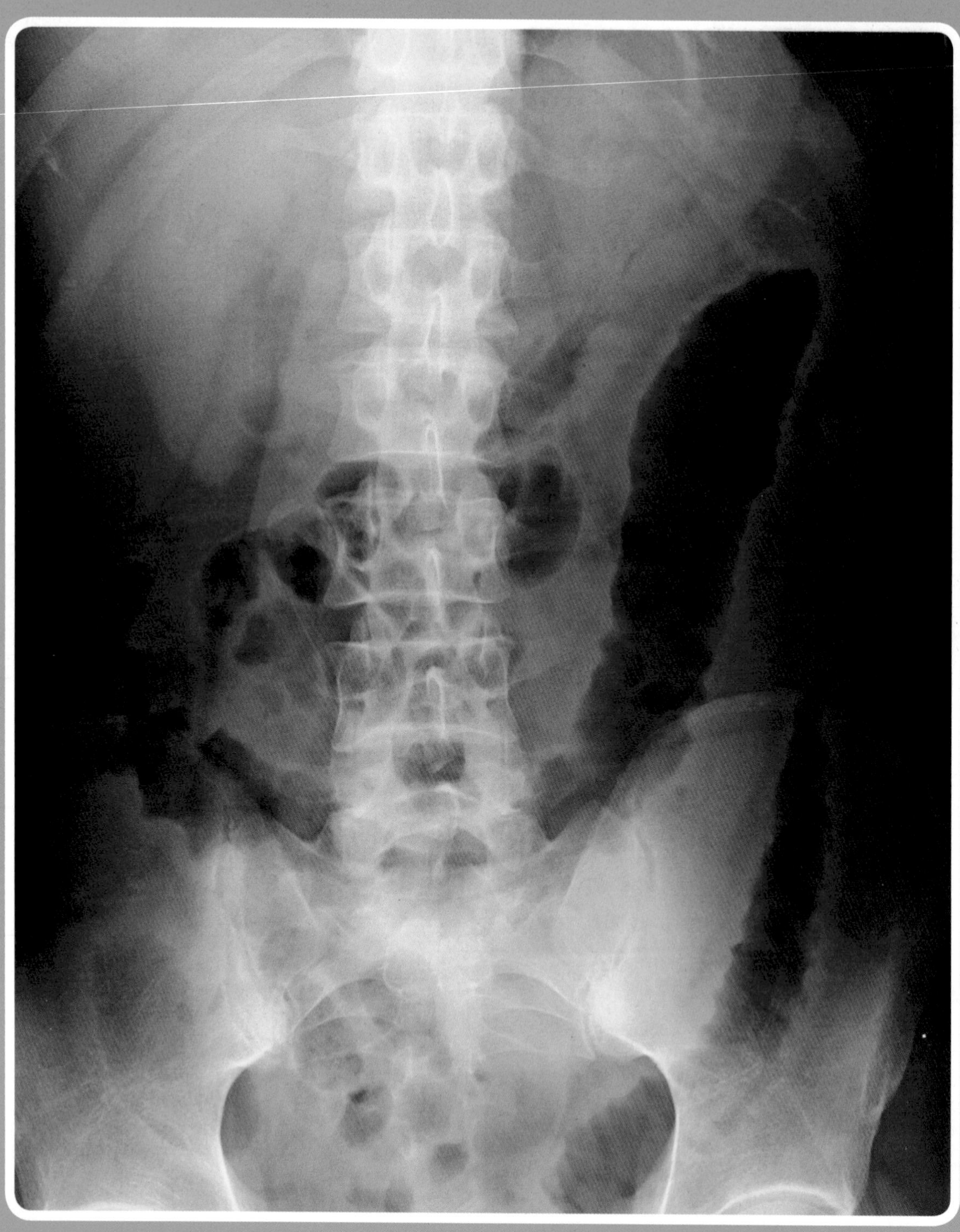

TECHNICAL INFORMATION

Patient ID: Anonymous.
Projection: AP supine.
Rotation: Adequate.
Penetration: Adequate – the spinous processes are visible.
Coverage: Inadequate – the pubic symphysis, inferior pubic rami, hip joints and hemidiaphragms have not been fully included.

BOWEL GAS PATTERN

The bowel gas pattern is normal.

BOWEL WALL

There is evidence of mural thickening of the transverse and descending colon in the left upper and lower quadrants, with loss of the normal colonic haustral folds and evidence of 'thumbprinting', in keeping with mural oedema.

There is no evidence of intramural gas within the large or small bowel.

PNEUMOPERITONEUM

There is no evidence of free intraabdominal gas.

SOLID ORGANS

The solid organ contours are within normal limits with no solid organ calcification.

VASCULAR

No abnormal vascular calcification.

BONES

There are no abnormalities of the imaged thoracic and lumbar spine, or within the pelvis.

SOFT TISSUES

The psoas muscle outline is visible bilaterally.

The extraabdominal soft tissues are unremarkable.

OTHER

There are no radiopaque foreign bodies.

There are no vascular lines, drains or surgical clips.

REVIEW AREAS

Gallstones/renal calculi: No radiopaque calculi.
Lung bases: Not fully included.
Spine: Normal.
Femoral heads: Not visualized.

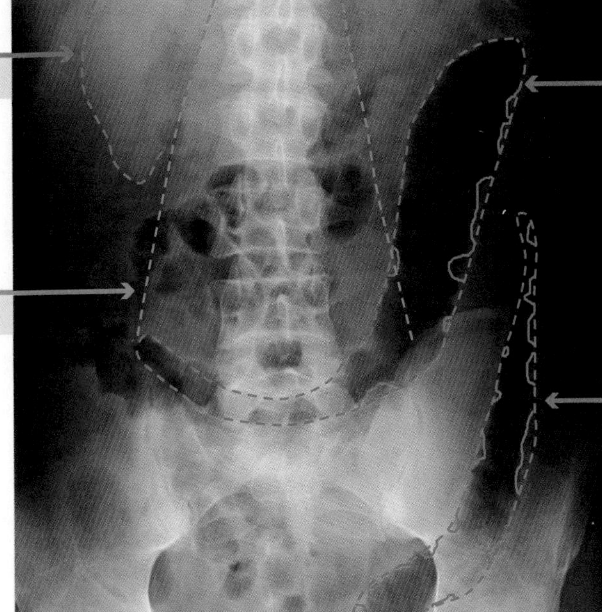

SUMMARY

This X-ray demonstrates mural oedema of the transverse and descending colon, with loss of the normal colonic haustral folds and evidence of 'thumbprinting' in keeping with colitis. Given the clinical history, this is most likely infective or inflammatory in nature.

INVESTIGATIONS AND MANAGEMENT

This patient should be resuscitated using an ABCDE approach.

Adequate analgesia and hydration should be provided.

Urgent bloods should be taken, including FBC, U&Es, LFTs, ESR, CRP, iron studies, folate, blood gas, and group and save. A stool sample should be sent.

Urgent referral to the gastroenterology team should be considered.

A CT scan of the abdomen/pelvis with IV contrast should be considered for better visualization of the anatomy and to assess for complications such as pneumoperitoneum and abscess formation.

Treatment will depend on the results of further investigations as well as the clinical state of the patient.

Case

98

A 10-day-old baby girl, born at 28 weeks' gestation, currently admitted to NICU develops severe abdominal distension and vomiting. She had bowel surgery on day 5 of life for Hirschsprung disease. On examination, she has oxygen saturations of 98% in room air and a temperature of 36.9°C. Her HR is 170 bpm and RR is 60. The abdomen is grossly distended and bowel sounds are absent.

An urgent abdominal X-ray is requested to assess for possible perforation.

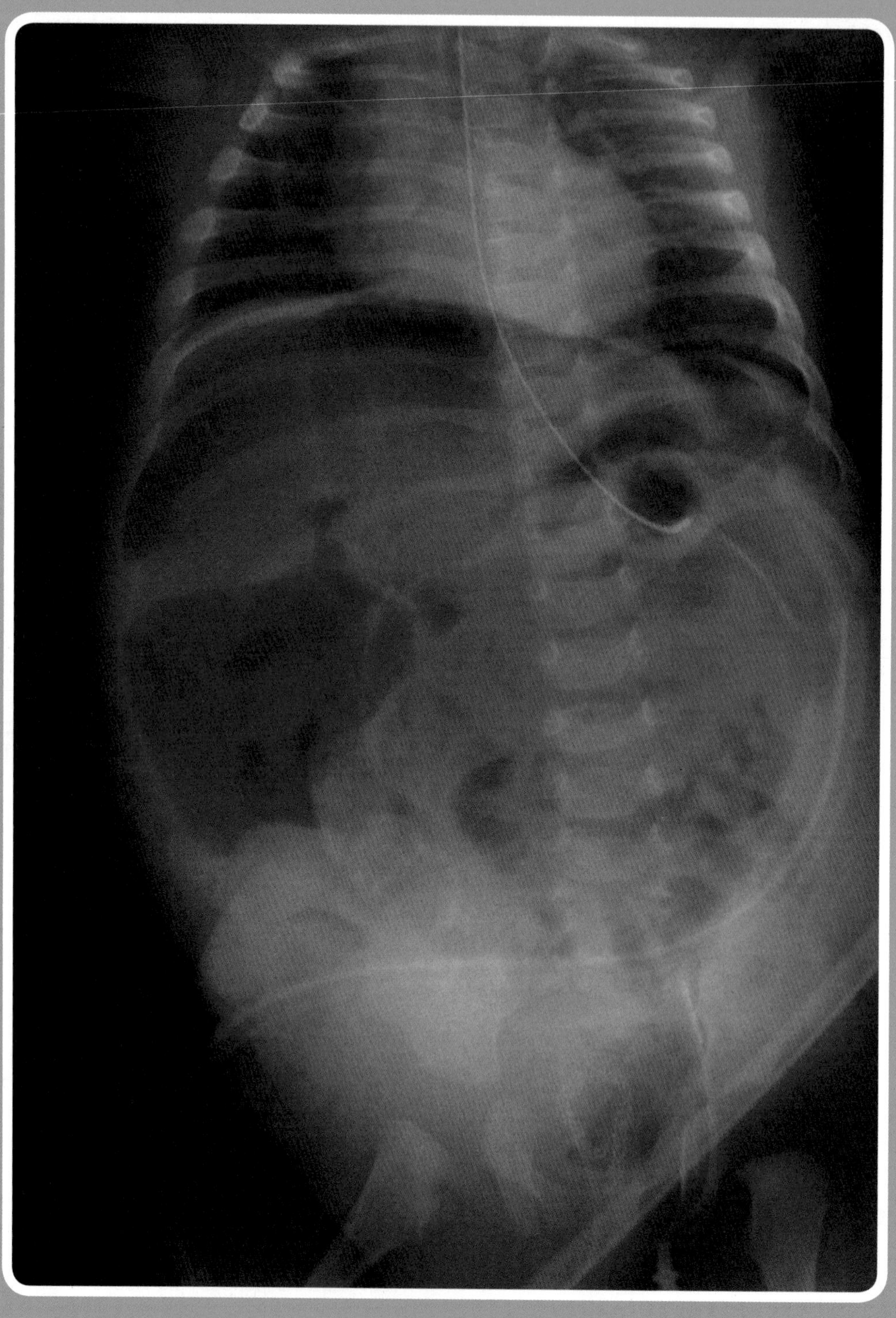

TECHNICAL INFORMATION

Patient ID: Anonymous.
Projection: AP supine.
Rotation: Asymmetrical pelvis and obturator foramina due to patient rotation to the right.
Penetration: Adequate – the spine is visible.
Coverage: Adequate – the anterior ribs are visible superiorly and the inferior pubic rami are visible.

BOWEL GAS PATTERN

The bowel gas pattern is normal.

BOWEL WALL

There is no evidence of mural thickening or intramural gas within the large or small bowel.

PNEUMOPERITONEUM

There is evidence of free intraabdominal gas, in keeping with pneumoperitoneum.

There is subdiaphragmatic free gas.

Rigler's sign (double-wall sign) can be seen, in keeping with air present on both the luminal and peritoneal sides of the bowel wall.

The falciform ligament sign can be seen, in keeping with air present within the abdomen outlining the falciform ligament of the liver.

The football sign can be seen, in keeping with a large amount of air present within the abdomen outlining the entire abdominal cavity.

The lucent liver sign can be seen, in keeping with a large amount of air present anterior to the liver.

SOLID ORGANS

The liver is outlined by free gas.

VASCULAR

No abnormal vascular calcification.

BONES

The spine is deviated to the left, which is due to patient rotation towards the right.

There are growth plates at the femoral head and acetabulum (triradiate cartilage) as the ossification centres have not yet fused, which is a normal finding in a child of this age.

There is cartilage seen between vertebrae, which is a normal finding in a child of this age.

SOFT TISSUES

The psoas muscle outline is not visible bilaterally, which is nonspecific, particularly in a child of this age.

Extraabdominal soft tissues are unremarkable.

OTHER

There is an NG tube in situ, with its tip appropriately projected over the stomach in the left upper quadrant.

There is a radiopaque line projecting across the abdomen with the tip in the left upper quadrant, likely to represent an abdominal drain.

There is a radiopaque line seen projected over the region of the left hemipelvis in keeping with a femoral venous catheter, with the tip appropriately sited in at the level of the inferior vena cava.

There are radiopaque surgical sutures seen within the rectum, in keeping with previous bowel surgery for Hirschsprung disease.

REVIEW AREAS

Gallstones/renal calculi: No radiopaque calculi.
Lung bases: Normal.
Spine: Deviated to the left due to patient rotation. There is cartilage between the vertebrae and the sacrum is not yet fused which is a normal finding in a child of this age.
Femoral heads: Normal – growth plates present.

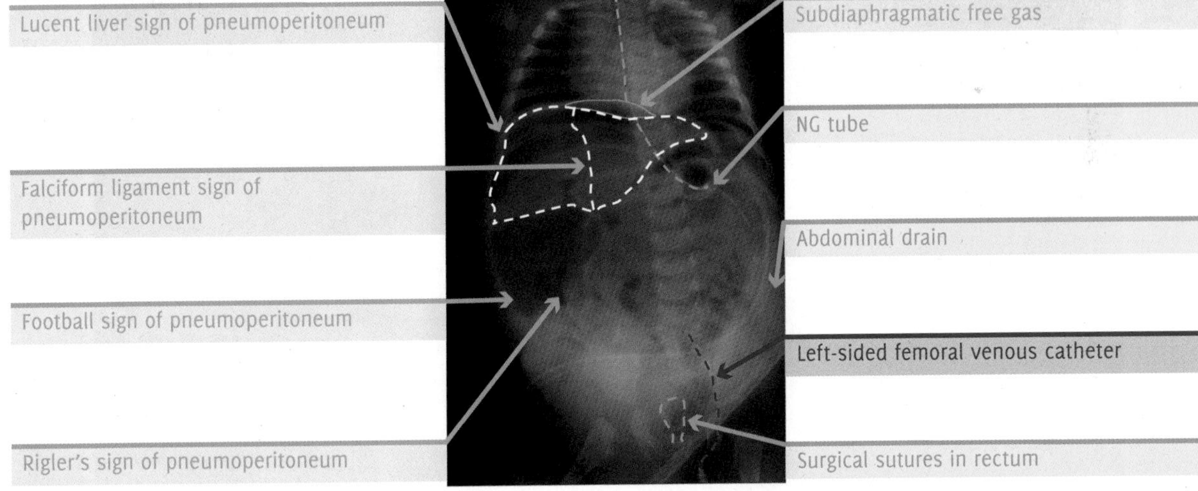

SUMMARY

This abdominal X-ray demonstrates extensive pneumoperitoneum. This may be out of proportion to expected postsurgical appearances suggesting possible bowel perforation. The NG tube, abdominal drain, femoral venous catheter and surgical sutures are incidental findings.

INVESTIGATIONS AND MANAGEMENT

The patient should be resuscitated using an ABCDE approach.

Adequate analgesia and hydration should be provided.

The baby should be started on broad-spectrum IV antibiotics, made NBM and started on IV fluids.

Intubation should be considered in view of possible perforation and severity of illness.

Urgent bloods should be taken, including FBC, U&Es, CRP, bone profile, LFTs, coagulation, blood cultures, blood gas and crossmatch.

The patient should be referred urgently to the neonatal surgeons for assessment.

Case

99

A 16-year-old female attends the gastroenterology outpatient clinic for an assessment of her bowel motility. Her past medical history is significant for chronic constipation and she is a nonsmoker. On examination, she has oxygen saturations of 98% in room air and a temperature of 37.1°C. Her HR is 75 bpm, RR is 16 and blood pressure is 110/65 mmHg. The abdomen is soft and there is no tenderness with normal bowel sounds. Urine dipstick is unremarkable and a pregnancy test is negative. A patency capsule is given, but it has not as yet passed.

An abdominal X-ray is requested to assess for the position of the patency capsule.

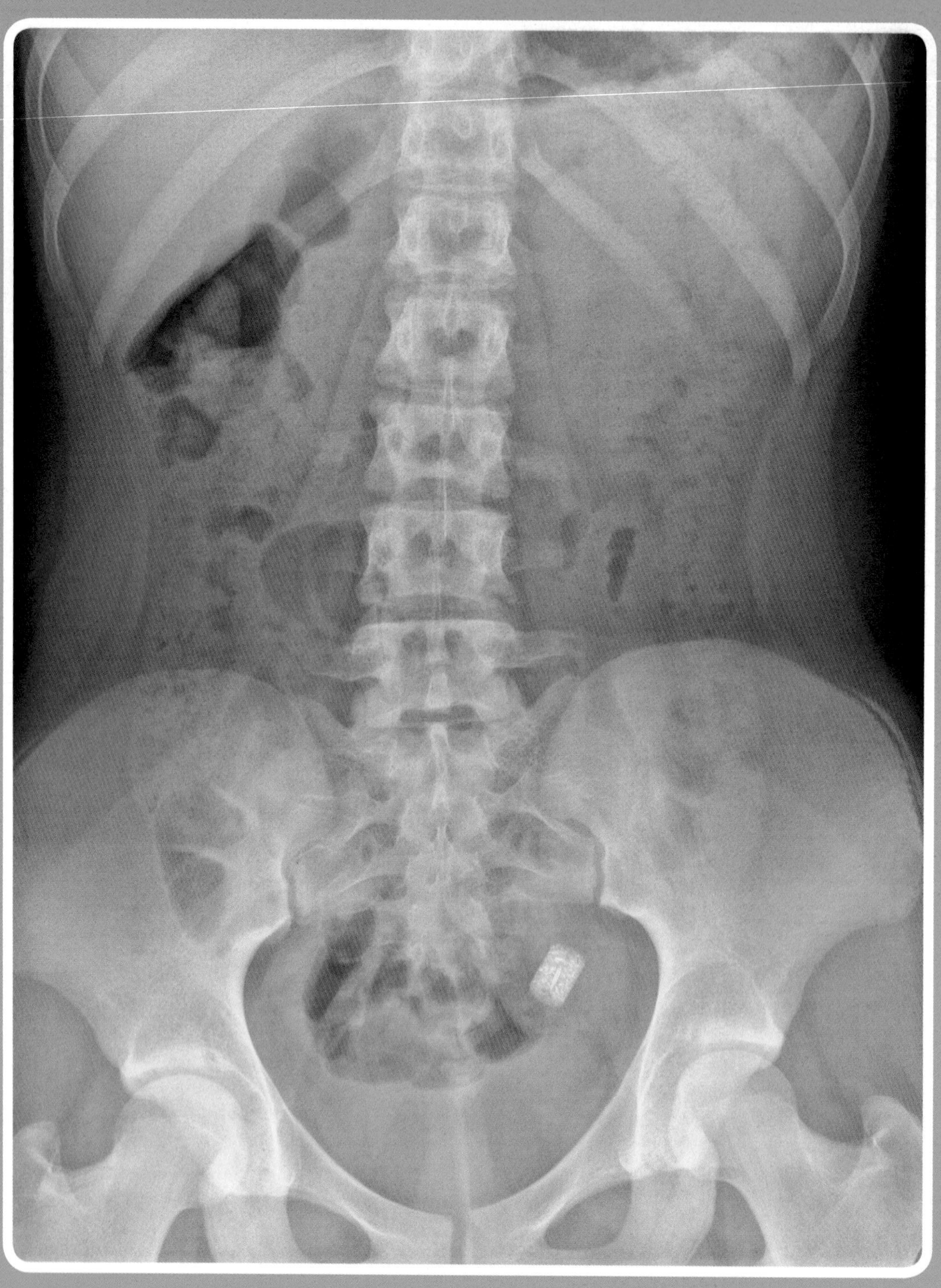

TECHNICAL INFORMATION

Patient ID: Anonymous.
Projection: AP supine.
Rotation: Adequate.
Penetration: Adequate – the spinous processes are visible.
Coverage: Inadequate – the inferior pubic rami have not been included.

BOWEL GAS PATTERN

The bowel gas pattern is normal.

There is a small volume of faecal residue present throughout the large bowel.

BOWEL WALL

There is no evidence of mural thickening or intramural gas within the large or small bowel.

PNEUMOPERITONEUM

There is no evidence of free intraabdominal gas.

SOLID ORGANS

The solid organ contours are within normal limits with no solid organ calcification.

VASCULAR

No abnormal vascular calcification.

BONES

There are no abnormalities of the imaged thoracic and lumbar spine, or within the pelvis.

An epiphyseal line can be seen at the femoral head where growth plate fusion has occurred. The iliac crests apophyses are visible bilaterally. These are normal findings in an adolescent of this age.

SOFT TISSUES

The psoas muscle outline is visible bilaterally.

The extraabdominal soft tissues are unremarkable.

OTHER

There is a cylindrical radiopaque object projected over the region of the left hemipelvis in keeping with the patency capsule, likely within pelvic small bowel or the sigmoid colon.

There are no vascular lines, drains or surgical clips.

REVIEW AREAS

Gallstones/renal calculi: No radiopaque calculi.
Lung bases: Not fully included.
Spine: Normal.
Femoral heads: Normal.

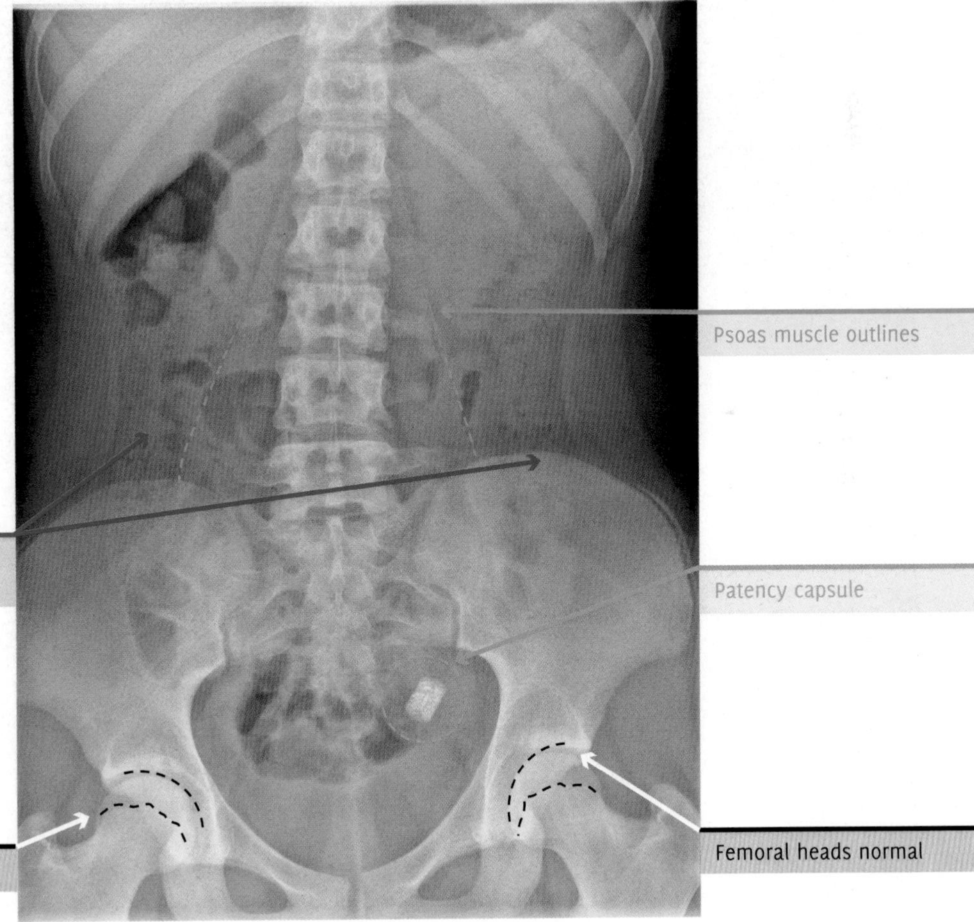

SUMMARY

This X-ray demonstrates a mild volume of faecal residue throughout the large bowel. The patency capsule is projecting over the left hemipelvis likely within pelvic small bowel or the sigmoid colon.

INVESTIGATIONS AND MANAGEMENT

The patient should be advised that the patency capsule is likely to appear within the stool and should be followed up by gastroenterology.

Case

100

A 68-year-old male presents to ED with peritonitic abdominal pain, worsening abdominal distension, nausea and bilious vomiting. He has not passed flatus or opened his bowels for over 24 hours. He has no significant past medical history and is a nonsmoker. On examination, he has oxygen saturations of 90% in room air and a temperature of 37.0°C. His HR is 110 bpm, RR is 25 and blood pressure is 125/77 mmHg. The abdomen is peritonitic and there are tinkling bowel sounds. Urine dipstick is unremarkable.

An abdominal X-ray is requested to assess for possible bowel obstruction.

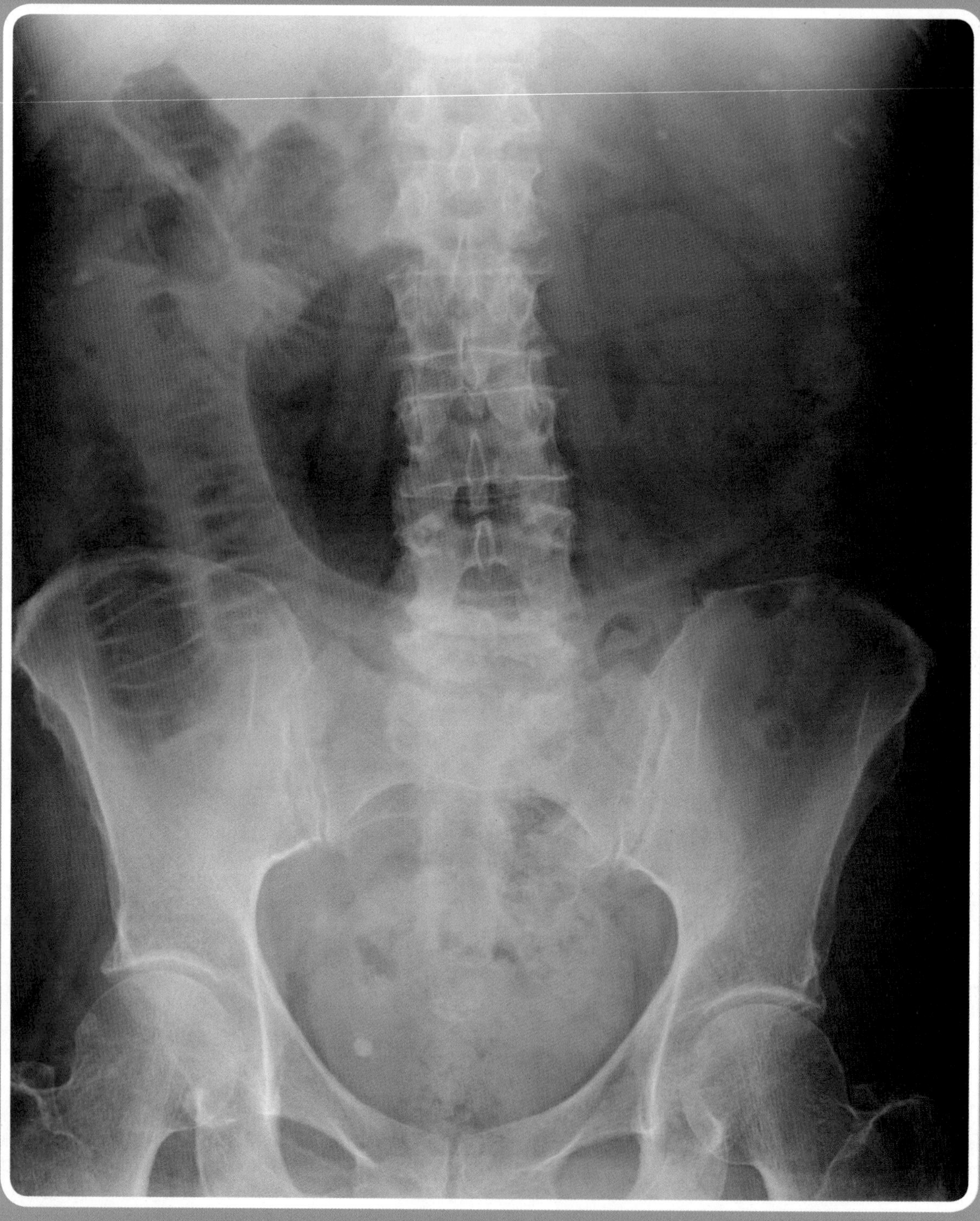

TECHNICAL INFORMATION

Patient ID: Anonymous.
Projection: AP supine.
Rotation: Adequate.
Penetration: Adequate – the spinous processes are visible.
Coverage: Adequate – the anterior ribs are visible superiorly and the inferior pubic rami are visible.

BOWEL GAS PATTERN

There is a large gas-filled loop of bowel in the left upper quadrant and epigastrium demonstrating haustra, in keeping with caecal volvulus (a normally positioned caecum in the right lower quadrant is not visible).

There are multiple loops of dilated bowel seen within the right upper quadrant and within the right paracolic gutter demonstrating valvulae conniventes in keeping with small bowel obstruction.

The location of the caecum in the left upper quadrant and small bowel in the right paracolic gutter raise the possibility of an underlying malrotation.

There is faecal material present within the distal colon and rectum.

BOWEL WALL

There is no evidence of mural thickening or intramural gas within the large or small bowel.

PNEUMOPERITONEUM

There is no evidence of free intraabdominal gas.

SOLID ORGANS

The solid organ contours are within normal limits with no solid organ calcification.

VASCULAR

No abnormal vascular calcification.

BONES

There are no abnormalities of the imaged thoracic and lumbar spine, or within the pelvis.

SOFT TISSUES

The psoas muscle outline is visible bilaterally.

The extraabdominal soft tissues are unremarkable.

OTHER

There are no radiopaque foreign bodies.

There are no vascular lines, drains or surgical clips.

There is a rounded radiopaque density projected over the region of the pelvis, most likely a phlebolith.

REVIEW AREAS

Gallstones/renal calculi: No radiopaque calculi.
Lung bases: Not fully included.
Spine: Normal.
Femoral heads: Normal.

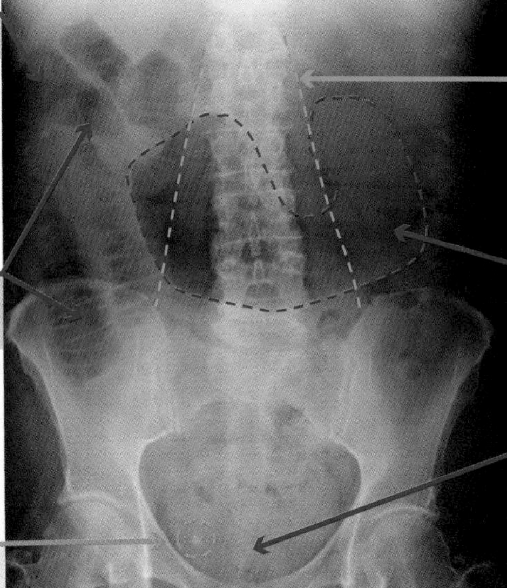

SUMMARY

This X-ray demonstrates a large gas-filled loop of bowel in the left upper quadrant and epigastrium, in keeping with caecal volvulus. There are multiple dilated small bowel loops in the right upper quadrant and right paracolic gutter in keeping with secondary small bowel obstruction. The location of the caecum in the left upper quadrant and small bowel in the right paracolic gutter raise the possibility of an underlying malrotation. The pelvic phlebolith in the pelvis is an incidental finding.

INVESTIGATIONS AND MANAGEMENT

The patient should be resuscitated using an ABCDE approach.

Adequate analgesia and hydration should be provided.

The patient should be kept NBM and an NG tube inserted on free drainage to relieve the pressure in the small bowel. IV fluids should be commenced.

Urgent bloods should be taken, including FBC, U&Es, CRP, LFTs, coagulation, blood gas, and group and save.

The general surgical team should be contacted urgently and a CT scan of the abdomen/pelvis with IV contrast should be considered for better visualization of the anatomy and further assessment. Management will be with either endoscopic decompression or surgical intervention via detorsion and caecotomy.

Case Questions and Answers

CASE 1: FAECAL RESIDUE

1. **What from the clinical history might be able to explain the aetiology of the constipation in this patient?**
Codeine is an opioid that acts on mu and delta receptors in the gut. This inhibits gastric emptying and gut peristalsis, leading to increased water absorption in the gastrointestinal tract and constipation.
2. **What clinical signs would be expected in this patient if her bowel was completely obstructed?**
Clinical signs of bowel obstruction include vomiting, particularly bilious vomiting, and a distended abdomen, without bowel motions or flatus.
3. **What diagnostic criteria can be used to assess functional constipation?**
The Rome IV criteria can be used to define functional constipation. Two criteria should have been met for at least 3 months, including fewer than three bowel movements a week and, at least 25% of the time, any of the following: lumpy or hard stool, straining, sensation of incomplete evacuation or manual manoeuvres to facilitate defecation.

CASE 2: MEDULLARY NEPHROCALCINOSIS

1. **What causes renal calculi?**
Urolithiasis (renal calculi) occur when solutes crystallize out of urine.
2. **What are the types of renal calculi?**
Renal stones can form from various solutes and each type has different risk factors. Types of calculi and their predisposing factors include calcium oxalate/phosphate (hyperparathyroidism, hyperoxaluria, hypomagnesaemia, hypocitraturia), struvite stones (Gram-negative urease positive organisms – pseudomonas, proteus, klebsiella), uric acid (high intake of purine foods (fish, legumes, meat) or gout) and cystine stones (cystinuria).
3. **What are the limitations of using an abdominal X-ray for the investigation of possible renal stones?**
Certain stones, such as uric acid, medication-induced (e.g. indinavir) and pure matrix stones, are radiolucent. A CT KUB is a more sensitive modality for detecting renal stones.

CASE 3: INFERIOR VENA CAVA FILTER

1. **What are the indications for an IVC filter?**
IVC filters are used to prevent PE in the setting of an absolute contraindication to anticoagulation, failure of anticoagulation or progression of a DVT despite anticoagulation.
2. **How is the filter placed and what variation in anatomy needs to be considered during placement?**
IVC filters are inserted by interventional radiologists via the femoral vein. Duplication of the IVC occurs in 0.7% of the population, which can complicate the insertion of the IVC filter.
3. **What factors from the clinical history might be contributing to the patient's degenerative spinal changes?**
Obesity is the most likely factor, leading to mechanical overload of normal joints.

CASE 4: OSTEOARTHRITIS OF HIP JOINTS

1. **What risk factors does this patient have for avascular necrosis of his femoral heads?**
This patient has vasculopathy and associated ischaemic heart disease. Smoking may have contributed to this.
2. **What cardiac investigation would be important to conduct in this patient before any operative intervention?**
An echocardiogram to look at cardiac function would be an important preoperative assessment to inform procedural risk.
3. **What other cause of pain related to vasculopathy should be considered in this patient?**
Chronic ischaemia of the gut can lead to abdominal pain. This would particularly be suggested if there was any history of bloody stools.

CASE 5: FAECAL RESIDUE RECTUM

1. **What is the mechanism of action of an SSRI?**
SSRIs increase the concentration of serotonin in the brain by inhibiting its reuptake in presynaptic neurons.
2. **What first-line laxatives could be used in this patient?**
Osmotic laxatives, such as lactulose or macrogol, could be started to help soften the stools.
3. **What lifestyle factors in the history might be relevant in assessing the cause of the constipation?**
Assessing for triggers for her change in bowel habit would be important. Examples of triggers include changes to diet, fluid intake, exercise pattern, mood or medication.

CASE 6: SMALL BOWEL OBSTRUCTION

1. **What is the most likely cause of bowel obstruction in this patient?**
Adhesions secondary to abdominal surgery are the most likely cause of bowel obstruction in this case.
2. **What are the common sites for metastasis of endometrial cancer?**
Common sites of metastasis of endometrial cancer are local pelvic metastasis, peritoneum and lungs.

3. **What are the different ways of performing a hysterectomy?**
   Approaches include laparoscopic, open (abdominal hysterectomy), vaginal and robotic-assisted hysterectomy.

CASE 7: SPINAL CORD STIMULATOR

1. **What are the indications for a spinal cord stimulator?**
   Spinal cord stimulators are used to treat chronic pain, including back pain, postsurgical pain and neuropathic pain.
2. **How is a spinal cord stimulator inserted?**
   Electrodes are inserted into the epidural space at any level of the spine, and the implantable pulse generator is sited via another incision on the back.
3. **What are the types of idiopathic scoliosis?**
   Infantile idiopathic scoliosis develops from birth to 3 years of age. Juvenile idiopathic scoliosis develops from 4 to 9 years of age. Adolescent idiopathic scoliosis develops from 10 to 18 years of age.

CASE 8: RIGHT JJ STENT AND BLADDER CALCULUS

1. **What medical therapy can potentially be started for treating the urinary tract calculi?**
   Oral alkalinizing agents (potassium citrate) can be used in calcium stones to maintain a higher urinary pH (6.5–7) and increase urine citrate levels. The citrate binds to calcium to prevent the formation of urinary crystals.
2. **What are the surgical treatment options for treating a bladder stone?**
   Surgical options for treating bladder stones include endoscopic surgery (lasers, mechanical crushing), ultrasound and extracorporeal shockwave lithotripsy (ESWL). Occasionally, open surgery is required.
3. **How could the ureteric stent be removed, if clinically indicated?**
   If the ureteric stent has an external thread, it can be removed by pulling on the thread; either by a nurse or the patients themselves. If there is no thread, the ureteric stent is removed using a flexible cystoscope in clinic.

CASE 9: LEFT NEPHROSTOMY WITH SCLEROTIC METASTASES

1. **What are the treatment options for prostate cancer?**
   Treatment options for prostate cancer depend on the staging of the cancer. Therapies include radiotherapy, brachytherapy, radical prostatectomy, chemotherapy, cryotherapy, high-intensity focussed ultrasound and hormonal therapy.
2. **Where does prostate cancer typically metastasize to?**
   Prostate cancer usually metastasizes to the regional lymph nodes, bones and lungs.
3. **What are the indications for insertion of a nephrostomy tube?**
   Indications for nephrostomy tube insertion include for relief of urinary obstruction, urinary diversion, access for interventional procedures and diagnostic testing.

CASE 10: LEFT JJ STENT AND RENAL CALCULI

1. **What are the indications for surgical intervention for renal calculi?**
   Stones >7 mm are unlikely to pass spontaneously, therefore often require surgical intervention. Other indications for removal include ongoing pain, infection or risk of urosepsis.
2. **What is the most common type of renal stones?**
   Calcium oxalate stones are the most common types of renal stone.
3. **When is a nephrostomy indicated in the treatment of renal stones?**
   Nephrostomy tubes are inserted when a stone is causing renal obstruction (gross hydronephrosis).

CASE 11: RIGHT RENAL CALCULI AND SURGICAL CLIPS

1. **What are the chances these stones pass spontaneously?**
   As these stones appear small and <7 mm in diameter, they are likely to pass spontaneously.
2. **What is the preferred treatment modality in this scenario?**
   Allowing the stones to pass spontaneously with adequate hydration and analgesia is the optimal management.
3. **What methods for bowel anastomosis could have been used in this patient?**
   Bowel anastomosis can be created by stapling or suturing.

CASE 12: FAECAL LOADING AND RIEDEL'S LOBE

1. **What is the most reassuring feature in this abdominal X-ray, given the clinical presentation?**
   There is no evidence of bowel dilatation (which would suggest bowel obstruction) or other pathology beyond constipation.
2. **What is the most appropriate investigation if the patient had delayed passage of meconium and long-standing constipation?**
   A rectal biopsy should be considered to rule out Hirschsprung disease.
3. **What are examples of red flags in the context of constipation?**
   Examples of red flags in constipation include persistent rectal bleeding, night sweats, severe abdominal pain and significant changes in weight (loss or gain).

CASE 13: ANTEGRADE COLONIC STOMA

1. **What clue in the neonatal history might make you worry about Hirschsprung disease?**
   Delayed first passage of meconium is suggestive of Hirschsprung disease.
2. **What types of enemas can be given via an ACE?**
   Simple saline enemas can be used alone via the ACE or they can be mixed with a phosphate enema (fleet) or glycerin.

3. **What is the advantage of an ACE over a rectal enema?**
ACE allows the patients to wash out the whole colon; retrograde washouts (rectal) are unlikely to reach the ascending colon.

CASE 14: PERCUTANEOUS ENDOSCOPIC GASTROSTOMY-JEJUNOSTOMY

1. **What are the indications for a jejunostomy tube?**
The indication for jejunostomy tube insertion is post-pyloric feeding for reflux. Other indications for jejunostomy tube insertion are gastric outlet obstruction and gastroparesis.
2. **How are jejunostomy tubes changed in a child?**
Jejunostomy tube changes are done under radiological guidance by an interventional radiologist.
3. **How is the position of a jejunostomy tube confirmed?**
Contrast is injected into the jejunostomy to confirm its position in the small bowel.

CASE 15: LARGE BOWEL OBSTRUCTION

1. **What are the causes of bowel obstruction?**
Causes of bowel obstruction can be classified as intraluminal (polyp, foreign body, faecal impaction), luminal (intussusception, stricture, mass, Meckel's diverticulum) and extraluminal (mass from external structures, hernias, adhesions, volvulus).
2. **What is the treatment of bowel obstruction?**
Initial treatment is bowel rest, IV fluids and a nasogastric tube placed on free drainage. If there is no improvement with these measures and/or there is suspicion of bowel ischaemia, surgical intervention would be indicated.
3. **Which procedure is it important to consent the patient for when going to theatre for a laparotomy in the case of bowel obstruction?**
The patient should be consented for the possibility of stoma formation. The surgical treatment would depend on the cause of obstruction and extent of bowel ischaemia or necrosis, but may necessitate colostomy formation in the acute setting.

CASE 16: CHOLECYSTECTOMY CLIPS

1. **What are the different types of gallstones?**
Gallstones can either be cholesterol stones or pigment (bilirubin) stones.
2. **What are the risk factors for gallstones?**
Risk factors for gallstone formation can be remembered with the mnemonic '5Fs': fair (white Northern European), fat (BMI >30), forty (age >30 years old), female and fertile (has one or more children).
3. **Are dietary changes needed following cholecystectomy?**
Most patients do not require a special diet following cholecystectomy, although a low-fat diet before the operation may reduce symptoms while awaiting surgery.

CASE 17: SMALL BOWEL OBSTRUCTION

1. **In general, what volume of fluid bolus should be given to a child?**
A child should be given a 10 mL/kg bolus of 0.9% sodium chloride.
2. **What are the potential causes of bowel obstruction in a previously well 5-year-old child?**
Differentials include obstruction secondary to delayed presentation of appendicitis, volvulus around a congenital band (Meckel's or patent vitello-intestinal duct), intussusception or hernia (groin or internal).
3. **How would an obstructed hernia be managed?**
Reduction can be attempted with, if required, analgesia and optimal patient positioning (Trendelenburg position). A herniotomy would be required, although this can be delayed if reduction is successful.

CASE 18: BOWEL OBSTRUCTION

1. **Where is the tip of the NG tube likely to be anatomically within the stomach?**
The tip of the NG tube is likely in the antrum or pylorus.
2. **What is likely to be aspirated from the NG tube?**
As the patient is obstructed you would expect bilious fluid (green) to be aspirated.
3. **What are reassuring signs on this X-ray?**
There is air in the rectum, which implies there isn't a complete obstruction. Additionally, there are no signs of perforation.

CASE 19: FAECAL RESIDUE

1. **What are the main respiratory manifestations of cystic fibrosis?**
Most commonly, recurrent chest infections are seen in cystic fibrosis. This may lead to lung damage and bronchiectasis. Cystic fibrosis is also associated with nasal polyps and pneumothoraces.
2. **What severe cause of bowel obstruction that is associated with rectal bleeding needs to be considered in patients with cystic fibrosis?**
Patients with cystic fibrosis at risk of intussusception, which can lead to bowel obstruction and rectal bleeding.
3. **What other causes of abdominal obstruction is often seen in patients with cystic fibrosis?**
Distal intestinal obstruction syndrome, where the small intestine gets blocked by thickened faecal matter, can develop in cystic fibrosis.

CASE 20: RIGHT RENAL CALCULUS

1. **What site is the pain of kidney stones typically felt?**
Kidney stones typically result in pain radiating from the loin to the groin.
2. **What is the most common bacterial cause of pyelonephritis?**
Escherichia coli is the most common bacterial cause of pyelonephritis.

3. **What are the surgical management options for ongoing fevers and pain if the kidney is obstructed secondary to a renal calculus?**
   A nephrostomy or ureteric stent can be used to relieve urinary obstruction from renal calculi.

CASE 21: ILEOSTOMY

1. **What test could be done on the patient's stool to quantify the degree of gut inflammation?**
   Faecal calprotectin can be tested as a biomarker of gut inflammation.
2. **What part of the bowel does Crohn's disease commonly affect?**
   Crohn's commonly affects the terminal ileum and colon, although it can affect any part of the gastrointestinal tract.
3. **What investigations are primarily used to diagnose Crohn's disease?**
   Colonoscopy and upper gastrointestinal endoscopy (with biopsies) are the main investigations used in diagnosing Crohn's disease.

CASE 22: NORMAL

1. **Can an abdominal X-ray rule out significant gut pathology?**
   An abdominal X-ray is not sensitive enough to completely rule out gut pathology. A CT scan of the abdomen would provide more detailed imaging of the gut should it be clinically indicated.
2. **How might the appendix cause left iliac pain?**
   In a nonrotated gut, the appendix would be found in the left side of the abdomen, so appendicitis in such a case would produce left iliac fossa pain.
3. **In an older patient presenting with left iliac fossa pain, fever and altered bowel habit, what would be the most likely diagnosis?**
   These symptoms in an older patient would suggest diverticular disease.

CASE 23: NORMAL

1. **What might you see on the abdominal X-ray if there was perforation?**
   Signs of perforation on an abdominal X-ray include air under the diaphragm (although this is better seen on an erect chest X-ray), Rigler's sign (visualization of both sides of the bowel wall) and visualization of the falciform ligament (football sign).
2. **What is the differential diagnosis of this patient's abdominal pain?**
   The differential diagnosis includes gastrointestinal (peptic ulcer, pancreatitis, appendicitis, gastroenteritis, obstructed hernia), renal (pyelonephritis, kidney stones) and vascular (mesenteric ischaemia) causes.
3. **If no cause is determined on CT imaging, and the pain is settling, what might be a reasonable next step?**
   Discharge with appropriate analgesia. Review lifestyle factors, including dietary intake, and consider modification. If pain worsens or persists, investigate for chronic causes of abdominal pain, such as inflammatory bowel disease, peptic ulcer disease or coeliac disease.

CASE 24: INTRAUTERINE CONTRACEPTIVE DEVICE AND TAMPON

1. **How does an IUCD prevent conception?**
   There are two main types of IUCD: copper-releasing (which is primarily spermicidal) and levonorgestrel-releasing (which thickens the cervical mucous plug and thins the endometrium to prevent implantation) devices.
2. **What would be the major concern if the patient had a positive pregnancy test?**
   An ectopic pregnancy is more likely in a patient with an IUCD and would need to be further investigated, such as with ultrasound imaging.
3. **What are the treatment options for an ectopic pregnancy?**
   The management for ectopic pregnancy depends on the woman's risk of tubal rupture. Management options include expectant management with close monitoring (if low risk for rupture and asymptomatic), medical management (e.g. methotrexate) and surgical management (e.g. laparoscopic surgery with either salpingostomy or salpingectomy).

CASE 25: PERITONEAL DIALYSIS CATHETER

1. **What are the types of peritoneal dialysis?**
   Peritoneal dialysis can be CAPD or APD. CAPD takes around 30 minutes and is done manually up to four times a day. APD can be done while asleep.
2. **What potential complication of peritoneal dialysis could this patient have developed?**
   Patients on peritoneal dialysis are at risk of developing peritonitis.
3. **What are the other options for dialysis in this patient?**
   An alternative method of dialysis would be haemodialysis via a central line.

CASE 26: NORMAL PAEDIATRIC ABDOMINAL RADIOGRAPH

1. **What further investigation should be requested?**
   Given the acute illness, stool cultures should be sent for MCS and virology.
2. **What is the most common cause of gastroenteritis in a toddler?**
   Rotavirus is the commonest cause of gastroenteritis in toddlers.
3. **How should the patient be monitored?**
   The child should have regular observations and careful monitoring of fluid balance, including any vomiting and diarrhoea.

CASE 27: SMALL BOWEL OBSTRUCTION

1. **What clinical examination findings may provide clues as to the cause of the small bowel obstruction?**
   Examination may show surgical scars, which would point to possible adhesions. Examination of the hernial orifices may reveal an obstructed hernia.
2. **What is a phlebolith?**
   A phlebolith is a calcification within a vein and is particularly common in the pelvis.

3. **What is the differential diagnosis for pelvic phleboliths?**
   Pelvic phleboliths are benign and commonly encountered on imaging. However, they may be confused for urinary tract calculi, which occur in distinct anatomical positions.

CASE 28: SMALL BOWEL OBSTRUCTION

1. **What is the most likely cause of this patient's bowel obstruction?**
   Adhesions following her appendicectomy is the most likely cause of this patient's small bowel obstruction.
2. **What percentage of patients have bowel obstruction following an open appendicectomy?**
   One to two percent of patients undergoing open appendicectomy develop small bowel obstruction.
3. **How long are conservative measures usually trialled for to relieve bowel obstruction before surgical intervention is considered?**
   If the patient is stable conservative measures for bowel obstruction are usually trialled for 48 hours before considering surgical intervention.

CASE 29: SACRALIZATION OF L5

1. **Which nerve roots are involved in the sciatic nerve?**
   A combination of nerve roots from L4 to S3 combine to form the sciatic nerve.
2. **What is the most common cause of sciatica?**
   A prolapsed intervertebral disc is the commonest cause of sciatica.
3. **What is the common level of sciatic nerve impingement in the spine?**
   Lesions most often occur at segments L4 to L5 or L5 to S1.

CASE 30: INGESTED FOREIGN BODIES

1. **What anatomical landmark signifies an increased likelihood of a foreign body passing naturally?**
   Once a foreign body passes beyond the stomach, it will often pass spontaneously in the stools. Therefore most of these cases can be left to pass without intervention.
2. **What would expedite surgical intervention in this patient?**
   Clinical features that would expedite surgical interventions include presence of corrosive foreign bodies, e.g. button batteries, ongoing pain or tenderness or evidence of obstruction or perforation.
3. **What are the narrowest points of the gastrointestinal tract where foreign bodies might get stuck?**
   The oesophagus is the commonest site of foreign body impaction. It has three points of narrowing where there is a higher risk of impaction: in the proximal oesophagus (cricopharyngeus muscle), at the aortic arch and at the gastro-oesophageal junction.

CASE 31: FAECAL RESIDUE

1. **What dietary changes might help address constipation?**
   Increase intake of water alongside a high-fibre diet, with increased intake of fruit and vegetables, can help in softening the stools.
2. **What oral laxatives may be prescribed?**
   Osmotic (e.g. macrogol) or stimulant laxatives (e.g. senna) can be prescribed to help relieve constipation.
3. **What category indicates constipation on the Bristol Stool Chart?**
   Type 1 or 2 stools on the Bristol stool scale indicate constipation.

CASE 32: INGESTED MAGNETS

1. **What is the normal transit time in the gut in adults?**
   Transit time through the gastrointestinal tract ranges from 12 to 72 hours.
2. **What is the main concern regarding the ingestion of magnets?**
   Magnets can separate while in the gut, resulting in adjacent loops being caught in-between magnets and thereby leading to perforation.
3. **What is the main aspect being reviewed on serial abdominal X-rays?**
   The progression of magnets along the gastrointestinal tract should be monitored on serial X-rays. Surgical intervention may be considered if magnets remain static.

CASE 33: INGESTED FOREIGN BODY

1. **Which feature of the foreign body suggests this is a button battery?**
   The 'halo' (or double-ring) sign is the hallmark of a button battery.
2. **Where are the commonest places for button batteries to get stuck?**
   The commonest places for button batteries to impact are in the oesophagus, including the thoracic inlet, region of the aortic arch and at the gastro-oesophageal junction. If impacted, they can form local electrical circuits that can damage surrounding organs with complications that include aorto-oesophageal and trachea-oesophageal fistulation.
3. **What is the optimal management plan for this patient?**
   As the button battery has left the stomach, it is likely to be passed in the stool and does not require surgical intervention. A repeat X-ray in 7 to 14 days to ensure passage is sufficient should be requested, with the child returning if there are any concerns in the meantime.

CASE 34: MULTIPLE FRACTURES WITH VASCULAR CALCIFICATION

1. **What are the commonest causes of pelvic fractures?**
   The commonest causes of pelvic fractures are high-impact trauma such as motor vehicle accidents, falls and sports injuries.
2. **What are the most worrying injuries that might be associated with a pelvic fracture?**
   Pelvic fractures can be complicated by pelvic haemorrhage, which can be severe, and rupture of the bladder or urethra.
3. **What arteries might be injured in a pelvic fracture?**
   The external iliac, obturator and internal iliac arteries are the most commonly injured arteries in pelvic fracture.

CASE 35: DRUG MULE

1. **What symptoms does cocaine produce?**
   Cocaine has sympathomimetic effects, causing tachycardia, agitation, sweating and dilated pupils. Hypertension and hyperthermia can result from high doses.
2. **What is the best possible clinical outcome a patient who has smuggled drugs in this manner?**
   The best possible outcome is spontaneously passing the drugs without rupture of the drug capsules.
3. **If needed, how would the drug capsules be surgically removed?**
   The surgical approach would be a laparotomy with enterotomies (incisions into intestine) to remove the foreign bodies.

CASE 36: COLITIS

1. **What are the causes of a 'lead pipe' colon?**
   A 'lead pipe' colon is classically caused by ulcerative colitis, signifying loss of the colonic haustra.
2. **What other sign on an abdominal X-ray is seen in the diagnosis of colitis?**
   Other signs of colitis include mural thickening and, in more severe cases, thumbprinting (where the normal haustra become thickened). Severe cases may show dilatation of the bowel, with toxic megacolon being particularly worrisome.
3. **What pathogens cause infective colitis?**
   Common bacterial causes of infective colitis include *Campylobacter jejuni*, *Shigella*, *E. coli*, *Salmonella* and *Clostridium difficile*.

CASE 37: ENDOVASCULAR ILIAC BRANCH AORTIC STENT WITH RENAL STENTS

1. **Which vessel provides access for endovascular aortic stents?**
   Interventional radiologists insert endovascular aortic stents via the femoral artery.
2. **What are the major complications of endovascular stent insertion?**
   Major complications of endovascular stents include endoleaks (blood flow outside the graft within the aneurysm sac), stent migration, stent occlusion, ischaemia (limb, renal, bowel, spinal cord), cerebrovascular accidents and graft infection.
3. **What is the indication for elective surgery on an AAA?**
   Elective surgery should be considered with symptomatic AAAs, asymptomatic AAAs with a diameter ≥5.5 cm, and asymptomatic AAAs with a diameter ≥4 cm and rapid expansion (grown >1 cm in 1 year).

CASE 38: SPLENOMEGALY AND BONE LESIONS

1. **What are the most common myeloproliferative disorders in this age group?**
   The most common myeloproliferative disorders are chronic myeloid leukaemia, polycythaemia vera, essential thrombocythaemia and primary myelofibrosis.
2. **What does a mottled bone appearance indicate?**
   Destructive bony lesions produce a mottled bone appearance on imaging.
3. **Why is the spleen enlarged?**
   Spleen enlargement is directly linked to splenic extramedullary haematopoiesis.

CASE 39: PSOAS ABSCESS AND SCOLIOSIS

1. **What are the three most likely bacterial causes of a psoas abscess?**
   Staphylococcus aureus, *E. coli* and *Streptococcus* are the commonest causes of a psoas abscess.
2. **How is a large psoas abscess typically treated?**
   Alongside drainage, a prolonged course (approximately 6 weeks) of broad-spectrum antibiotics is required to treat a psoas abscess.
3. **What advice would you give regarding the scoliosis?**
   Surgical intervention of scoliosis is very rarely required in adults. If back pain is an issue, regular analgesia and exercise should be encouraged to strengthen and stretch the back.

CASE 40: PELVIC MASSES

1. **What genetic association is important to know about in ovarian cancer?**
   Women with BRCA1 (40%–60% lifetime risk) and BRCA2 (10%–30% lifetime risk) gene mutations have an increased risk of developing ovarian cancers.
2. **What are the primary sites of metastasis in ovarian cancer?**
   Ovarian cancer can locally spread to the pelvis, abdominal cavity, lymph nodes, lungs and the liver.
3. **What tumour marker is commonly associated with ovarian cancer?**
   Ovarian cancer is associated with increased CA-125 serum levels.

CASE 41: APPENDICOLITH

1. **What clinical signs are associated with acute appendicitis?**
   Other than right iliac fossa tenderness, other signs of acute appendicitis include Rovsing's sign (right lower quadrant pain after palpating left lower quadrant), obturator sign (right lower quadrant pain with flexion and internal rotation of right hip) and psoas sign (right lower quadrant pain with the patient in left decubitus position and right leg extended).
2. **What is the most common age of presentation for appendicitis?**
   Appendicitis most commonly occurs in 10- to 19-year-olds.
3. **What key features help differentiate appendicitis from mesenteric adenitis?**
   Mesenteric adenitis is more likely to be associated with cervical lymphadenopathy and a preceding viral infection. Appendicitis is more likely to present with vomiting, elevated inflammatory markers, severe abdominal pain and tachycardia.

CASE 42: PNEUMOPERITONEUM

1. **What name is given to the clinical sign where gas is seen outlining both sides of the bowel wall on an abdominal X-ray?**
   This is known as Rigler's sign.
2. **Which part of the bowel does spontaneous intestinal perforation typically affect in a neonate?**
   The terminal ileum is the most frequently affected area in spontaneous intestinal perforation.
3. **What are the two main surgical management options in necrotizing enterocolitis?**
   Peritoneal drain which can be placed at the bedside or laparotomy.

CASE 43: SPINA BIFIDA OCCULTA

1. **What are the different types of spina bifida?**
   The three most common types of spina bifida are spina bifida occulta (isolated posterior body fusion defect), meningocele (protrusion of the meninges through the skull, the posterior arches of the vertebra or the sacrum) and myelomeningocele (protrusion of the spine and spinal cord through the vertebra).
2. **What antenatal intervention is helpful in preventing spina bifida?**
   Maternal folic acid supplementation reduces the risk of neural tube defects.
3. **Why is it important for urologists to be involved in myelomeningocele cases?**
   Children with myelomeningoceles have a neurogenic bladder, increasing the risk of developing urinary tract infections and renal failure because of bladder dysfunction. The risk of these complications can be reduced with intermittent catheterization.

CASE 44: ENDOVASCULAR ILIAC BRANCH AORTIC STENT

1. **What early complications could occur following EVAR?**
   EVAR insertion can be complicated by renal, bowel, spinal and leg ischaemia, as well as contrast-induced nephropathy. Femoral access can be complicated by pseudoaneurysm, haematoma and distal embolism.
2. **When is the main contraindication for EVAR?**
   The main contraindications to EVAR relate to unsuitable anatomy (e.g. tortuous aorta, small iliac arteries).
3. **What is the difference between a true aneurysm and a pseudoaneurysm?**
   In a true aneurysm, all three layers of the arterial wall are dilated. Pseudoaneurysms form when blood collects outside the blood vessel but without all three layers of the arterial wall; it is usually bound by the tunica adventitia or surrounding soft tissue.

CASE 45: DIABETIC PATIENT WITH PENILE IMPLANT

1. **What are the indications for a penile implant?**
   Indications for penile implant include erectile dysfunction that has not responded to other therapies, penile fibrosis and Peyronie disease.
2. **What are causes of calcification of the vas deferens?**
   Calcification of the vas deferens is most commonly caused by diabetes mellitus, although other causes include aging and chronic infections (e.g. tuberculosis, syphilis).
3. **How does a penile implant reservoir work?**
   Inflatable implants can be inflated to create an erection using a fluid-filled reservoir implanted under the abdominal wall. Fluid is pumped into inflatable cylinders to achieve an erection; fluid can then be drained back into the reservoir using a valve.

CASE 46: COLITIS

1. **What are the most common viral causes of infective colitis?**
   Common viral causes of infective colitis include norovirus, rotavirus, adenovirus and cytomegalovirus.
2. **What is the relationship between smoking and inflammatory bowel disease?**
   Smoking increases risk of Crohn's disease but decreases risk of ulcerative colitis.
3. **What clinical features are more common in ulcerative colitis as opposed to Crohn's disease?**
   Ulcerative colitis is more likely to be associated with bloody diarrhoea and left lower quadrant tenderness. Terminal ileum disease, mouth ulcers and perianal disease are more common in Crohn's disease.

CASE 47: COLITIS

1. **What region of the gut is typically affected by Crohn's disease compared to ulcerative colitis?**
   Crohn's disease typically affects the terminal ileum but can affect anywhere from mouth to the anus. Ulcerative colitis affects the rectum and extends proximally to the colon.
2. **What extraintestinal manifestations related to disease activity are associated with Crohn's disease?**
   Extraintestinal features of Crohn's disease that are related to disease activity include aphthous mouth ulcers, pauci-articular arthritis, erythema nodosum, episcleritis and metabolic bone disease.
3. **What endoscopic features are seen in ulcerative colitis?**
   Ulcerative colitis begins in the rectum and spreads proximally in a continuous and symmetrical pattern. There is formation of crypt abscesses and mucosal ulceration. Pseudopolyps are more common than in Crohn's disease.

CASE 48: SCOLIOSIS AND DISLOCATED LEFT HIP

1. **What are the indications for VP shunt?**
   A VP shunt is indicated for hydrocephalus. Causes of hydrocephalus include intraventricular haemorrhage, spina bifida or as a complication of meningitis.
2. **How can ventricular dilatation be measured in a newborn baby?**
   In the neonatal period, when the fontanelle is open, cranial ultrasound can be used to measure ventricular dilatation.
3. **What are the indications for operating on a patient with scoliosis?**
   Most cases of scoliosis do not require surgery. However, it may be indicated in patients with severe curvature (≥45 degrees) as these cases can progress even after skeletal maturity and impact on respiratory function.

CASE 49: OSTEOPETROSIS

1. **How is a PEG tube inserted?**
PEG insertion requires an oesophagogastroscopy to guide a single percutaneous stab of a needle into the stomach. A guidewire is passed through the needle entry site via a trocar and then attached to the endoscope to be pulled out through the mouth. The PEG tube is then fed over to the stomach via the guidewire.
2. **What is osteopetrosis?**
Osteopetrosis results from osteoclast failure. This leads to a failure in bone resorption, leading to an increase in bone density.
3. **What is the inheritance pattern of osteopetrosis?**
Osteopetrosis can be autosomal recessive or dominant. Rarely, it is X-linked recessive.

CASE 50: MIXED SMALL AND LARGE BOWEL OBSTRUCTION

1. **What is the most worrying possible cause of obstruction in this patient?**
Large bowel obstruction in an 80-year-old smoker may be related to malignancy.
2. **What important findings may be seen on rectal examination?**
Rectal examination would demonstrate an empty rectum because of the bowel obstruction. An obstructing mass may also be palpable.
3. **What in her history increases this patient's anaesthetic risk?**
Risk factors for this patient include her age, diabetes mellitus, smoking and hypertension.

CASE 51: MIXED LYTIC AND SCLEROTIC BONE LESIONS

1. **Apart from bone, where else does RCC typically metastasize?**
The most common site of RCC metastasis is the lungs, where it typically produces cannonball metastases.
2. **What are the presenting symptoms for RCC?**
RCC is often asymptomatic and most cases are detected incidentally. The classical triad of haematuria, flank pain and palpable abdominal mass are uncommon and suggest advanced disease.
3. **What are the stages of RCC?**
RCC is assigned stages I to IV. Stage I/II are localized to the kidney, stage III has regional spread and stage IV has more distant metastases.

CASE 52: FAECAL RESIDUE AND SACROILIAC JOINT FUSION

1. **What extraintestinal manifestations NOT related to disease activity are associated with Crohn's disease?**
Extraintestinal features of Crohn's disease that are not related to disease activity include axial and polyarticular arthritis, pyoderma gangrenosum, psoriasis, uveitis and hepatobiliary conditions (e.g. primary sclerosing cholangitis, steatosis and autoimmune hepatitis).
2. **At what age does Crohn's disease most commonly first present?**
Crohn's disease affects people of all ages but most commonly first presents between 15 and 30 years of age.
3. **What symptoms may she have from sacroiliac joint fusion?**
Sacroiliac joint fusion can cause lower back pain.

CASE 53: HEPATOSPLENOMEGALY

1. **What is the likely diagnosis for this patient?**
In a male with night sweats, lymphadenopathy and hepatosplenomegaly, a myeloproliferative disorder (e.g. leukaemia, lymphoma) should be considered, although infections (e.g. viral hepatitis, malaria, Leishmania) should also be considered.
2. **What is the treatment of massive hepatosplenomegaly?**
Hepatosplenomegaly does not itself require treatment; management should be focussed on treating the underlying cause.
3. **What is most common cause of portal hypertension?**
Cirrhotic liver disease is the commonest cause of portal hypertension.

CASE 54: LEFT INGUINAL HERNIA WITH BOWEL OBSTRUCTION

1. **How can the obstruction be relieved?**
Manual reduction of the inguinal hernia should initially be attempted to relieve the obstruction.
2. **How is an inguinal hernia repaired in neonates?**
Inguinal hernias can be repaired with either an open groin approach and herniotomy or laparoscopic closure of the deep inguinal ring.
3. **How common are inguinal hernias?**
There is a 5% lifetime risk of inguinal hernia in males, the majority of which occur in the first year of life. Males are affected 5 to 10 times as often as women.

CASE 55: CAECAL VOLVULUS

1. **What are the risk factors for caecal volvulus?**
Risk factors for caecal volvulus include advanced age, chronic constipation and diets rich in fibre.
2. **What radiographic features are suggestive of caecal volvulus as opposed to sigmoid volvulus?**
A caecal volvulus has the following features on imaging that distinguish it from sigmoid volvuli: extends towards the left upper quadrant, maintains colonic haustral pattern and distended small bowel with collapsed distal colon.
3. **What are the chances of success with endoscopic management?**
Endoscopic decompression is rarely successful and there is a high risk of perforation, so surgical intervention is required in most cases.

CASE 56: DERMOID CYST

1. **What is the differential diagnosis for a calcified mass in the pelvis?**
   Differential diagnosis of calcified pelvic masses include appendiceal calculus, urinary stones, calcified lymph nodes, fallopian tube calcification, calcified vascular structures (e.g. arterial, phlebolith) and calcified leiomyoma or dermoid cyst.
2. **What is the prognosis of a teratoma?**
   Teratomas are usually benign masses with a high survival rate. However, they have the potential to malignantly transform, which consequently severely reduces survival rate.
3. **What is the histology of an ovarian mature cystic teratoma?**
   An ovarian mature cystic teratoma is composed of at least two embryonic layers (ectoderm, mesoderm or endoderm).

CASE 57: OSTEOARTHRITIS WITH VERTEBRAL COMPRESSION FRACTURES

1. **What is the differential diagnosis for rectal bleeding in this patient?**
   Differentials include ischaemic or inflammatory colitis, anal polyp, anal fissure and colorectal malignancy.
2. **What are the treatment options for longstanding atrial fibrillation?**
   Longstanding atrial fibrillation can be pharmacologically managed with rate-controlling drugs (e.g. β-blockers, digoxin) and anticoagulation should be started to reduce the risk of thromboembolism. Catheter ablation should be considered in cases refractory to pharmacological treatment.
3. **What risk factors for general anaesthetic are present in this patient?**
   Risk factors include age, hypertension and atrial fibrillation.

CASE 58: LEFT FEMORAL VENOUS CATHETER

1. **How long can a femoral vein catheter remain in situ?**
   Given the risk of infection at these sites, femoral lines should be taken out as soon as possible. In adults usually they can be left in for up to 7 days, but policies vary between units.
2. **What other checks would confirm NG tube position?**
   An aspirate from the NG tube can be obtained to check the pH; an acidic pH confirms positioning in the stomach.
3. **Why might a patient with sepsis fail to pass stool?**
   Sepsis can induce ileus, thereby stopping the passing of stools.

CASE 59: NEONATAL LINES

1. **How many umbilical arteries and veins does a neonate typically have?**
   Neonates typically have two umbilical arteries and one umbilical vein.
2. **How long can a UVC remain in situ?**
   Using UVC for more than 7 days should be avoided.
3. **What is the thoracic level of the carina?**
   The carina is at the level of the 4/5th thoracic vertebrae.

CASE 60: COLITIS

1. **What medical therapies are available for ulcerative colitis?**
   Medical treatment options include corticosteroids, 5-aminosalicylates (e.g. mesalamine, sulfasalazine), thiopurines (e.g. azathioprine) and biological agents (e.g. infliximab).
2. **What would be the indications for surgery?**
   Surgery should be considered if, for example, there is failure of medical therapy or development of toxic megacolon.
3. **What is the risk of doing a colonoscopy in this patient?**
   Colonoscopy in an acute flare-up should be avoided because of the risk of perforation.

CASE 61: INCARCERATED INGUINAL HERNIA WITH SMALL BOWEL OBSTRUCTION

1. **What is the cause of tinkling bowel sounds in bowel obstruction?**
   The tinkling sound is produced when fluid drips from one distended and tympanic bowel loop into another.
2. **What is the significance of phleboliths?**
   Phleboliths are calcification within a vein and are a common incidental finding on imaging. It is important to differentiate them from urinary tract calculi.
3. **What should be the initial management in this patient?**
   Reduction of his inguinal hernia should initially be attempted as this would resolve the obstruction.

CASE 62: SIGMOID VOLVULUS

1. **What are the risk factors for sigmoid volvulus?**
   Risk factors for sigmoid volvulus include old age, previous abdominal surgery, constipation and living in a nursing home.
2. **What are the complications of a bowel anastomosis?**
   The most common complications of bowl anastomosis are bleeding, dehiscence, leaks, strictures and fistulas.
3. **If the patient requires emergency surgery, what potential intervention (apart from bowel resection) should the consent include?**
   Consent should include the possibility of stoma formation in case gangrene is present and/or extensive bowel resection is required.

CASE 63: FAECAL RESIDUE AND STERILIZATION CLIPS

1. **What sterilization methods are available for female patients?**
   Sterilization is performed by fallopian tube occlusion, which can be achieved by applying clips or rings, or resection of a small piece of fallopian tube.
2. **How effective is female sterilization at preventing pregnancy?**
   The procedure is over 99% effective at preventing pregnancy.
3. **What other contraception options could be offered to the patient?**
   Other contraceptive options include an IUCD, oral contraceptive pills or advice on barrier methods.

CASE 64: VENTRICULOPERITONEAL SHUNT

1. **Apart from VP shunts, what other shunts are available for treating hydrocephalus?**
   Ventriculopleural shunting or ventriculoatrial shunts are possible alternatives to VP shunts.
2. **What are the complications of a VP shunt?**
   The most common complications of VP shunts are shunt obstruction and infection. Abdominal pseudocyst is a late complication, which presents with a palpable abdominal mass and abdominal pain.
3. **What would you expect to see on abdominal ultrasound secondary to the shunt in the peritoneal cavity?**
   There may be more free fluid than expected due to the CSF draining into the peritoneal cavity.

CASE 65: SMALL BOWEL OBSTRUCTION WITH MURAL OEDEMA

1. **What are the possible causes of bowel obstruction in a 3-year-old patient?**
   Causes of bowel obstruction at this age would include volvulus, intussusception, obstructed congenital band and a groin hernia.
2. **What is the mainstay of treatment for intussusception in stable patients?**
   Contrast enema reduction is the initial treatment option in clinically stable patients with intussusception.
3. **What would you expect the child to be vomiting?**
   As there is small bowel obstruction, the vomitus is likely to be bilious in nature.

CASE 66: LARGE BOWEL OBSTRUCTION AND COMPRESSION FRACTURES

1. **What is the most common cause of large bowel obstruction in older adults?**
   The most common cause of large bowel obstruction in adults is colorectal cancer.
2. **What percentage of colorectal malignancy presents with bowel obstruction?**
   Between 8% and 40% of colorectal cancers initially present with bowel obstruction.
3. **What other physical examination is necessary in this patient?**
   A rectal examination to check for bleeding and masses would be indicated in this case.

CASE 67: SIGMOID VOLVULUS

1. **What percentage of bowel obstructions are caused by a sigmoid volvulus?**
   Sigmoid volvulus accounts for approximately 8% of all intestinal obstructions.
2. **What common, long-term, bowel disorder might put an individual at risk for sigmoid volvulus?**
   Chronic constipation is a risk factor for sigmoid volvulus.
3. **In what cases would definitive surgical intervention be avoided?**
   If the patient has significant comorbidities with high surgical risk, they may be managed expectantly.

CASE 68: BILATERAL MEDULLARY NEPHROCALCINOSIS AND STAGHORN CALCULUS

1. **What complications are associated with a renal ultrasound?**
   There are no complications with this procedure.
2. **What is the significance of a staghorn calculus?**
   Staghorn calculi occupy the majority of the renal collecting system and have high morbidity. They need to be treated surgically and fragments removed as otherwise they can lead to recurrent infections and stone formation.
3. **What is the management of a septic patient with an obstructed kidney?**
   This constitutes a urological emergency and should be treated urgently. Patients should be resuscitated, analgesia provided and surgical intervention performed with percutaneous nephrostomy or ureteric stent insertion to decompress the kidney.

CASE 69: RIEDEL'S LOBE

1. **What is Reidel's lobe of the liver?**
   Riedel lobe is an anatomical variant where there is a downward projection of the anterior edge of the right lobe of the liver.
2. **How many segments is the liver divided into?**
   The Couinaud classification divides the liver into eight functional segments each with its own vascular supply, biliary drainage and lymphatic drainage.
3. **What is the blood supply to the liver?**
   The liver receives oxygenated blood from the hepatic artery and deoxygenated blood from the hepatic portal vein.

CASE 70: POSTOPERATIVE HIRSCHSPRUNG DISEASE

1. **What is Hirschsprung disease?**
   Hirschsprung disease refers to bowel aganglionosis whereby parts of the intestine are missing a nerve supply.
2. **Which part of the gastrointestinal tract does Hirschsprung disease most commonly affect?**
   Hirschsprung disease most commonly affects the distal to proximal colon, usually the rectosigmoid (85% of cases).
3. **What is the surgery required in the neonatal period for Hirschsprung disease?**
   If the neonate is generally well, rectal washouts are started to achieve abdominal decompression. Several operations are described to remove the aganglionic segment in an elective setting before 1 year of age. If the patient is unwell, a staged operation may be offered whereby a stoma is initially fashioned until the patient's condition sufficiently improves for a subsequent pull-through operation.

CASE 71: SMALL BOWEL OBSTRUCTION WITH MURAL THICKENING

1. **How is abdominal abscess drainage performed?**
   Abdominal abscesses can be drained percutaneously or with open surgical drainage. Percutaneous drains are inserted by interventional radiologists under image guidance, be it ultrasound, CT or fluoroscopy.

2. **What are the different types of surgical drains?**
Drains can be classified by different systems. Whether they are open (drain onto a gauze or stoma bag) or closed (drain into a bottle or bag), and whether they are passive drains (allowed to drain freely) or active drains (suction applied).
3. **What is the most likely cause of obstruction in this patient?**
Adhesions secondary to intraperitoneal infection are the most likely cause of bowel obstruction in this case.

CASE 72: ASCITES

1. **What tests should be ordered on ascitic fluid?**
The ascitic fluid should be sent for bacterial culture and sensitivity, biochemical analysis (protein, glucose, amylase, LDH, glucose) and cytology.
2. **What malignancy presents with gross ascites and a lower abdominal mass in an older female?**
These clinical features would be concerning for an ovarian cancer.
3. **What would a cirrhotic liver look like on ultrasound imaging?**
Ultrasound imaging of a cirrhotic liver usually shows a nodular liver surface, coarsened echotexture and signs of portal hypertension.

CASE 73: LARGE BOWEL OBSTRUCTION AND PAGET DISEASE

1. **What is Paget disease?**
Paget disease is characterized by overactivity of osteoclasts, leading to increased bone resorption and bone remodelling.
2. **What parts of the body are usually affected by Paget disease?**
Paget disease most commonly affects the pelvis, spine, skull and proximal long bones.
3. **What is the main drug treatment for Paget disease?**
Bisphosphonates (risedronate) inhibit osteoclasts to reduce bone resorption and are the main treatment option for symptomatic patients. Patients should also be offered analgesics, including NSAIDs.

CASE 74: SMALL BOWEL OBSTRUCTION AND INFERIOR VENA CAVA FILTER

1. **What are the two types of IVC filters?**
IVC filters can be permanent or retrievable. Permanent filters are used in patients who need long-term prophylaxis against PE with a contraindication to anticoagulation. Retrievable filters are used in patients who need temporary prophylaxis or where the contraindication to anticoagulation is expected to resolve.
2. **What is the effectiveness of an IVC filter in preventing PE?**
Currently, there are limited high-quality studies on the effectiveness of IVC filters. Current evidence is suggestive that IVC filters may reduce the risk of PE, although may increase the risk of recurrent DVT.
3. **During laparoscopic cholecystectomy, what is Calot's triangle of safety?**
Calot's triangle is a small anatomical space that is carefully dissected during laparoscopic cholecystectomies, allowing safe ligation of the cystic duct and cystic artery while protecting the right hepatic artery. Its boundaries are the inferior surface of the liver (superior), cystic duct (right) and common hepatic duct (left).

CASE 75: COLONIC TRANSIT MARKERS

1. **What is the normal gut transit time in children?**
There is a gradual decrease in bowel movement frequency with advancing age. On average, infants pass around three stools per day, toddlers around two stools per day and children over age 4 years pass around one stool per day. However, there is a lot of variation in normal pattern.
2. **In a constipated child, what is the significance of time of first passage of meconium?**
The passage of meconium in the first 48 hours reduces the chances of the patient having Hirschsprung disease.
3. **What are the options for bowel management in this patient?**
The constipation can be treated with oral laxatives, rectal suppositories and/or rectal washouts.

CASE 76: FAILED RENAL TRANSPLANT

1. **What is renal osteodystrophy?**
Renal osteodystrophy is metabolic bone disease secondary to chronic renal insufficiency.
2. **How is vascular access obtained for HD?**
Short-term haemodialysis can be done via a central venous catheter. Long-term options for HD include a tunnelled line or arteriovenous fistula.
3. **What is the life expectancy on HD in the setting of CKD?**
Average life expectancy on dialysis is 5 to 10 years.

CASE 77: CRANIECTOMY BONE FLAP

1. **What are the indications for craniectomy?**
Decompressive craniectomy is used in the management of refractory intracranial hypertension, cerebral swelling (e.g. following subarachnoid haemorrhage or trauma) and malignant infarction of the middle cerebral artery.
2. **Where is the craniectomy bone flap stored?**
The bone flap needs to be stored in a sterile environment to permit restoration. This is typically done by either cryopreservation or temporary placement in a subcutaneous pocket (usually in the abdomen).
3. **What other options are available for cranial reconstruction?**
Aside from autologous bone, methyl methacrylate, calcium hydroxyapatite, titanium mesh and polyetheretherketone implants have been used.

CASE 78: ABDOMINAL AORTIC ANEURYSM

1. **What are the possible symptoms of a nonruptured AAA?**
A nonruptured AAA can present with abdominal/back/flank pain, thromboembolism, aortic infection or inflammatory aneurysm.

2. **What are the surgical options available for AAA repair?**
   AAA repair can be done with either endovascular stent insertion or open repair. In the setting of haemodynamic instability, open repair is usually necessary.
3. **What is the survival of an emergency AAA repair?**
   Emergency AAA repair has a mortality rate greater than 50%.

CASE 79: ASCITES

1. **What are some of the causes of ascites?**
   Causes of ascites include alcohol abuse, hepatitis, steatosis, cirrhosis, congestive heart failure, portal vein thrombosis, constrictive pericarditis, malignancy (e.g. colorectal, ovarian, pancreatic, hepatic), infection (e.g. tuberculosis), nephrotic syndrome and pancreatitis.
2. **What are the risk factors for developing ovarian cancer?**
   Risks factors for developing ovarian cancer include older age, early menarche, late menopause, genetic mutations, e.g. BRCA1, BRCA2, Lynch syndrome, and nulliparity.
3. **How is ovarian cancer staged?**
   The International Federation of Gynaecology and Obstetrics (FIGO) staging system is used to stage ovarian, fallopian tube and peritoneal cancers according to their spread. It includes stage I – growth confined to ovaries, stage II – growth confined to pelvis, stage III – growth spread to peritoneum or its lymph nodes and stage IV – distant metastatic present.

CASE 80: INTUSSUSCEPTION

1. **What is the most common site of intussusception?**
   Ileocolic intussusception is the most common site and accounts for 90% of cases.
2. **What is the most common age of presentation for intussusception?**
   Intussusception typically presents between ages 6 and 36 months, although most cases occur before 2 years of age.
3. **Why does intussusception occur?**
   The majority of cases of intussusception are idiopathic and often attributed to hypertrophied lymph nodes (Peyer's patches) in the bowel wall. Occasionally a lead point, an intestinal variation that can be trapped by peristalsis, can be identified, e.g. Meckel's diverticulum, polyp or duplication cysts.

CASE 81: CHRONIC PANCREATITIS

1. **What are the causes of acute pancreatitis?**
   The commonest causes of acute pancreatitis are alcohol and gallstones. Other causes include hypertriglyceridaemia, postendoscopic retrograde cholangiopancreatography, corticosteroids, infections (e.g. mumps), scorpion sting and drugs (e.g. tetracyclines, furosemide).
2. **What are some of the complications of chronic pancreatitis?**
   Complications of chronic pancreatitis include pseudocysts, exocrine insufficiency (and its associated complications, such as osteopaenia) and diabetes.
3. **What is the effect of chronic alcohol abuse on the liver?**
   Alcohol causes steatosis and hepatitis. Chronic alcohol use leads to fibrogenesis and ultimately cirrhosis of the liver.

CASE 82: BLADDER EXSTROPHY AND BLADDER CALCULI

1. **What is the initial treatment of bladder exstrophy in the newborn period?**
   The bladder exstrophy should be covered in 'cling film' to protect the bladder surface, and the patient should be referred to a specialist centre for surgical management.
2. **What are the long-term complications of surgical treatment for bladder exstrophy?**
   Complications following surgical correction of bladder exstrophy include chronic kidney disease and urinary incontinence.
3. **What are the management options for bladder calculi?**
   Medical therapies include attempting dissolution of the bladder stones, such as with oral alkalinizing agents. Endoscopic procedures, such as cystolitholapaxy, can be used to treat stones. Open cystostomy is used in cases of extremely large stones.

CASE 83: NEONATAL LINES

1. **How many umbilical veins are present in the normal neonatal umbilicus?**
   The neonatal umbilicus has one umbilical vein.
2. **What structure within the umbilical cord drains the foetal urinary bladder?**
   The urachus extends through the umbilical cord and drains the urinary bladder of the foetus.
3. **What complications are associated with a low-lying UVC?**
   Low-lying UVCs are associated with a higher risk of extravasation and infection.

CASE 84: BILATERAL JJ STENTS AND RETROPERITONEAL FIBROSIS

1. **How are JJ ureteric stents inserted?**
   JJ ureteric stents are threaded into the ureter via cystoscopy.
2. **What are the complications of JJ stents?**
   Ureteric stent complications include infection, blockage, migration, encrustation and stone formation.
3. **What are the risk factors for renal calculus formation?**
   Risk factors for renal calculi include older age, low fluid intake, impaired urinary drainage (e.g. hydronephrosis), hypercalciuria (e.g. hyperparathyroidism), hyperoxaluria (e.g. vegetarian diet), hyperuricaemia (e.g. gout) and urinary tract infection.

CASE 85: ABDOMINAL AORTIC ANEURYSM AND FAECAL RESIDUE

1. **What are the risk factors for developing AAA?**
   Risk factors for AAA include older age, smoking, male, family history, hypertension and atherosclerosis.

2. **What are the indications for a dynamic hip screw?**
   Dynamic hip screws are used for the fixation of extracapsular neck of femur fractures.
3. **What materials can a dynamic hip screw be made from?**
   Dynamic hips screws can be made from stainless steel and titanium alloys.

CASE 86: ABDOMINAL AORTIC ANEURYSM AND VASCULAR CALCIFICATION

1. **What is the approximate 30-day mortality from elective AAA repair?**
   Thirty-day mortality rates are approximately 1% for elective AAA repair.
2. **What is the approximate yearly rupture rate for untreated AAA larger than 5.5cm?**
   Untreated AAA larger than 5.5cm have approximately a 5% chance of rupture per year.
3. **Where is the aorta in relation to the peritoneal cavity?**
   The abdominal aorta is retroperitoneal.

CASE 87: ILEOSTOMY WITH DILATED SMALL BOWEL

1. **What are the complications of ileostomy?**
   Complications of ileostomies include obstruction, skin excoriation, high output stoma, vitamin B12 deficiency, stoma prolapse or retraction.
2. **How can an ileostomy be clinically differentiated from a colostomy?**
   An ileostomy is a stoma made from the small bowel. Therefore its contents tend to have a liquid consistency and the stoma has a spout to reduce skin irritation. In addition, ileostomies are typically fashioned in the right iliac fossa, as opposed to colostomies which are usually placed in the left iliac fossa.
3. **Give some examples of extraintestinal manifestations of Crohn's disease.**
   Extraintestinal manifestations include erythema nodosum, pyoderma gangrenosum, peripheral arthropathy, uveitis, nephrolithiasis, obstructive uropathy, primary sclerosing cholangitis and musculoskeletal pain.

CASE 88: RETROPERITONEAL MASS

1. **What are the retroperitoneal structures in the abdomen?**
   The major retroperitoneal structures include the distal oesophagus, duodenum (second and third part), colon (ascending/ descending), rectum, adrenal glands, kidneys, pancreas, abdominal aorta and inferior vena cava.
2. **What are the potential causes of a retroperitoneal collection?**
   The main causes of retroperitoneal collections to consider are abscesses and haematomas.
3. **What are the risk factors for developing a psoas muscle abscess?**
   Risk factors for psoas muscle abscess include diabetes mellitus, immunosuppression, IV drug use and renal failure.

CASE 89: PROSTHETIC AORTIC VALVE AND LEFT LOWER LOBE COLLAPSE

1. **What are the two main types of aortic valve replacements?**
   Aortic valve replacements can either be mechanical (metal, plastic, pyrolytic carbon) or biological (human donor or xenograft) valves.
2. **What anticoagulation will be required following valve replacement?**
   Patients with mechanical valves are typically on long-term anticoagulants (e.g. warfarin). Patients with biological valve replacements do not routinely require long-term anticoagulation although will likely be on long-term aspirin.
3. **What are the indications for aortic valve replacement in aortic stenosis?**
   Indications for aortic valve replacements include symptomatic aortic stenosis or asymptomatic patients with severe aortic stenosis and reduced (<50%) ejection fraction.

CASE 90: DUODENAL ATRESIA

1. **What is the association between Down syndrome and duodenal atresia?**
   Around 30% to 50% of patients with duodenal atresia have Down syndrome.
2. **What are the types of duodenal atresia?**
   Type 1 duodenal atresia is the commonest type, accounting for >90% of cases, and have a web formed by mucosa and submucosa but no defects in the muscle. Type 2 duodenal atresia has atretic proximal and distal ends with a cord connecting both ends. Type 3 also has atretic ends but with no cord attached.
3. **What is the operation to correct duodenal atresias?**
   Duodeno-duodenostomy is the definitive treatment for duodenal atresia.

CASE 91: BOWEL OBSTRUCTION AND PNEUMOPERITONEUM

1. **What key event has happened that has led to a significant deterioration in the baby's condition?**
   Intestinal perforation secondary to bowel obstruction.
2. **What is the ideal position of an ET tube on a neonatal X-ray?**
   The ET tube should ideally be around 1 cm above the carina, or around T2/3 if the carina is not clearly visible.
3. **What is the main concern in any term baby with bilious vomiting?**
   Bilious vomiting in newborns is suggestive of intestinal obstruction, including malrotation with volvulus, duodenal atresia or meconium ileus.

CASE 92: PNEUMOPERITONEUM

1. **How long is pneumoperitoneum visible on abdominal X-ray after a laparotomy?**
   Most postoperative free gas will resolve by 5 days postoperatively.

2. **What is the purpose of a surgical drain in this setting?**
   This is a contaminated operation, so a surgical drain will allow any residual collection or fluid to drain out and reduce the probability of infection.
3. **What is the most common major trauma to adults in the UK?**
   The most common cause of major trauma in the UK is falls from a height less than 2 m.

CASE 93: MURAL OEDEMA WITH PSEUDOPOLYPOSIS

1. **What is an inflammatory pseudopolyp?**
   An inflammatory pseudopolyp is seen in ulcerative colitis. It is an island of normal colonic mucosa that appears raised due to surrounding atrophic tissue.
2. **What is the surgical treatment of ulcerative colitis?**
   A proctocolectomy is the definitive treatment for ulcerative colitis, which can be performed with either an ileal pouch-anal anastomosis or with an end ileostomy.
3. **What percentage of patients with ulcerative colitis require surgery?**
   Approximately 23% to 45% of people with ulcerative colitis eventually require surgery.

CASE 94: DILATED BOWEL WITH PERCUTANEOUS ENDOSCOPIC GASTROSTOMY-JEJUNOSTOMY

1. **What are the indications for PEG-J tubes?**
   PEG-J tubes are usually indicated for postpyloric feeding if there are issues with gastric feeding, such as delayed gastric emptying, significant reflux or recurrent aspirations.
2. **What confirms malrotation on an upper gastrointestinal contrast study?**
   There is abnormal positioning of the duodenojejunal junction: to the right of the midline and inferior to the duodenal bulb.
3. **What is the most common presentation of intestinal malrotation in neonates?**
   The most common presentation in infancy is a bilious vomiting.

CASE 95: LYTIC BONE LESIONS WITH PAUCITY OF BOWEL GAS

1. **What are the risk factors for developing multiple myeloma?**
   Risk factors for developing multiple myeloma include older age, male sex and a family history.
2. **What is the pathogenesis of multiple myeloma?**
   Multiple myeloma refers to monoclonal proliferation of malignant plasma cells. These produce immunoglobulins, usually IgG, and occur principally in the bone marrow, causing diffuse infiltration. Myeloma cells secrete osteoclast-stimulating factors, leading to derangement of bone remodelling and lytic lesions.
3. **What is the life expectancy of patients diagnosed with multiple myeloma?**
   Median survival from diagnosis is approximately 5.5 years.

CASE 96: RADIOLOGICALLY INSERTED GASTROSTOMY

1. **What are the risk factors for nasopharyngeal cancer?**
   Risk factors for developing nasopharyngeal cancer include Epstein–Barr virus, male sex, a diet that includes salted fish, family history, alcohol use and smoking.
2. **What is the indication for a RIG tube in this patient?**
   RIG tubes can be inserted to manage inadequate oral intake due to dysphagia, which in this case is caused by nasopharyngeal carcinoma.
3. **What are the complications of a RIG tube?**
   Complications of RIG tubes include leaks, dislodgement and a buried bumper.

CASE 97: COLITIS

1. **What are the main types of colitis?**
   Colitis can be inflammatory, infective, ischaemic or radiation-induced.
2. **What is the commonest age of presentation of ulcerative colitis?**
   Most patients present between 15 and 25 years old.
3. **What bacterial organisms cause infective colitis?**
   Common bacterial causes of infective colitis include *C. jejuni, Shigella, E. coli, Salmonella* and *C. difficile*.

CASE 98: PAEDIATRIC PNEUMOPERITONEUM

1. **What conditions are associated with Hirschsprung disease?**
   A number of syndromes are associated with Hirschsprung disease such as Down syndrome, neurocristopathy syndromes (e.g. Waardenburg–Shah syndrome), multiple endocrine neoplasia IIa and neuroblastomas are also associated with Hirschsprung disease.
2. **What is a major complication of patients with Hirschsprung disease?**
   A life-threatening complication of Hirschsprung disease is enterocolitis.
3. **What is the relationship between biological sex and Hirschsprung disease?**
   Hirschsprung disease is more likely to affect males (4:1).

CASE 99: PATENCY CAPSULE

1. **When are patency capsule used?**
   Patency capsule tests are used to check for a stricture before proceeding to capsule endoscopy.
2. **What are patency capsules made from?**
   Patency capsules are mainly composed of barium (which makes it radiopaque) and lactose.
3. **What is the purpose of patency capsule tests?**
   Patency capsules are used to test for intestinal luminal patency. If they leave the body before dissolving, this confirms the intestine is patent before a capsule endoscopy is performed. If they do not leave the body before dissolving (which takes approximately 30 hours), it suggests a risk that a capsule endoscopy could be retained if used (and thereby require surgical intervention to remove).

CASE 100: CAECAL VOLVULUS WITH SMALL BOWEL OBSTRUCTION

1. **What are the two main predisposing factors for developing caecal volvulus?**
   The two key predisposing factors to developing caecal volvulus are a free, mobile proximal colon and presence of a fulcrum/fixed point such as an adhesion to facilitate twisting.
2. **What proportion of bowel obstructions do colonic volvulus account for?**
   Colonic volvulus is rare and accounts for approximately 2% of all cases of bowel obstruction.
3. **What is the definitive management of caecal volvulus?**
   Endoscopy is rarely successful in patients with caecal volvulus, so a laparotomy is required in most cases with potential right hemicolectomy if there is bowel ischaemia.

Case Index

Index

Note: Page numbers followed by *f* indicate figures.